Midwifery: Best Practice Volume 5

For Elsevier:

Commissioning Editor: Mairi McCubbin
Development Editor: Michèle le Roux
Project Manager: Joannah Duncan
Design Direction: George Ajayi

Midwifery: Best Practice Volume 5

Edited by

Sara Wickham RM MA BA(Hons) PGCert
Independent Midwifery Lecturer and Consultant

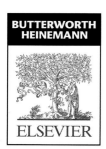

EDINBURGH LONDON NEW YORK OXFORD PHILADELPHIA ST LOUIS SYDNEY TORONTO 2008

BUTTERWORTH
HEINEMANN
ELSEVIER

First edition 2003
Second edition 2004
Third edition 2005
Fourth edition 2006
Fifth edition 2008

ISBN: 978 0 7506 7540 6

British Library Cataloguing in Publication Data
A catalogue record for this book is available from the British Library

Library of Congress Cataloging in Publication Data
A catalog record for this book is available from the Library of Congress

Note

Knowledge and best practice in this field are constantly changing. As new research and experience broaden our knowledge, changes in practice, treatment and drug therapy may become necessary or appropriate. Readers are advised to check the most current information provided (i) on procedures featured or (ii) by the manufacturer of each product to be administered, to verify the recommended dose or formula, the method and duration of administration, and contraindications. It is the responsibility of the practitioner, relying on their own experience and knowledge of the patient, to make diagnoses, to determine dosages and the best treatment for each individual patient, and to take all appropriate safety precautions. To the fullest extent of the law, neither the Publisher nor the Editor assumes any liability for any injury and/or damage to persons or property arising out or related to any use of the material contained in this book.

The Publisher

Working together to grow
libraries in developing countries

www.elsevier.com | www.bookaid.org | www.sabre.org

ELSEVIER   BOOK AID International   Sabre Foundation

your source for books, journals and multimedia in the health sciences
www.elsevierhealth.com

Printed in China

The publisher's policy is to use **paper manufactured from sustainable forests**

Contents

Introduction

Welcome to the fifth volume of *Midwifery: Best Practice*, which, as usual, contains a gathering of articles designed to inform, entertain, educate or simply provide food for thought and reflection. Most of the articles in this book have been written by midwives for midwives, and, while some have a timeless quality, many also reflect the interesting times that midwifery is experiencing around the world.

This fifth volume includes articles from *The Practising Midwife*, *Midwifery* and *The Journal of Midwifery & Women's Health*, and I would like to begin by extending a big thank-you to the past and present editorial teams of these journals for their help in making this book possible, as well as a thank-you to each of the authors of the articles. This volume also contains six longer original articles written especially for this book, and more thanks go to the authors of these articles for taking time out of their busy lives to share their thoughts and knowledge.

As always, the articles are grouped into nine sections, and five of these are similar to those in each of the other volumes: 'Women and Midwives', 'Pregnancy', 'Labour and Birth', 'Life After Birth' and 'Stories and Reflection'. We have tried to do something slightly different with each edition of *Midwifery: Best Practice* and this volume is no exception. Previously, we have included an introduction to each of the main sections, and then suggested a few professional development activities at the end of these sections. This time around, all of the discussion has been focused around ideas for further thinking and professional development, and there is a page of suggested topics for further reflection at the end of each of the first eight sections. It is almost impossible to make every suggested topic or question relevant to every midwife or student because of the diversity that exists in the ways that we learned and the environments in which we practice, so you are invited to take what is useful, skim over what isn't and adapt what you can for your own use! The final 'Stories and Reflection' section offers, as previously, a selection of the more narrative and reflective pieces which celebrate anecdotes, storytelling and women's ways of thinking, being and knowing; ways which often contrast with the current trend towards a more scientific approach to writing and thinking about midwifery.

It is with great sadness that I need to tell you of the deaths of two of the midwives who contributed to this book: Tricia Anderson and Jeanne Raisler. I had always intended – as I have in past volumes – to give the 'last word' to one of the editorial staff of *The Practising Midwife*, and Tricia's words of inspiration, in closing this book, are more poignant now than ever.

Finally, huge thanks as ever to the team at Elsevier; most especially to Mairi McCubbin, Fiona Conn, who was growing her own baby while also midwifing this literary one, Michèle le Roux, Joannah Duncan and Mary Seager, who may have retired from her Elsevier post, but who was the original midwife of this series and, as such, has remained very much in my thoughts as I edited this latest volume.

Sara Wickham 2008

Acknowledgements

We would like to thank all those who have contributed to this volume of *Midwifery: Best Practice*:

Deirdre Amos, Tricia Anderson, Kathleen Baird, Kirsten Baker, Alison Baum, Nils Bergman, Karsten Bidstrup, Belinda Blake, Sarah J Buckley, Ethel Burns, Susan Burvill, Sarah Bush, Irene Calvert, Jennifer Cameron, Sue Carfoot, Jean Chapple, Usa Chuahorm, Kirstin Clark, Suzanne Colson, Lorna Davies, Fiona Dickinson, Rumona Dickson, Nerissa Fields, Valerie E M Fleming, Caroline Flint, Ina May Gaskin, Anne Haines, Kay Hardie, Barbara Hastings-Asatourian, Anna Hewitt, Tracey Hodgson, Phil Hogan, Virginia Howes, Pamela Hunt, Billie Hunter, Kate Jackson, Rosie Kacary, Holly Powell Kennedy, Linda Kimber, Jeanette Kinsey, Mavis Kirkham, Sandy Kirkman, Sheila Kitzinger, Diane Kornbrot, M Kathryn Kravetz, Tina Lavender, Sue Lennox, Ans G Luyben, Kath McKay, Rosemary Mander, Marianne M P Mead, Lisa M Mitchell, Jo Morgan, Mary Nolan, Claire Patterson, Sharon Phillips, Sally Price, Siew Quek, Jeanne Raisler, Becky Reed, Sonia Richardson, Debra Salmon, Maureen T Shannon, Ishvar Sheran, Hora Soltani, Sue Spencer, Mary Stewart, Sarah Stewart, Judith Tanner, Jane Wallsworth, Denis Walsh, Bette L Waters, Paula Williamson, Claire Wood.

Women and Midwives

SECTION CONTENTS

Women, midwives, partnership and power

Sarah Stewart

Introduction

Midwives have long since recognized that the relationships they have with women during the childbirth continuum are very important, both for the outcome of the woman's birthing experience and for their own personal satisfaction and professional growth. It is only recently that we have come to understand more about the relationship between the woman and the midwife, how it works and the effect on both participants. Partnership has been espoused as the ideal way for midwives to work with women, where power is shared and both partners are equal. However, there have been discussions about whether partnership is truly possible and that developing a relationship is the more realistic approach for a midwife to take in her dealings with women. Using a personal story from practice, I will consider how midwives work in relationships with women and how reflection can broaden our understanding and thinking around the issues.

Working with women

The work of a midwife is demanding and challenging. Not least of the midwife's responsibilities is the development of a relationship between herself and the woman she cares for, be it in the space of an 8-hour shift in a birthing facility or over a period of months in a 'one-to-one' model of maternity care. The quality of that relationship can have direct effects on the outcomes of the woman's childbirth experience (Hallgren et al 2005; Homer et al 2002). The way we are with women may resonate with them for years, long after we have forgotten them. This was brought home to me a few years ago when a very elderly lady told me about the experience she had with the midwife who had 'delivered' her baby. The lady became so angry as she remembered the midwife who had abused her, I thought she was going to physically attack me. A number of authors have explored what women want from their relationships with midwives and have found that shared values, trust, respect, friendship, and reciprocity are among the desired elements of the relationship (Edwards, 2000; Hunter, 2006). Effective communication is considered to be very important, with the midwife giving information in a way that can be understood and in turn, listening and empathizing with the woman (Thomas 2000).

From the midwife's point of view, the relationship with the woman is considered to be one of equality, with each person bringing something of value to the relationship (Powell Kennedy et al 2004). Powell Kennedy et al investigated the meaning of relationships with 14 midwives using narrative analysis to explore their stories about their practice in the USA. The midwives articulated a personal connection with women that often entailed friendship. This enabled them to tailor their care to meet the individual needs of the woman, which in turn gave them a sense of accomplishment. The outcomes for the midwives were personal growth and learning as a result of reflection and the desire to change when required. This was tied up with the midwives' beliefs that the woman would make the right decisions for herself. In the research carried out by Hunter (2006), reciprocity was the theme of three focus groups carried out with 19 community midwives in the UK. Six midwives were also observed in practice. The midwives described their relationships with women as emotionally rewarding, especially when the women affirmed that the midwives were doing a good job. Relationships that were reciprocal with 'give and take' between the midwife and woman were considered by the midwives to be in 'balance'. Interactions were warm and friendly with disclosure from both parties about families and social events that were not directly related to the woman's maternity care (Hunter 2006).

Pairman (1999, 2000, 2006) has written at length about the relationship between the midwife and woman as one of partnership, which echoes the findings of Powell Kennedy et al (2004). Pairman (2006) interviewed six midwives and their clients in New Zealand. The midwives were self-employed midwives who provided total midwifery care to women throughout their birthing experience from conception to six weeks postpartum as lead maternity carers (LMC). The participants described their relationships to be one of equality, where each person brought different aspects to the relationship and were valued for it. The woman brought to the partnership the knowledge of her body, family and situation as well as her expectations for trust and openness from the midwife. Within the partnership the woman was autonomous, taking responsibility for her decisions and control of her experience. The midwife brought her professional knowledge and skills, whilst supporting the woman in a way that shared power and control, respecting the woman's autonomy (Pairman 1999, 2000, 2006).

The concept of partnership underpins midwifery practice in New Zealand at legislative, educational and professional levels, and with it comes the supposition that the woman is the focus of midwifery care (Stewart 2006). Continuity of carer is imperative, as is the belief in normal birth. Partnership is ingrained in the New Zealand College of Midwives Ten Standards of Practice and Code of Ethics (New Zealand College of Midwives 2002). As a midwife working as a LMC in New Zealand I have always strived to work in a way that facilitates partnership with the women I care for. Yet, the following story I am about to tell describes how partnership did not exist between myself and the woman I was caring for, and how I struggled to respect her autonomy. It is not an earth-shattering story, but I was left with a feeling of guilt and powerlessness that impacted on me for some time following. I have used reflection as a tool to help me better understand how relationships between women and midwives work and broaden my thinking around the issue.

The story of Hene

Once I had a client named Hene who was referred to me by her general practitioner (GP) at about 16 weeks gestation. She was a 17-year-old Maori woman expecting her second baby. She came from a poor background and lived with her boyfriend and family. The labour and birth of her first child, a little boy, had been difficult and she did not want that to happen again. Her labour had been induced at 39 weeks gestation because her son was thought to be small, and she ended up having an epidural and forceps delivery. The baby was in fact a normal size. It took me a few weeks to make contact with her as she was never in when I visited, she was not on the phone and she did not respond to the letters I sent her. To add insult to injury, I had had a near-death experience with her ferocious dog. As with all the women I work with, I gave her information about her care and encouraged her to make choices accordingly.

Hene was quite clear that she did not wish for any medical interventions because she did not want a similar outcome to her previous pregnancy and labour. During her pregnancy Hene developed several medical conditions that had the potential to affect the outcome of the pregnancy and birth. However, she would not take medications prescribed despite being warned that the effects of the untreated condition could result in medical intervention. I always had difficulty in locating Hene. She was never in although I had made appointments, and she moved twice without telling me. Yet when she was acutely sick she always managed to get hold of me and expected me to drop everything and attend her. On one occasion I gave her the option of having another midwife. However, she declined this offer, and told me that she was happy having me as her midwife.

Eventually, I referred Hene to the obstetrician because I was concerned about her health and the baby's growth. He thought the baby was small and Hene's labour should be induced at 39 weeks. However, I negotiated that I would frequently monitor the baby's heart and movements for a week, in an effort to prevent induction of labour and consequently facilitate a natural birthing experience for Hene. She 'complied' with this monitoring and went into spontaneous labour just before 40 weeks gestation. She had a rapid labour and vaginal birth with no interventions and a healthy baby boy. She went home very early the next morning.

I attempted to visit Hene at home daily but only managed to find her once. At 10 days post partum, I found out that she was an in-patient on the surgical ward – she had seen her GP twice and had been referred to the surgical ward with severe haemorrhoids. I went to see her whilst she was in hospital, and told her that because she obviously did not need me to visit her, I was discharging her back into her GP's care. This was in spite of the expectation that the LMC visit until 4–6 weeks post partum (New Zealand Ministry of Health 2002). So why did I feel so unhappy about what happened? What were the issues that I needed to resolve? After all, this story is not one of difficult 'life and death' dilemmas, but rather of everyday midwifery practice. I resented the fact that I had wasted a lot of time chasing around after Hene when I had other clients who did want me to spend time with them. I did not feel she appreciated me or recognized the importance of my role. When she wanted something, such as when she was very ill and needed to be admitted to hospital, she would find a way to communicate with me. Yet she would never contact me when she wanted to break appointments or had changed address. I had worried about her and expended a lot of emotional energy in an attempt to provide quality care that would counterbalance the experience she had had with the birth of her first child. I felt as if I was doing all of the giving and she did not respond in any way. In failing to respect Hene's autonomy and not accepting the decisions she made, I failed to work in partnership with her, which not only contravened my own midwifery philosophy but that of the profession (New Zealand College of Midwives 2002). Finally, I felt guilty that I had discharged her much earlier than I should have done, and had not provided adequate postnatal care. I felt I had acted in an unsympathetic manner, which is not usually how I behave.

Understanding relationships between midwives and women

The first step in my reflection was to understand why I felt disempowered as a midwife. It is difficult to find literature that deals with midwifery relationships that are not based on the professional ideal. Indeed, Hunter (2006) found the midwives in her study were very reluctant to criticize clients, describing this as 'taboo'. It is almost as if you are not a good midwife if you admit you have a poor relationship with a woman that is not based on equality or mutuality. It was only when the midwives were given 'permission' to speak that they revealed the emotional toll it took when working in difficult relationships (Hunter 2006). My personal feelings of anxiety and lack of fulfilment were reflected in the findings of McCrea and Crute (1991). They carried out a study that looked at midwives' experiences of relationships with women by interviewing 16 hospital-based midwives in the UK. They established that midwives considered relationships to be 'poor' if there was no recognition of the midwife's role or affirmation by the woman. The midwives found it difficult to work with women if there was no feedback from the women about their performance. This in turn created a lack of confidence because there was no assurance that they were doing the right thing for the woman (McCrea & Crute 1991). This importance of reciprocity is mirrored in the work of Hunter (2006). Midwives found the relationship to be emotionally rewarding if there was reciprocal exchange between the woman and midwife. However, if the woman was hostile and rejected the midwife's advice, was overly familiar or had unrealistic expectations of the midwife, the emotional toll for the midwife was high and the relationship was out of balance.

I could relate to the midwives in both studies because my advice was rejected and I had no sense that I was valued by Hene. In fact, straight after the birth of the baby, Hene turned to her GP for help with her haemorrhoids which echoes McCrea and Crute's (1991) findings that midwives felt resentment when women turned to doctors for information, which inspired a feeling of not being needed. What was of concern to me as I reflected at length was my need to be 'needed' by Hene and the threat to my professional identity by her rejection of my role and advice. Whilst it is only human to enjoy the sense of being valued, it is not the role of the midwife to encourage the woman to be 'needy'. Rather, the midwife works to ensure the woman is independent and autonomous. The midwife walks alongside the woman in the childbirth journey, pointing out the way as she goes (Leap 2000). The midwife is not the walking stick that the woman leans on. Expecting women to take our advice and being offended when they do not smacks of paternalism, which is something that midwives should strive against (Walsh 2005). I had to recognize that it was not my role to rescue Hene or 'mother' her as described by Hunter (2006). I had to recognize her autonomy and right to make her own decisions within the context of her own life.

Partnership or relationship?

When I analysed our relationship, I believed it was not a partnership. Partnership implies an equality within the relationship although there may be times that the balance of power changes according to the needs of the participants of the partnership (Guilliland & Pairman 1995). Partnership evokes shared power and responsibility, however, I feel that the power often lay with me, the health professional. As Hene's pregnancy progressed, it was complicated by iron deficiency anaemia. She declined oral medication so I insisted that she have intramuscular medication which she agreed to have. I could not accept Hene's right to decline treatment. It did not make sense to me. By refusing to take her medication, I believed she may have been compromising her ability to have a natural birth. Rather than acknowledging Hene's autonomy, I took a paternalistic approach which is the anthesis to midwifery partnership (Walsh 2005). To act in such a manner is untenable. Promoting informed choice and supporting the woman in her choice should be at the heart of midwifery practice (New Zealand College of Midwives 2002).

Did Hene want a partnership with me? She said she was happy to have me as her midwife, but then she would have needed a lot of nerve to tell me to my face that she did not want me as her midwife. Did Hene want to make choices for herself – was she able to? She was quite clear that she did not want to have her labour induced because she believed that would increase her chances of having an epidural and instrumental delivery. She also showed an interest in labouring in water and articulated an understanding of the process of labour. Hene had a careplan which included an immediate return home after she had given birth. She did not fulfil her end of the partnership 'bargain' because she did not recognize her responsibilities to me. Missing appointments might not seem like a big deal but it was an important issue to me. I expended a lot of time and energy trying to ensure that Hene was 'empowered' but made the mistake of not paying attention to the context of Hene's life. Most likely what she was concerned about was living her day-to-day life in what were often difficult circumstances. Developing a 'fulfilling' relationship with me was the last of her priorities. Recognizing this makes me understand that her interactions with me were not a personal rejection of me, and allowed me to maintain my professional credibility whilst empathizing with Hene.

I would argue that we had a relationship rather than a partnership. I would concur with authors that in some cases partnership is an unachievable goal because of the inequality of power within the relationship (Skinner 1999). Skinner (1999), who was a midwife in New Zealand, believed that partnership is mostly an ideal that cannot work at practice level because of the differing knowledge bases and experiences that the midwife and woman have. Partnership presumes that informed consent is always possible when in reality it is not. Skinner (1999) was concerned that this left both midwife and woman exposed and was not necessarily desired by all women. Flemming (1998) examined the relationship between midwives and women in New Zealand by interviewing 12 LMCs and 20 women who had LMC midwives. She found that there was a difference in expectations between midwives and women. The midwives defined partnership as their philosophy of practice and were most concerned that they worked in a way that facilitated the woman's equal involvement. Yet the women saw their relationships with the midwives in a different way, believing that the midwives were there to provide medical input and did not consider the relationship they had with the midwives. Some of the women were quite passive, expecting that they would do what the midwife told them (Flemming 1998). This research was carried out some time ago when women had not been exposed to the concept of informed choice in quite the same way that they are today, so it may be that women's expectations about their involvement in their care have changed. Recent research supports the notion that there does not need to be equality within the relationship for it to work effectively (Freeman 2004). In a study carried out in New Zealand, Freeman et al (2004) interviewed and surveyed 41 midwives who were either LMC or hospital-based midwives and 37 nulliparous women who were cared for by those midwives in labour. The researchers discovered that the relationship could work effectively even though there was an inequality of power between participants. It was explained by participants that decisions were made co-jointly with midwives and women sharing information and working together toward a common aim, rather than in terms of equality and shared power as described by Pairman (2006). Decisions concern-

ing low-risk issues were made by the woman; medium-risk decisions were made jointly by the midwife and woman; decisions concerning high-risk issues that might have required medical input were made by the midwife (Freeman et al 2004). Nevertheless, midwives did not ignore their responsibilities to include the woman in her care, and explained the rationale for the decisions they made and kept the woman informed of their actions.

Lessons to be learnt from reflection

Reflection remains as vital as ever in ensuring responsive and appropriate midwifery practice. After reflecting on my interactions with Hene I have had to accept that I am not the 'be all and end all' for every woman I meet. I only pass through their lives for a relatively short time. Some of the women I have cared for have become great friends, but the majority of women I have dealt with have continued to live their lives without much thought of me. This was a hard lesson for me to learn. I recognized that this was an issue about my pride. I wanted to do a good job. I wanted women to remember me with fondness, and I wanted to have made a difference in women's lives. Having said that, women do remember midwives and the effects of the midwives' actions can stay with them for many years. So it is vital that midwives continually reflect on their practice to ensure that they are working in a way that impacts positively on the woman's life.

Peer review is invaluable for reflecting on practice. I used my midwifery colleagues as sounding boards and they helped me to work through this situation. I believe it is vital that midwives have a safe place to reflect and obtain support, with someone who is non-judgemental. This may be with a mentor, supervisor, or in an informal context with midwifery friends (MacGuiness 2006). By being open about your practice with colleagues, not only does it give you the opportunity to grow but it brings issues to the fore for colleagues to explore and learn. This is one way that midwifery practice can develop as we broaden our understanding of what we do and why. I also presented this story when I underwent my annual practice review with the New Zealand College of Midwives Standards Review Committee (Stewart 1999). The result of this was that I developed a leaflet that I gave out to women. It detailed who I was, what services I provided and what my responsibilities were. I detailed what times it was convenient for the woman to call me at home; what hours I worked; what to do if she could not keep an appointment and so on. It also catalogued the woman's responsibilities so she knew what I expected of her (Homebirth Australia). This has proved to be a very useful resource for the woman and me.

Another element of reflection on midwifery practice is getting regular feedback from women about your performance. This can be very difficult depending on the context in which you work, but it is very worthwhile in that it offers a different perspective on your actions. As a LMC working in New Zealand, it is a requirement for me to give women written feedback forms which they return at their convenience (Stewart 1999). Generally, responses are very positive but occasionally issues will crop up that make me reflect and change my practice.

Partnership is an ideal that I will always strive to achieve. Nevertheless, on the occasions when I work with women who do not participate in that way with me I will endeavour to work in a way that is sensitive to the woman's needs, working to facilitate informed choice whilst recognizing the woman's personal autonomy. Skinner (1999) sums it up:

What I have found in my practice however, is a great sense of enjoyment and privilege as I build relationship with women whose lives I would never have otherwise touched and who have come to know me enough to trust that I will treat them with respect and honesty. It is not a partnership, it is a relationship.

I would suggest that more research is required to look at how relationships work between midwives and women. In particular, we need to look at how we work with women of different cultures, ethnicity, social status and so on, as well as how we work in different models of care, i.e. how is the relationship of midwives with women different if they work in hospitals compared to the community (Powell Kennedy et al 2004)? Another area that needs to be considered is the effect on partnership when the expectations of women or legal requirements lead to a practice or ethical dilemma. For instance, how can a midwife maintain partnership when she is asked by the woman to practise in a way that is contrary to her personal philosophy, experience or outside professional or legal requirements (Freeman et al 2004)?

Conclusion

The story of my dealings with Hene has led me to question partnership in my midwifery practice and to learn more about how relationships function. I valued the opportunity to reflect on partnership in my practice as I have never done so before. Thinking in terms of having a relationship with women as opposed to having a partnership made my every-day working life more manageable, especially when it came to working with women like Hene who did not want to interact with me in that way. I do not ask too much of myself or the woman but take her for who she is and provide the care she requests, not what I think she should have. It was about 12 months after Hene had her baby that I bumped into her again. She cheerfully informed me that she was just pregnant, and asked me to be her midwife again. The joys of being a midwife!!

REFERENCES

Edwards N 2000 Women planning homebirths: their own views on their relationships with midwives. In: Kirkham M (ed.) The midwife-mother relationship. MacMillan Press, Basingstoke, p 55–91

Flemming V 1998 Women and midwives in partnership: a problematic relationship? Journal of Advanced Nursing 27:8–14

Freeman L, Timperley H, Adair V 2004 Partnership in midwifery care in New Zealand. Midwifery, 20(1):2–14

Guilliland K, Pairman S 1995 The midwifery partnership: a model for practice. Department of Nursing and Midwifery, Victoria University of Wellington, Wellington

Hallgren A, Kihlgren M, Olsson P 2005 Ways of relating during childbirth: an ethical responsibility and challenge for midwives. Nursing Ethics 12(6):605–621

Homebirth Australia (no date) The pregnant women's homebirth Bill of Rights and Responsibilities. Online. Available: http://www.homebirthaustralia.org/homebirth.html 20 January 2007

Homer C, Davis G, Cooke M, Barclay L 2002 Women's experiences of continuity of midwifery care in a randomised controlled trial in Australia. Midwifery 18(2102–112)

Hunter B 2006 The importance of reciprocity in relationships between community-based midwives and mothers. Midwifery 22:308–322

Leap N 2000 Less we do, the more we give. In: Kirkham M (ed.) The midwife-mother relationship. MacMillan, Basingstoke, p 1–18

MacGuiness F 2006 Mothers need support as much as mothers. British Journal of Midwifery 14(2):60

McCrea H, Crute V 1991 Midwife/client relationships: midwives' perspectives. Midwifery 7:189–192

New Zealand College of Midwives 2002 Midwives handbook for practice, 2nd edn. New Zealand College of Midwives, Christchurch

New Zealand Ministry of Health 2002 Notice Pursuant to Section 88 of the New Zealand Public Health and Disability Act 2000: New Zealand Ministry of Health

Pairman S 1999 Partnership revisited: towards midwifery theory. New Zealand College of Midwives Journal (21):6–12

Pairman S 2000 Partnerships or professional friendships? In: Kirkham M (ed.) The midwife-mother relationship. Macmillan Press, Basingstoke, p 207–226

Pairman S 2006 Midwifery partnership: working with women. In: Page L, McCandlish R (eds) The new midwifery: science and sensitivity in practice, 2nd edn. Churchill Livingstone, Philadelphia, p 73–96

Powell Kennedy H, Shannon M, Chuahorm U, Kravetz K 2004 The landscape of caring for women: a narrative study of midwifery practice. Journal of Midwifery and Women's Health 49(1):14–23

Skinner J 1999 Midwifery partnership: individualism, contractualism or feminist praxis? New Zealand College of Midwives Journal 21:14–17

Stewart S 1999 Midwifery standards review in New Zealand: a personal view. British Journal of Midwifery 7(8):511–514

Stewart S 2006 Informed choice: the challenge for midwives in New Zealand. British Journal of Midwifery, 14(10):574

Thomas G 2000 Be nice and don't drop the baby. In: Page L (ed.) The new midwifery: science and sensitivity in practice, 1st edn. Churchill Livingstone, Edinburgh, p 173–183

Walsh D 2005 Professional power and maternity care: the many faces of paternalism. British Journal of Midwifery 13(11):708

Conflicting ideologies as a source of emotion work in midwifery

Billie Hunter

Summary

Objective: to explore how a range of midwives experienced and managed emotion in their work.

Design: a qualitative study using an ethnographic approach. Data were collected in three phases using focus groups, observations and interviews.

Setting: South Wales, UK.

Participants: *Phase One*: self-selected convenience sample of 27 student midwives in first and final years of 18-month (postnursing qualification) and 3-year (direct entry) programmes. *Phase Two*: opportunistic sample of 11 qualified midwives representing a range of clinical locations and clinical grades. *Phase Three*: purposive sample of 29 midwives working within one NHS Trust, representing a range of clinical locations, length of clinical experience and clinical grades.

Findings: community and hospital environments presented midwives with fundamentally different work settings that had diverse values and perspectives. The result was two primary occupational identities and ideologies that were in conflict. Hospital midwifery was dominated by meeting service needs, via a universalistic and medicalised approach to care; the ideology was, by necessity, 'with institution'. Community-based midwifery was more able to support an individualised, natural model of childbirth reflecting a 'with woman'

ideology. This ideology was officially supported, both professionally and academically. When midwives were able to work according to the 'with woman' ideal, they experienced their work as emotionally rewarding. Conversely, when this was not possible, they experienced work as emotionally difficult and requiring regulation of emotion, i.e. 'emotion work'.

Key conclusions: unlike findings from other studies, that have located emotion work primarily within worker/client relationships, the key source of emotion work for participants was conflicting ideologies of midwifery practice. These conflicts were particularly evident in the accounts of novice midwives (i.e. students and those who had been qualified for less than 1 year) and integrated team midwives. Both groups held a strong commitment to a 'with woman' ideology.

Implications for practice: understanding the dilemmas created by conflicting occupational ideologies is important in order to improve the quality of midwives' working lives and hence the care they give to women and families. In the short term, strategies involving education and supervision may be of assistance in enabling midwives to reconcile these conflicting perspectives. However, in the long term more radical solutions may be required to address the underpinning contradictions.

Introduction

Pregnancy and childbirth have an emotional impact not only on parents but also on midwives (Kirkham, 2000; Mander, 2001). Providing emotional support to women and their families is acknowledged as a key aspect of midwifery work (Berg et al., 1996; Halldorsdottir and

Karlsdottir, 1996). There is little discussion, however, of the emotional experiences of midwives themselves. This is a surprising anomaly, given the emphasis on the psychosocial aspects of midwifery practice in current UK maternity service policy and midwifery education (House of Commons Select Committee, 1992; Department of Health (DoH), 1993; Standing Nursing and Midwifery Advisory Committee (SMMAC), 1998; United Kingdom Central Council's Commission for Nursing and Midwifery Education, 1999; Page, 2000).

Reported in this paper are the findings from a larger study (Hunter, 2002), that sought to explore how a range of midwives studying and working in South Wales experienced emotion in their work, and how they managed the emotions generated. Questions were asked regarding situations that midwives experienced as emotionally rewarding or emotionally difficult, whether there were differences in the emotional experiences of student and qualified midwives, and what impact clinical setting and level of occupational responsibility had.

Emotion in the workplace

There has been a rapidly growing interest in the 'emotional arena' of the wider workplace over the past 20 years (Fineman, 1993, p. 10). This was triggered by the groundbreaking work of Arlie Russell Hochschild (1979, 1983), who drew attention not only to the significance of emotion in the workplace, but also to the work expended in managing emotion. Hochschild (1983) coined the terms 'emotional labour' or 'emotion work' (p. 7) to describe this work, proposing that regulation of emotion is essential for the effective functioning of organisations, particularly those engaged in 'people work' of some kind. Hochschild (1979) argued that emotions are managed in accordance with 'feeling rules' (p. 563), that is social norms relating to feeling and display of emotion. These feeling rules will be subject to occupational and professional norms.

Subsequent studies of work and occupations have explored the concept further, investigating a variety of occupations, developing and refining Hochschild's theories. It is notable that the majority of studies have tended to locate emotion work primarily within relationships between workers and clients. As will be seen, the evidence from this study indicates that this may be a rather narrow conceptualisation.

Of particular interest to health-service research are the studies by Smith and Kleinman (1989) who explored how medical students learn to manage their feelings in relation to the human body; Smith (1992), who explored the emotional aspects of the socialisation of student nurses and James (1989, 1992), whose study of hospice nurses identified the gendered nature of emotion work. These studies offer some insights for midwifery, but their focus on ill-health settings limits their relevance.

Emotion in midwifery

Although this study is the first to focus explicitly on the emotion work of midwives, other recent studies have

described aspects of the emotional nature of practice. For example, research into stress and burn-out in midwifery (Sandall, 1997, 1998; Mackin and Sinclair, 1998) indicates that stress is a significant feature of midwifery work and identifies worryingly high levels of poor psychosocial health in the midwifery population. Kirkham (1999) and Kirkham and Stapleton (2000) argue that the culture of midwifery in the UK has a profound (and often negative) effect on midwives' experiences, and this finding is reiterated in the recent investigation into why midwives leave the profession (Ball et al., 2002). Chronic staff shortages and low morale in British midwifery have been widely documented (Carvel, 2001; Ball et al., 2002; House of Commons Select Committee, 2003; Walter, 2003) and are of ongoing concern. Greater understanding of midwives' emotion work may assist in addressing these issues.

Moreover, it is particularly important to understand the emotional aspects of midwifery, as the ways in which midwives manage emotion potentially affect not only midwives themselves, but also the women for whom they are caring. There is a wealth of research evidence demonstrating that the midwife is highly significant in determining the quality of childbirth experiences, and that emotional support is central to this relationship (Niven, 1994; Oakley, 1994; Halldorsdottir and Karlsdottir, 1996; Walsh, 1999). It is also evident that the quality of this support is variable. Why is it that some midwives (or some midwives at some times) are able to 'be there' for women, or conversely are experienced by women as 'absently present' (Berg et al., 1996, p. 13)? The answer may well relate to the ways in which midwives manage their emotions.

Methods

A qualitative research design, incorporating focus groups, observation and interviews, was used to obtain data from a range of midwives. The study adopted an ethnographic approach as opposed to undertaking a traditional ethnography, as it was not possible to spend extended periods of time immersed in the life of the participants (Morse and Field, 1996). Nevertheless, from the perspective of Hammersley and Atkinson (1995), who argue for a liberal interpretation of the term 'ethnography', the study has all the key elements of an ethnographic approach: that is, it explored an aspect of midwifery culture from the emic perspective, using a variety of data collection methods in order to gain as many insights as possible. In line with an inductive approach to theory generation, the early imposition of a theoretical framework was avoided by not introducing the concept of emotion work to participants. Instead, very general questions were asked relating to emotionally rewarding and emotionally difficult experiences.

Box 1.2.1   Research design
Phase One • Dates: November 1997–September 1998 • Population: Student midwives at a Welsh university, first and final years of 18-month and 3-year programmes • Sample: Self-selected convenience sample ($n = 27$) • Method: Focus groups (4)
Phase Two • Dates: November 1998–March 1999 • Sample: Opportunistic sample of qualified midwives, representing a variety of clinical locations and clinical grades ($n = 11$) • Method: Focus groups (2)
Phase Three • Dates: November 1999–July 2000 • Population: All qualified midwives working within one Welsh NHS Trust • Sample: Purposive sampling ($n = 29$) • Method: Focus groups (4), observation (12), interviews (12)

Phase One of study

The study was conducted in three phases between November 1997 and July 2000 (see Box 1.2.1). In Phase One, four focus groups were conducted with a self-selected convenience sample of student midwives at a Welsh university. Students were in the first and final years of the 18-month midwifery programme (for qualified nurses) and the 3-year (direct-entry) midwifery programmes ($n = 27$). All students were invited to participate, and it was emphasised that non-participation would not affect educational experiences in any way. Convenience sampling was used for ease of access (due to my role as lecturer in the department). Convenience sampling is considered an acceptable qualitative sampling strategy; the sample needs to be relevant to the research aims rather than representative, as there is no aim of generalising from the findings (Morse and Field, 1996; Bryman, 2001).

Briefings were given to student groups prior to sending out personal invitations to participate, together with a written consent form. My dual role as lecturer and researcher meant that close attention to ethical issues was necessary, to ensure that students felt under no pressure to participate and were assured of confidentiality. Focus groups were held on campus and lasted on average 2 h, with myself as facilitator, and an academic colleague in the role of observer. A combination of questions and visual triggers (photos of midwives at work) was utilised to generate discussion. Discussions were tape-recorded, transcribed and thematically analysed (Coffey and Atkinson, 1996). Themes generated were then explored further with qualified midwives in Phase Two ($n = 11$) and Phase Three ($n = 29$).

Phase Two of study

In Phase Two, two further focus groups were conducted using an opportunistic sample of qualified midwives ($n = 11$), all of whom had expressed interest in taking part. Such flexibility of research design is an advantage of a qualitative approach, enabling incorporation of unanticipated data sources (Bryman, 2001). The first of these focus groups consisted of qualified midwives undertaking undergraduate studies at the University; the second was comprised of newly qualified midwives, who had previously participated as students and wanted to contribute their different experiences of emotion work since qualification. Participants represented a broad range of clinical locations, length of clinical experience and clinical status. The same questions and visual cues were utilised as with student midwives, to facilitate comparison. It became clear from early analysis of this data that the emotion work undertaken by qualified midwives differed from that of students, and appeared to be influenced by clinical context and status.

Phase Three of study

A more substantive period of investigation was thus undertaken in Phase Three of the study, which consisted of an in-depth study of qualified midwives working within one NHS Trust, over a period of eight months. The research design was adapted to include observation and interviews in order to obtain further insights into how midwives 'do' emotion work, rather than how it is 'talked' in focus groups.

Phase Three was conducted in a regional maternity unit undertaking approximately 3600 births per annum. The caesarean section rate during the period of data collection was 25.4% (National Assembly for Wales (NAW), 2003). One hundred and fifty midwives were employed by the Trust, of whom 86 were hospital-based, 51 were community-based and four were in senior management posts. Community midwives worked either in 'integrated' teams (whose members provided antenatal, intrapartum and postpartum care in both community and hospital, with the aim of increasing continuity of care for mothers) or in 'traditional' teams who provided antenatal and postnatal care in the community setting, but rarely attended births. The integrated team midwives were required to work 1 day a week in the maternity unit, 1 day 'on call' for the labour ward and also to be on-call (for both community and unit) one or two nights per week. Integrated practice had been implemented 10 months prior to the study, and was thus a relatively new innovation.

All midwives working for the NHS Trust (with the exception of those on maternity and long-term sick leave, those due to retire and those in senior management posts) were invited to take part in the study. Following briefings by the researcher at team meetings and shift handovers, information letters and consent forms were sent to midwives' work addresses. The initial response rate was disappointing and attempts were taken to redeem this by further attendance at staff meetings and by displaying posters in the unit. This led to the inclusion of several additional participants.

Out of a possible sample size of 137, 36 midwives consented to participate. As a result of illness and work commitments, only 29 of these actually took part.

Of the final sample ($n = 29$), seven were employed as E-grade midwives, 14 as F-grade midwives and eight as G-grade midwives (these clinical grades relate to UK pay scales linked to level of clinical responsibility and seniority; E-grade midwives have the least clinical experience and responsibility, and G grades the most). There was a notable bias in the sample towards community-based practice: 19 participants worked in the community, as opposed to 10 who were hospital-based. Only one hospital G-grade midwife participated, and this is acknowledged as a limitation of the study. Length of clinical experience as a midwife varied between 18 months and 25 years.

Participants were allocated either to focus groups or to be individually observed and interviewed. Purposive sampling (Bryman, 2001) was used to ensure that participants in each of these situations represented a range of clinical contexts and clinical status. Four focus groups were conducted, with a total of 17 midwives; composition of groups was determined by clinical location (i.e. hospital or community-based) and clinical grade (see Box 1.2.2), as homogeneity of focus groups is considered to

enhance cohesion and thus facilitate discussion (Krueger, 1994). The focus groups were held in a side room away from the main maternity unit, and conducted as previously described.

Following this, 12 periods of observation followed by 12 semi-structured interviews were undertaken with six midwives working in hospital-based practice and six in community-based practice (see Box 1.2.3). Of the six hospital-based midwives who were observed, four were employed as E-grade midwives, one as an F grade and one as a G grade; observation took place whilst these midwives were working in the maternity wards, labour ward and antenatal clinic. The six community-based midwives included four F-grade midwives and two G-grade midwives: four worked in integrated teams and two in 'traditional' teams. Four were observed working in community settings, and two whilst they were working within the unit as part of their integrated practice.

Observations were undertaken by 'shadowing' midwives for several hours whilst they worked. Each midwife was observed on one occasion, usually for the duration of a shift and at least for several hours. Detailed fieldnotes of the observation were kept, which focused on the emotional aspects of the midwife's work. The period of

---

Box 1.2.2 Phase Three: data collection: details of focus groups

Focus Group 1
Integrated team midwives, G grades
All white, female
Five participants from three different teams
Length of midwifery experience: 11–25 years

Focus Group 2
Integrated team midwives, F grades
All white, female
Four participants from two different teams
Length of midwifery experience: 4–10 years

Focus Group 3
Integrated team midwives, F grades
All white, female
Four participants from three different teams
Length of midwifery experience: 4–16 years

Focus Group 4
Hospital-based midwives, three E grades, one F grade
All white, female
Four participants working throughout unit
Length of midwifery experience: 3–7 years

Box 1.2.3 Phase Three: data collection; observations and interviews

Community-based midwives (6)

Type of practice
Integrated team midwives: 4
Traditional team midwives: 2

Employment details
Full-time: 5
Part-time: 1
F grade: 4
G grade: 2
Length of midwifery experience: 10–20 years

Demographic details
All female. All white

Location of observation
Four observed working in the community
Two observed working in the maternity unit

Hospital-based midwives (6)

Data collected: March 2000–May 2000
Clinical grade
E grade: 4
F grade: 1
G grade: 1
Length of midwifery experience: 18 months–21 years

Demographic details
All female. All white

Location of observation
Four observed working on maternity wards
One observed working on labour ward
One observed working in antenatal clinic

observation was followed by a semi-structured interview. This enabled a comparison to be made between the researcher's observation of the midwife's emotion work and the midwife's lived experience of this. Hand-written fieldnotes and analytic memos were recorded during the periods of observation and written up in full shortly after, in order to provide as detailed a record as possible. The interviews were conducted in private, tape-recorded and later transcribed.

Permission to undertake the study was received from the Director of the University Department, the Head of Midwifery in the NHS Trust and ethical approval obtained from the Local Research Ethics Committee. Participants were assured at the recruitment stage that all data would be anonymised, and confidentiality maintained. Ground rules relating to confidentiality of group discussions were agreed at the start of each focus group and participants had the right to withdraw from the study at any time. Transcription was undertaken by myself and an assistant unrelated to the maternity unit or midwifery education department, and all data were stored securely. These measures applied throughout the study.

Verbal consent was gained from the women for whom midwives were caring during the observation periods. Clients were informed of the nature of the study prior to the observation, and their voluntary participation was requested. It was emphasised that the focus of the study was on the work of the midwife. Anonymity and confidentiality were explained and assured.

Data analysis

As is common in qualitative research, data analysis was undertaken concurrently with data collection (Silverman, 1993, Hammersley and Atkinson, 1995). Following each focus group, the facilitator and observer met to 'debrief', in order to compare observations (Morgan and Krueger, 1998). Debriefing notes, together with observational fieldnotes and transcriptions of focus group discussions and interviews, were then analysed using a form of thematic analysis (Hammersley and Atkinson, 1995; Coffey and Atkinson, 1996). Transcriptions and fieldnotes were read and coded manually. These codes were then interlinked using a 'mind-mapping' approach; this visual display facilitated identification of key concepts and the relationships between them. The transcripts were then re-read to ensure that all the original codes were covered by the wider categories. The coded data were recontextualised according to thematically based files and explored again, this time with interpretation in mind, looking for patterns and meanings (Dey, 1993, Coffey and Atkinson, 1996).

Attention was also paid to the possible existence of 'deviant cases' (Silverman, 2000, p. 44): that is, negative cases not consistent with the hypothetical explanation being developed. When such examples are encountered, the researcher must either reformulate the explanation to include the deviant case, or alternatively, adapt the hypothesis to exclude the case (Silverman, 1993; Bryman, 2001). The search for such cases, and the peer validation provided by the research supervisor throughout the data analysis, enhanced the 'trustworthiness' of the findings (Lincoln and Guba, 1985).

Findings

Data analysis indicated that midwifery was commonly described as highly emotional work, with participants experiencing many work-related conflicts and dilemmas. Both student and qualified midwives frequently described having to work on their emotions in order to maintain the appropriate 'professional performance' (Goffman, 1969). However, the source of this emotion work was unexpected. Unlike many other studies, in which worker/client relationships have been identified as the primary site of emotion work (see for example, Hochschild, 1983; Smith, 1992), it was more often interactions with colleagues and 'the organisation' that required management of emotion. At the nub of such situations was a common ingredient: the coexistence of contradictory ideologies of midwifery practice, which created dissonance for midwives.

Two primary ideologies of midwifery were evident, which were linked to the context in which midwives worked. Hospital and community environments presented fundamentally different work settings with diverse values and perspectives. Hospital-based midwifery was driven by the needs of the institution. The imperative of providing universal and equitable care to large numbers of women and babies 24 h a day, 7 days a week, resulted in a pragmatic response aimed at standardisation of care, risk reduction, efficiency and effectiveness. Within such a model, minimal attention could be given to the needs of individuals and to all intents, the occupational ideology was 'with institution'.

In contrast, community-based midwives were more likely to work according to a 'with woman' approach to practice. This approach was characterised by an individualised, woman-centred model of care, informed by a belief in the normal physiology of childbirth. This model was held as an ideal of practice by many participants in the study, and is reflected in contemporary UK midwifery education and maternity policies (Department of Health (DoH), 1993; Welsh Assembly Government (WAG), 2002; House of Commons Select Committee, 2003).

When midwives were able to work according to the ideal of the 'with woman' model, there was congruence between ideals and practice, and work was experienced as emotionally rewarding. However, it was frequently impossible for midwives to maintain this approach, and the dissonance that this created led to a variety of negative emotions, such as frustration, anxiety and anger, which required emotion work.

This was particularly true of the integrated team midwives and novice midwives (that is, student midwives and those who had been qualified for less than 1 year). It was notable that both of these groups held strong commitments to a 'with woman' approach to care. In addition, integrated team midwives were required to work in both hospital and community settings. They were thus in the ambiguous situation of attempting to adopt a 'with woman' style of practice within an institutional context that represented its antithesis.

The interrelationships between context of practice, occupational identity, occupational ideology and emotion work are described in a framework provided in Table 1.2.1. This framework will be discussed in more detail, using data extracts to illustrate.

'With institution' ideology

At the time of the study most hospital midwives were employed as core staff, working shifts in order to provide a homogenous and efficient service over a 24 h period. As long as the skill mix was appropriate for organisational demands, midwives were largely interchangeable. As Goffman (1968) has observed, the focus on the needs of the institution results in a restricted orientation towards clients. The emphasis was on successful completion of tasks, in order to ensure the physical safety of mothers and babies. The following data extract illustrates this task-orientated approach:

I just love that challenge of having to continually prioritise, who you've got on the monitor, who's your blood pressure, who's your normal delivery. (Phase Three: Interview 6, E-grade hospital midwife)

Integrated team midwives, who were able to compare the influence of hospital and community settings on practice, were particularly aware of this focus on tasks rather than clients:

You know it was unsettling because (. . .) I didn't get to know anyone properly. I was flitting about . . . go and discharge this one, go and admit that one (. . .) can you do a monitoring on this one (. . .) so that was very unsettling. (Phase Three: Interview 12, F-grade integrated team midwife)

At the end of a shift, the work was handed over to the next group of midwives. As frequently noted during the observational fieldwork, the emphasis was on 'getting through the work', so that few tasks were left for the next shift. The following account illustrates some of the key characteristics of hospital midwifery identified in this study: the dominance of organisational needs, the subsequent focus on task completion and the significance of relationships with colleagues rather than clients. As will be seen, these elements differed significantly from the characteristics of community-based midwifery:

You feel that you have to get round all your allocation in that one shift and sometimes you can't do it and everybody feels a bit guilty when you're handing over work to whoever's coming behind . . . we all try not to stand in report (staff handover) and say 'well I haven't done this and I haven't done that' because you feel that you've failed on your shift. (Phase Three: Interview 9, G-grade hospital midwife)

A medicalised approach to childbirth appeared to dominate hospital midwifery practice, despite many midwives' apparent criticisms of this. Medicalisation restricted midwifery autonomy: observation of hospital midwives indicated that practice was controlled by obstetric protocols and policies, designed to 'manage' pregnancy and childbirth and reduce birth-related pathology. In the wards particularly, the role of the midwife was observed to be largely that of a nurse: carrying out

Table 1.2.1 A model of the interrelationships between context, occupational ideology and emotion work in midwifery practice

Context	Aspects of occupational indentity	Occupational ideology	Emotion work
Hospital-based practice	• Medicalised approach • Universal provision of equitable care • Decreased autonomy • Midwives interchangeable • Decreased significance of relationships with clients • Increased sense of affiliation to colleagues and organisation	'With institution'	To resolve disparity between 'with woman' ideal and 'with institution' necessity
Integrated practice	Occupational identity = ambiguous	Ideologies incompatible →	Increased emotion work
Community-based practice	• Natural approach • Individualised provision of care • Increased autonomy • Increased emphasis on use of self • Increased significance of relationships with clients • Decreased sense of affiliation to organisation	'With woman'	To resolve conflicts (a) between 'with woman' ideal and institutional demands (b) related to sustainability of ideal

doctors' instructions for care and treatment of clients, arranging for tests and referrals and acting as a go-between in communications between clients and medical staff. This inevitably decreased the amount of time available for postnatal care, which was frustrating for midwives as this was acknowledged as being midwifery 'territory', in which midwives were more able to exercise some degree of occupational autonomy.

For many hospital-based midwives, job satisfaction tended to be measured in terms of organisational goals: work was described as emotionally rewarding when tasks were finished, women and babies were discharged home and midwives could leave knowing that their work was finished:

(It's) satisfying if you've had a good shift . . . and if you've managed to achieve the workload you've been given and managed that with time . . . you've actually managed to meet the needs set before you, whether it's one on labour ward, or whether it's eight women on the ward . . . you know nothing's been missed. (Phase Three: Focus Group 4, Hospital E-and F-grade midwives)

However, the more junior midwives (especially students) expressed frustration with hospital work, as it did not reflect their ideals of practice. Clashes with senior midwives were described, which were often underpinned by ideological conflicts. Senior midwives were commonly criticised for assuming a medicalised approach to childbirth, and for focusing more on the needs of the institution than the woman and her family:

Their focus is a sterile birth or a procedure – a mechanistic procedure that has to be undergone to have a live healthy infant (. . .) it isn't about how the woman feels about it (. . .) that's like an added frilly bit, it's not essential – I suppose that's how they cope with the workload – they don't cope with it because they don't deal with it. (Group agreement) (Phase 1: Focus Group 1, Final-year 18-month student midwives)

On the labour ward, there's (. . .) often an underlying pressure 'oh we've got to get this woman moving, she's been here too long' (strong group agreement) or 'the last one's delivered an hour and a half ago, let's rush her down to the ward' – and it's this 'clear the board' mentality. (Group agreement) (Phase Three: Focus Group 4, E-and F-grade hospital midwives)

Emotion work was therefore needed in order to reduce the disparity between the 'with woman' ideal and the 'with institution' reality. Although the findings suggested that some midwives were able to overcome this by adopting a variety of strategies aimed at restoring emotional balance (for example, finding emotional rewards in collegial relationships and doing 'real midwifery' wherever possible), many midwives felt alienated and frustrated by these ambiguities:

I got to a stage where I thought 'I hate it – I don't want to go to work at all' – because I was so fed up – I felt I was being bullied all the time to do things I didn't want to do, it wasn't in the woman's best interest and I thought, this wasn't what I came into midwifery for – to put up with all this nonsense. (Phase Three: Focus Group 4, E-and F-grade hospital midwives)

'With woman ideology'

In contrast to hospital-based practice, community-based midwifery provided many more opportunities to work in ways that were 'with woman' and thus ideologically congruent. Community-based midwives generally adopted a 'natural' approach to maternity care, demonstrated not only by their expressed confidence in physiological processes, but also by their focus on the psychosocial aspects of care. Many midwives were observed during home visits chatting about the social aspects of the woman's life, and appeared to have considerable knowledge about her family and wider community. This was frequently explained as a strategy to make the contact less formal and relaxed, and hence allow the woman to 'open up'. The midwife would explain that she was assessing the woman's psychological and physical needs informally during this time, and would base her subsequent care on this:

It's not so much a physical job is it? You're picking up signs that things could be physically wrong by what you're asking them. (Phase Three: Interview 2, G-grade traditional midwife)

Being able to 'pick up signs' in a covert way was perceived to be a key skill of midwifery. Midwives considered that 'knowing the woman' made their work easier, although it was also observed that this aspect of work was relatively undervalued and unrecognised:

It's possible to spend a great deal of time doing things that wouldn't be counted as work – the emotion bit can't be measured. (Phase Three: Fieldnotes 4, F-grade integrated team midwife)

Consequently, relationships with clients and their families assumed much greater significance than they did for hospital-based midwives. When asked about what made midwifery emotionally rewarding, variations on the answers: 'Oh the women! Getting to know them, them getting to know you!' (Phase Three: Interview 3, F-grade traditional midwife) 'They're the ones who keep you going' (Phase Three: Interview 4, F-grade team midwife), were notable in their immediacy and enthusiasm. In Lipsky's (1980, p. 47) words, clients formed the 'primary reference group' for midwives; that is they were a key source of support and affirmation, in contrast to hospital midwives for whom colleagues assumed this role. Both Brodie (1996) and Sandall (1997) have similarly observed the value community-based midwives place on client relationships.

The findings suggested that community midwives found their work rewarding when they were able to work in a way that was congruent with a 'with woman' ideology. Although such work was emotionally demanding, it was fulfilling and hence not experienced as emotionally difficult. For example:

I mean when you're called at three o'clock in the morning and it's one of your women, it's completely different than being called by somebody else's woman – you just don't mind! (Group agreement) (Phase Three: Focus Group 2, F-grade integrated team midwives)

Emotion work was needed to manage the negative emotions experienced when midwives could not work in this ideal way or when work was experienced as unsustainable. Ironically, it was the integrated team midwives who were most likely to experience these difficulties. This occurred particularly when they were working within the maternity unit, i.e. when the context of their practice was altered. In addition to feeling geographically dislocated, as noted in other studies (Ball et al., 2002), they also found that their autonomy was compromised and it became difficult to maintain a natural, woman-centred approach. In the following account, an integrated team midwife describes how her ideals were challenged by senior, hospital-based midwives, and the impact that this had on her relationship with the woman:

Midwife: Recently there was a woman not wanting a VE (vaginal examination) – she's got every reason to – didn't seem to need one but it was 'oh well, she should have one . . . can you not persuade her to have one?' On and on and on about it until in the end I felt like I didn't know which way I was going – I felt less able to be with her and say 'yes don't have it if you don't want it' and more like 'well she's being a stroppy little madam and I've really had enough now'. BH: so it undermined your relationship with her? Midwife: yeah. (Phase Three: Interview 12, F-grade integrated team midwife)

Other integrated team midwives described similar compromising situations. Common to these accounts were feelings of divided loyalty and ambiguous autonomy. Integrated team midwives frequently found themselves playing 'piggy in the middle' between the women, senior midwives, doctors and organisational policies (Murphy-Lawless, 1991):

Midwife 1: this is supposed to be my case load, I'm supposed to be responsible for these women, and yet I've got somebody up there saying, 'oh, no, you can't do that'. And that is very frustrating, and I feel that they're not respecting my position – (Group agreement) because I'm not giving these women what they want. I am really doing what they want me to do. (. . .) And that, to me, is very frustrating and I think will be the ruin of midwifery, really (. . .) As far as your job is concerned, it makes it much more difficult . . . Midwife 2: and very stressed. (Phase Three: Focus Group 2, F-grade integrated team midwives)

Although many integrated team midwives held strong beliefs regarding the importance of a 'with woman'

approach to care regarding themselves as pioneers in establishing a partnership approach to care, in reality the dominance of institutional needs over community work led to frequent compromise and disappointment.

Discussion

This study has some limitations, related to location and sample, which limit the potential for theoretical generalisation. At the time of data collection, the research site had a relatively stable workforce and there were few problems with recruitment and retention, in contrast to the wider national situation (Ball et al., 2002). The study population had specific characteristics, as it was predominantly white and all female, thus differing from other urban maternity units. The sample size was smaller than anticipated and consisted largely of E-and F-grade midwives; only one G-grade hospital midwife took part, thus the experiences of senior hospital-based midwives is relatively unknown.

However, the findings of this study raise important issues of relevance to contemporary UK midwifery, particularly related to key sources of emotion work. Issues that create emotional difficulty for midwives have been identified, which are likely to be of relevance to understanding the low morale and difficulties with staff retention currently evident in UK midwifery (Ball et al., 2002; House of Commons Select Committee, 2003; Walter, 2003).

The findings do not support the assumption found in much of the literature that emotion work is primarily situated in the worker/client relationship. Rather, for midwives it was the co-existence of conflicting ideologies of practice that created most dissonance and need for subsequent emotion work. This led not only to personal frustration, but also to disharmony between colleagues. It was evident that hospital-based midwives in particular divided themselves into 'us and them' groups on the basis of ideology; this finding may go some way to explaining the tensions within midwifery culture that have been identified by other authors (Leap, 1997; Kirkham, 1999; Kirkham and Stapleton, 2000; Ball et al., 2002).

The presence of conflicting ideologies also appeared responsible for much of the dissatisfaction with the new system of integrated practice. It appeared that midwives were prepared to meet the physical and emotional demands inherent in this way of working, as long as they were able do 'real midwifery' by working in a manner that was congruent with their ideals. Frustration at not being able to accomplish the full role of a midwife has been identified as the key reason for midwives leaving the profession (Ball et al., 2002).

Concerns have been expressed in the midwifery literature regarding the sustainability and desirability of integrated midwifery practice (Anderson, 2002, 2003), with some researchers citing integration as a cause of potential risk to client safety (Ashcroft et al., 2003). The system of integration present in the unit under study appeared to be problematic for midwives not only because of the physical demands of on-calls and long hours, but also because the focus on institutional needs was incompatible with a 'with woman' approach to care.

These differing ideologies have an historical legacy. The past 100 years have seen midwifery develop from a community-based 'craft', via a highly technocratic, hospital-based and medically controlled occupation in the 1970s, to current attempts to return to aspects of 'old style' practice, with midwives working 'flexibly' between community and institutional settings and attempting to reclaim their role as lead professionals in maternity care. Thus, the 'with institution' ideology has its roots in the high-tech maternity care of the 1970s, whilst 'with woman' ideology represents an attempt to return to the perceived essence of midwifery. The difficulty appears to arise because there is no acknowledgement of the co-existence of these two ideologies.

The current ethos within UK maternity care, as evident in educational philosophies, professional statements and national policy recommendations (Department of Health (DoH), 1993; Standing Nursing and Midwifery Advisory Committee (SMMAC), 1998; Royal College of Midwives (RCM), 2000; Welsh Assembly Government (WAG), 2002), rejects a 'with institution' approach as anachronistic and advocates a 'with woman' approach as ideal practice. For example, the recent Welsh maternity service strategy (Welsh Assembly Government (WAG), 2002) recommends that 'integration of maternity services has to be maintained, to include a visible base for midwives in a community setting, where midwives can be the first point of contact' (p. 6). The emphasis is on promoting normality in childbirth and providing a 'seamless service where midwives can use all their skills and provide continuity of care' (Welsh Assembly Government (WAG), 2002, p. 6).

This perspective, however laudable, appears to presume that all midwives will be able to work according to a shared 'with woman' ideology, regardless of context. There is no apparent questioning of the rationale of applying a shared ideology to two such diverse settings as hospital and community environments. It is assumed that 'a midwife is a midwife is a midwife' (Midwives Information and Resource Service (MIDIRS), 1989) and that midwives can be 'all things to all women' (Dennett, 2001, p. 454). The findings of this study, however, indicate that this is at odds with the lived experiences of midwives, who appear to have different occupational identities related to work location. Moreover, the findings also indicate that it is the unsustainability of this shared ideology that creates emotion work: it is rarely achievable within the hospital setting, and has varying degrees of success in community settings.

Implications for practice

It is important for midwives to acknowledge these conflicting ideologies as a primary source of emotional difficulty and address them explicitly. As it is, the dilemmas experienced are rarely articulated; universal issues thus become interpreted as personal dilemmas or even personal failings. This may well account for the guilt and self-blame that has been noted in midwifery (Kirkham, 1999; Kirkham and Stapleton, 2000), and is likely to be a contributory factor in low morale and poor retention (Ball et al., 2002).

These issues clearly need addressing. In the short term, midwives require strategies to enable them to retain their ideals, whilst acknowledging the reality of contemporary practice. Education, of both student and qualified midwives, could play a role in this, making use of innovative teaching methods such as participative theatre (Baker, 2000) and critical theory (Porter, 1998).

Workplace support is essential; a clinical supervision model (Kirkham, 1999), either on a one-to-one or peer support group basis could provide a forum in which these dilemmas could be aired.

These measures, however, are unlikely to be more than superficially successful unless attention is paid to the underpinning contradictions identified in this study: that is, the conflicting beliefs regarding the nature of childbirth and hence the nature of midwifery. Addressing these issues will require a fundamental challenge to accepted norms. It seems unlikely, however, given the current trends in reproductive medicine (e.g. assisted conception, fetal medicine, genetic screening) that there will be a paradigm shift away from a medicalised model of childbirth. Rather, it is argued that midwives need to conserve their energies and find more pragmatic solutions.

It may be that we need to accept that there are different types of midwife, whose work is underpinned by different ideals and values, and who would prefer to work in different settings. For example, it would be possible to have midwives practising solely in the community, holding their own caseloads of 'low risk' women and attending normal births at home or in a midwife-led birthing centre (in fact, following the model adopted by independent midwives). There would also be hospital midwives, who would be the experts in abnormal midwifery, skilled in managing technology and providing care for women experiencing complications. Since the study was undertaken, this approach to organising midwifery services has been debated by several authors (Mason, 2000; Dennett, 2001; Anderson, 2003).

Alternatively, it may be possible to remove the basis of these contradictions by shifting the location of birth from hospital to midwife-led birth centre. In doing so, it should be possible not only to shift occupational jurisdiction to midwives, but also eventually to change cultural attitudes towards childbirth (Wagner, 2001). However, it is acknowledged that shifting the location of birth could also be problematic. Midwives have developed expertise in differing areas of practice; for those who have acquired more technological skills, and prefer working in an obstetric unit, return to a more 'natural' focus is likely to be frustrating if not inappropriate. This returns us to the previous argument for creating different types of midwife.

Conclusion

In this study, I explored how a range of student and qualified midwives in South Wales experienced and managed emotion in their work. A theory is proposed that the key source of emotion work is the dissonance created by the co-existence of conflicting ideologies of practice, which has potential application to other midwives in the UK. It may also be of potential relevance to midwives internationally, in particular those who work within a dominant medicalised paradigm. It would therefore be valuable to undertake further research in other geographical locations, particularly those with differing demographic features and where there are workforce shortages, in order to further develop these concepts and theories.

By increasing our understanding of the sources of emotion work in midwifery, it may be possible to improve the working lives of midwives and hence the care that they give to women and their families.

Acknowledgements

This research was partly funded by a Welsh National Board Research Training Fellowship (1997–1998) and the Iolanthe Midwifery Trust Research Fellowship (1999–2001). The author wishes to thank all the midwives and women who participated in this study. Thanks also to Dr Lesley Griffiths and independent referees for their comments on this paper.

REFERENCES

Anderson, T., 2002. Integration or disintegration? The scandal of the integration of midwifery services. MIDIRS Midwifery Digest 12 (4), 445–447.

Anderson, T., 2003. Integration or disintegration? The scandal of the integration of midwifery services Part 2. MIDIRS Midwifery Digest 13 (1), 122–124.

Ashcroft, B., Elstein, M., Boreham, N., Holm, S., 2003. Prospective semi-structured observational study to identify risk attributable to staff deployment, training and updating opportunities for midwives. British Journal of Medicine 327, 584–600.

Baker, K., 2000. Acting the part: using drama to empower student midwives. Practising Midwife 3 (1), 20–21.

Ball, L., Curtis, P., Kirkham, M., 2002. Why do Midwives Leave? Women's Informed Childbearing and Health Research Group, University of Sheffield.

Berg, M., Lundgren, I., Hermansson, E., et al., 1996. Women's experience of the encounter with the midwife during childbirth. Midwifery 12, 11–15.

Brodie, P., 1996. Being with women: the experience of Australian team midwives. Unpublished Masters Thesis, University of Technology, Sydney, Australia.

Bryman, A., 2001. Social Research Methods. Oxford University Press, Oxford. Carvel, J., 2001. Mothers get one-to-one childbirth care. The Guardian June 16, 4.

Coffey, A., Atkinson, P., 1996. Making Sense of Qualitative Data. Sage, London.

Dennett, S., 2001. Midwifery practice – time for radical change? MIDIRS Midwifery Digest 11 (4), 454–456.

Department of Health (DoH), 1993. Changing Childbirth: Part 1: Report of the Expert Maternity Group. HMSO, London.

Dey, I., 1993. Qualitative Data Analysis: A User-Friendly Guide for Social Scientists. Routledge, London.

Fineman, S. (Ed.), 1993. Emotion in Organizations. Sage, London.

Goffman, E., 1968. Asylums. Essays on the Social Situation of Mental Patients and Other Inmates. Penguin, Harmondsworth.

Goffman, E., 1969. The Presentation of Self in Everyday Life. Allen Lane, The Penguin Press, London.

Halldorsdottir, S., Karlsdottir, S.I., 1996. Journeying through labour and delivery: perceptions of women who have given birth. Midwifery 12, 48–61.

Hammersley, M., Atkinson, P., 1995. Ethnography: Principles and Practice, 2nd Edition. Routledge, London.

Hochschild, A.R., 1979. Emotion work, feeling rules and social structure. American Journal of Sociology 85 (3), 551–575.

Hochschild, A.R., 1983. The Managed Heart. Commercialization of Human Feeling. University of California Press, Berkeley, California.

House of Commons Select Committee, 1992. Second Report: Maternity Services. HMSO, London.

House of Commons Select Committee, 2003. Fourth Report: Provision of Maternity Services. Stationary Office, London.

Hunter, B., 2002. Emotion work in midwifery: an ethnographic study of the emotional work undertaken by a sample of student and qualified midwives in Wales. Unpublished Ph.D. Thesis, University of Wales, Swansea.

James, N., 1989. Emotional labour: skill and work in the social regulation of feelings. Sociological Review 37, 15–42.

James, N., 1992. Care = organisation + physical labour + emotional labour. Sociology of Health and Illness 14 (4), 489–509.

Kirkham, M., 1999. The culture of midwifery in the National Health Service in England. Journal of Advanced Nursing 30 (3), 732–739.

Kirkham, M. (Ed.), 2000. The Midwife-Mother Relationship. Macmillan Press, Basingstoke.

Kirkham, M., Stapleton, H., 2000. Midwives' support needs as childbirth changes. Journal of Advanced Nursing 32 (2), 465–472.

Krueger, R.A., 1994. Focus Groups: A Practical Guide for Applied Research, 2nd Edition. Sage, London.

Leap, N., 1997. Making sense of 'horizontal violence' in midwifery. British Journal of Midwifery 5, 689.

Lincoln, Y.S., Guba, E., 1985. Naturalistic Inquiry. Sage, Beverley Hills, California.

Lipsky, M., 1980. Street-Level Bureaucracy: Dilemmas of the Individual in Public Services. Russell Sage Foundation, New York.

Mackin, P., Sinclair, M., 1998. Labour ward midwives' perceptions of stress. Journal of Advanced Nursing 27, 986–991.

Mander, R., 2001. Supportive Care and Midwifery. Blackwell Science, London.

Mason, J., 2000. Defining midwifery practice. AIMS Journal 12 (4), 5–6.

MIDIRS (Midwives Information and Resource Service), 1989. Editorial. A Midwife is a midwife is a midwife. MIDIRS Information Pack No 10, April 1989.

Morgan, D.L., Krueger, R.A., 1998. The Focus Group Kit. Sage, London.

Morse, J.M., Field, P.A., 1996. Nursing Research: The Application of Qualitative Approaches. Chapman & Hall, London.

Murphy-Lawless, J., 1991. Piggy in the middle: the midwife's role in achieving woman-controlled childbirth. The Irish Journal of Psychology 12 (2), 198–215.

National Assembly for Wales (NAW), 2003. Maternity Statistics, Wales: Method of Delivery 1995–2002 www.wales.gov.uk/ statistics.

Niven, C., 1994. Coping with labour pain: the midwife's role. In: Robinson, S., Thomson, A.M. (Eds.), Midwives, Research and Childbirth, Vol. 3. Chapman & Hall, London.

Oakley, A., 1994. Giving support in pregnancy: the role of research midwives in a randomised controlled trial. In: Robinson, S., Thomson, A.M. (Eds.), Midwives, Research and Childbirth, Vol. 3. Chapman & Hall, London.

Page, L.A. (Ed.), 2000. The New Midwifery. Science and Sensitivity in Practice. Churchill Livingstone, Edinburgh.

Porter, S., 1998. Social Theory and Nursing Practice. Macmillan, Basingstoke.

Royal College of Midwives (RCM), 2000. Vision 2000. RCM, London.

Sandall, J., 1997. Midwives' burnout and continuity of care. British Journal of Midwifery 5 (2), 106–111.

Sandall, J., 1998. Midwifery work, family life and wellbeing: a study of occupational change. Unpublished Ph.D. Thesis. University of Surrey, Guildford.

Silverman, D., 1993. Interpreting Qualitative Data: Methods for Analysing Talk, Text and Interaction. Sage, London.

Silverman, D., 2000. Doing Qualitative Research: A Practical Handbook. Sage, London.

Smith, A.C., Kleinman, S., 1989. Managing emotions in medical school: students' contacts with the living and the dead. Social Psychology Quarterly 52 (1), 56–69.

Smith, P., 1992. The Emotional Labour of Nursing. Macmillan, London.

Standing Nursing and Midwifery Advisory Committee (SMMAC), 1998. Midwifery: Delivering our Future. February 1998. Department of Health, London.

United Kingdom Central Council Commission for Nursing and Midwifery Education (UKCC), 1999. Fitness for Practice. (Chair: Sir Leonard Peach) UKCC, London.

Wagner, M., 2001. Fish can't see water: the need to humanize birth. International Journal of Gynecology and Obstetrics 75 (Suppl. 1), S25–S37.

Walsh, D., 1999. An ethnographic study of women's experience of partnership caseload midwifery practice: the professional as friend. Midwifery 15, 165–176.

Walter, N., 2003. Expect the worse. The Guardian: Comment and Analysis 28 May.

Welsh Assembly Government (WAG), 2002. Delivering the Future in Wales: A Framework for Realising the Potential of Midwives in Wales. Briefing Paper 4. Realising the Potential: A Strategic Framework for Nursing, Midwifery and Health Visiting in Wales into the 21st Century.

Midwifery 2004; 20(3): 261–272

Advice on advice

Mary Nolan

A client asked me at a recent antenatal class whether I could advise her on vaginal birth after caesarean. I replied automatically that I could not do so because I am not a health professional and therefore not qualified to give advice. All NCT antenatal teachers (and doubtless educators from other charitable organisations involved in maternity care) have drummed into them from the first day of their Diploma course that they cannot give advice. The word has to be expunged from students' written work and must not cross teachers' lips during classes.

Many years ago, I was a health professional and doubtless gave a lot of advice. I have an uneasy feeling, with the wisdom of hindsight and perhaps greater awareness of what makes myself and my fellow human beings tick, that none of it was very helpful. When did you last act on a piece of advice, act on it without modifying in any way what you were told to do? People – adults and children – don't tend to take advice.

The world of healthcare has moved on since I was a part of it. Now clinicians are educated to be reflective practitioners. They learn how to 'bend back' (re-flect) their thoughts in order to explore significant experiences in their personal lives or in their professional practice so they can understand what makes them act as they do, and how their own experiences might affect the way in which they care for others. We reflect so that the people for whom we care are free to make their own decisions – free of our emotional baggage and prejudices.

We are never going to be in a position to advise a single client, because we can never stand in their shoes, live in their world, think with their brain. We can only help people make their own decisions.

Making decisions

The process by which people make decisions varies according to their learning/living styles. Some people are analytical thinkers, who like to break a problem down into its component parts. They focus their attention on the details. They like to work through the problem logically, one step at a time, perhaps noting the key points on a list.

Holistic thinkers are very different. They like to confront the big picture; they are not interested in the details. They like to solve their problems while out for a walk, swimming or doodling. They make decisions impulsively and may not be able to analyse how they have reached their conclusions. They rely on insight and hunches.

We all know people who favour one or other of these approaches to life. It is very difficult for analytical thinkers to be patient with crazy holistic thinkers, and holistics think analytics are boring.

So there is a problem in giving advice if the way we would approach a decision is very different from the way our client does.

As health professionals or lay people with a specialist interest in healthcare, we are immersed in academic and clinical research, the statistics and the accumulated and interacting experiences of perhaps many years of practice. We have a global perspective on maternity care and the issues that confront our clients as they travel through the system.

Our concern may be keeping up to date with the wealth of information now available through electronic sources, the plethora of journals and all the documents coming from government. Any single issue may raise questions in our minds such as, 'Is there a Cochrane Review about that?' 'Has the RCOG published Green Top Guidelines?' 'What does NICE recommend?' These are not questions that hold any interest for most of our clients.

Context, not content

The human brain can only deal with limited amounts of information; it is not good at doing content, but it is extremely good at doing context. That is, it seizes on information and filters it through our life experiences, viewing it from the perspective of events that happened when we were children and since we have become adults.

It examines the information from the point of view of our religious and moral convictions. It weighs it up in our own particular risk scales – some of us are risk inclined and some of us are risk averse. It listens to what our mother has to say on the subject, our partner, our best friend and the media. It applies the insights of *The Sun* or *The Independent*, according to personal preference. Finally, when the information is firmly embedded in the rich and unique context of our own life, the brain reaches a judgement about its relevance or otherwise and decides whether any action is required.

That is why women continue to bottle-feed despite the overwhelming evidence of the superiority of breast-feeding, why they fail to demand home births despite the overwhelming evidence of the safety of home birth, why they continue to ask for epidurals when you know that they would have a better birth experience without.

The next generation

It takes a long time to embed accurate information in society, and for sufficient women to have had a range of experiences different from those of their mothers and sisters (and the soap stars) so that the next generation of women coming to childbirth can make decisions within a different social and personal context.

In the meantime, we cannot force anyone's hand. All we can do is provide a few facts, as simple or as complex as the woman can accommodate, choose our words carefully so that the facts aren't weighted with our own meanings, and ask the woman the right questions. How does she feel about what the two of you have discussed? (No information reaches the cortex or thinking part of the brain without passing through the limbic or emotional centre.) How does it fit in with other things that she knows? How does it fit in with what the people closest to her have told her? Is it information that sits comfortably with her understanding of her life? Is it information on which she will act?

Combs (cited in Prashnig 2004: 24) said that learning (or 'decision making') always consists of two parts:

First – confrontation with new information or
     experience;
Second – discovery of personal, individual meaning.

However frustrating it is, we can't advise people as to what their personal, individual meanings should be; we can only confront them with a little new information and stand by, empathising and encouraging, providing more information if needed, while they discover their own meanings. Our care follows in the wake of the clients' decisions; it doesn't fly ahead.

REFERENCE

Prashnig B (2004). The Power of Diversity, Stafford: Network Educational Press.

The Practising Midwife 2005; 8(6): 4–5

Developing a maternity unit visiting policy

Hora Soltani, Fiona Dickinson, Judith Tanner

Southern Derbyshire Acute Hospitals NHS Trust has a policy of open visiting for people who wish to visit ward-based patients. The maternity unit, however, has adopted a slightly different approach, in which the visiting policy loosely consists of set hours with a degree of flexibility for mothers and visitors who wish to have extended visiting or want visitors outside the set hours. This article describes research undertaken to formulate a policy within the trust.

Many studies have been undertaken evaluating open visiting, although these have focused primarily on children (Bradley 2001) and critically ill patients in intensive care areas (Carlson et al 1998; Ramsey et al 2000). Open visiting is intended to improve the quality of care for patients and their visitors by allowing visitors access to wards at any time. While it is widely considered to be a positive intervention (Clarke 2000), concerns raised by the local Maternity User Group, as well as informal feedback from staff, suggest that mothers and staff may prefer to have a visiting policy where hours are restricted rather than open. Within maternity wards, in addition to the mother and baby's comfort, the issue of security complicates the process of policy making. To date, there is little research evidence as to what women, their families and the staff think about visiting hours within maternity services. The only identified maternity-related study was by Malcolmson et al (1999), showing that women and staff preferred a more liberal open visiting policy for partners.

The study

The aim of this study was to ascertain mothers', visitors' and ward staff's preferences relating to the hospital visiting times and to provide evidence for the development of a maternity ward visiting policy.

Method

A questionnaire was distributed to mothers and visitors during one week, and all ward staff working on the Derbyshire Maternity Suite (DMS). DMS provides care and support for women who are admitted for antenatal or postnatal care.

Sample

Questionnaires were distributed to 100 women and visitors over the week; 26 and 25 responses respectively were received. All midwives and healthcare assistants (a total of 90 staff) received the questionnaire; 29 were returned.

Questionnaire

The focus of the questionnaire was to ask participants for their opinions of the visiting times and to identify their preferences for a visiting policy. The questionnaires were orientated to make them appropriate for mothers, visitors and ward staff and colour coded for each group, to assist with the analysis. The questionnaires were piloted using ward staff, mothers and visitors on one ward prior to the start of the study, and amendments made where appropriate. The questionnaire was adapted from one designed for use in a larger study of visiting hours throughout the hospital.

Ethical approval was sought and obtained from the Local Research Ethics Committee and Southern Derbyshire Acute Hospitals NHS Trust.

Distribution and collection of questionnaires

The questionnaires were distributed by allocated staff and researchers on DMS. To encourage compliance, the researcher informed staff of the study at the ward meeting.

A sealed collection box was placed on the ward for completed questionnaires.

Formal consent was not sought, as consent was implied through completion and return of the questionnaire. The questionnaires were anonymous to ensure confidentiality.

Analysis

The information collected included both quantitative and qualitative data. The data were entered using the Formic data capture system (version 3.4) and transferred to SPSS (Statistical Package for Social Sciences, version 11.5) for analysis. For the qualitative data we used thematic content analysis to identify indepth practical information to be reflected in the visiting policy. The quantitative data was analysed using simple descriptive statistics.

Results

There was a comparable response rate from all three groups: women 26 per cent (n = 26), visitors 25 per cent (n = 25) and staff 32 per cent (n = 29).

Open versus restricted visiting

A number of questions were asked to elicit views on the nature of visiting – whether it should be open to all or restricted and in what way.

The initial questions asked respondents to tick boxes indicating whether they agreed or disagreed with given statements. A number of statements were common across all three groups, with appropriate wording. Table 1.4.1 gives a summary of these findings.

There were four statements to which the majority of respondents strongly agreed or disagreed.

A majority of staff and mothers agreed that they did not like people visiting during meal times. However, although a significant number of visitors felt this way, more than half indicated that they should be able to visit during meal times.

Staff and visitors were asked if visitors should be able to stay overnight, of which 100 per cent of staff and 62.5 per cent of visitors said that they did not want this.

The most significant result obtained from these questions was relating to the option of having open visiting for the women's partner (or one identified visitor) and restricted visiting times for others. A large majority of all three groups agreed with this statement, suggesting a possible way forward for future policy.

The idea of having a quiet time, without visitors, was also popular with both mothers and staff.

Visiting times

All three groups of respondents were broadly asked when they thought visiting hours should be (Table 1.4.2). The majority of mothers and visitors thought that visiting should be in both the morning and afternoon, but the majority of staff thought that it should be restricted to the afternoon.

The respondents were then asked to be more specific about visiting times, given a range of options (Tables 1.4.3 and 1.4.4).

The largest proportion of all three groups thought that visiting should start at 10am, although a significant number of mothers and staff felt that it should be delayed

Table 1.4.1 Perceptions on the nature of visiting arrangements

	Agree (%)			Disagree (%)		
	Visitors	Staff	Mothers	Visitors	Staff	Mothers
Visitors should be able to visit at any time	88.0	3.6	56	12.0	96.4	44.0
Embarrassing/difficult to have visitors present when having midwifery care	16.0	100.0	34.6	84.0	0	65.4
Don't like visiting during mealtimes	44.0	89.7	61.5	56.0	10.3	38.5
Visitors should be able to visit during the night	37.5	0	#	62.5	100.0	#
Open visiting for the partner (or identified visitor) and restricted hours for others	79.2	92.9	80.8	20.8	7.1	19.2
Some (of my) visitors stay too long	#	100.0	11.5	#	0	88.5
Other people's visitors stay too long	#	#	34.6	#	#	65.4
There should be a quiet time with no visitors	#	89.7	73.1	#	10.3	26.9
Other people's visitors disturb me	#	#	26.9	#	#	73.1
Visitors can be helpful with maternity care	#	46.2	#	#	56.8	#
I find visiting time tiring	#	#	23.1	#	#	76.9

#Question was not asked of this group

Table 1.4.2 Should visiting time be in the morning or afternoon? (%)

	Morning	Afternoon	Both
Mothers (n = 26)	0	26.9	73.0
Visitors (n = 25)	0	28.0	72.0
Staff (n = 29)	0	65.5	34.5

Table 1.4.3 When should visiting time start? (%)

	6am	7am	8am	9am	10am	11am	No restriction
Mothers (n = 25)	4.0	4.0	4.0	4.0	40.0	36.0	8.0
Visitors (n = 21)	9.5	0	9.5	9.5	42.9	14.3	14.3
Staff (n = 16)	6.3	0	6.3	0	50.0	37.5	0

Table 1.4.4 When should visiting time end? (%)

	8pm	9pm	10pm	11pm	No restriction
Mothers (n = 26)	19.2	53.8	11.5	3.8	11.5
Visitors (n = 25)	20.0	44.0	20.0	0	16.0
Staff (n = 28)	71.4	21.4	7.1	0	0

Table 1.4.5 Should there be a maximum number of visitors? (%)

	Yes	No
Mothers (n = 26)	73.1	26.9
Visitors (n = 25)	80.0	20.0
Staff (n = 29)	100.0	0

Table 1.4.6 What should be the maximum number of visitors? (%)

	2	3	4	5	6
Mothers (n = 20)	0	40.0	45.0	10.0	5.0
Visitors (n = 21)	28.6	23.8	42.9	4.8	0
Staff (n = 28)	28.6	32.1	35.7	3.6	0

until 11am. Although small relative to the overall responses, the largest proportion of people who thought there should be no restriction was in the visitors group and this was the same for both the start and end of visiting.

Most staff thought that visiting should end at 8pm, but the largest proportions of mothers and visitors preferred it to continue until 9pm. Across all three groups, the totalled percentages showed that 9pm was slightly more popular (119.2 total %), compared with 8pm (110.6 total %).

Number of visitors

All three groups were asked if there should be a maximum number of visitors each woman can have at a time and what the maximum number should be. This was considered to be of importance, as the vast majority of women have to share six-bedded bays as well as having cots and other equipment, limiting available space. Their responses are given in Table 1.4.5.

All three groups were strongly in favour of there being a maximum number of visitors 'per bed'. However, there was wide variation in relation to what that number should be (Table 1.4.6).

The majority of mothers thought that the maximum number should be either three or four, with only 15 per cent thinking it should be anything else. Visitors indicated a majority preference of between two and four, with only 5 per cent wanting five visitors per bed. Staff also showed a majority preference for between two and four,

with only 3.6 per cent wanting five visitors. It is interesting to note that the only group to show a preference for a maximum of six visitors per bed, were the mothers themselves.

Qualitative findings

The staff questionnaire was slightly different from the others in that it included two extra qualitative questions. These explored the reasons why staff had asked visitors to leave the ward, and what they thought was important in planning visiting hours. A number of the responses given were similar in both questions.

One of the most commonly cited reasons why staff asked visitors to leave was so that the women could get some rest – 'Some women have been overtired but did not want to offend their visitors therefore requested that we ask them to leave or restrict them' (7); 'After 10pm and ladies wanting to sleep' (16). They also asked them to go because they had over stayed visiting hours or it was very late – 'Have stayed long after visiting times' (24); 'Because it was late and the mother was tired' (29); – and because there were too many visitors: '10 visitors round one bed, very noisy not allowing other visitors to visit other patients' (16); 'Too many with first day c/s' (15).

When asked what they thought were important issues when planning visiting hours, staff responded with a wide range of issues. One of these was visiting at meal times: 'Meals are left uneaten when visitors arrive' (8); '. . . you get either the scenario where the patient doesn't eat their meal or the visitor eats the meal for them' (11).

These comments are in line with what the majority of respondents expressed in the quantitative responses, ie not wanting visitors at meal times.

Others included routine care such as:

Hygiene needs or drug rounds
'Having chance to shower and bath baby in morning' (2)
'Drug rounds, doctors rounds' (20)

Safety
'Health and safety, eg, if fire, how many can safely exit: 62 mothers, 62 babies, staff, 62 × 1 visitor is a lot of people to move safely and quickly' (16)

Privacy to breastfeed
'Reluctance to feed their babies by breast' (26)

Difficulty in getting rest
'Rest time for mums and babies' (5)

Number of people in a limited space
'No space for the 8–10 people some patients would have' (22)

Opportunity for women and their partners to spend time with their new baby
'Time for husband to be with wife (partner) and baby on their own' (12)

External arrangements, eg having to pick other children up from school
'Afternoon visitors being able to visit before picking up own children from school' (6)

Staff workload
'Workload re discharge procedures' (25)

Arrangements on the ward, eg lounge area where people could take their visitors away from beds and other resting women
'Flexible area away from bed, family area' (14)

All three groups were given an opportunity to make any further comments they wished to. Two of the women and one visitor added extra comments and these all expressed a desire for combination visiting:

'I have found some (not all) visitors of other parents to be noisy when I have been trying to rest. I understand the need to have company – I have that need, too, but I think that the restrictions in place now are good and that only partners should have open visiting' (7, patient)

Open visiting for partners, restricted for others
'This is important' (13, patient)
'Filled in as a husband wishing to have open visiting but with other visitors restricted to pm and evenings' (19, visitor)

A number of members of staff took this opportunity to further express their opinions with regard to visiting arrangements. As well as comments in line with those stated previously, three further points were raised as key issues. These were:

There should be a set policy and all staff should keep to it
'We should be able to make times for visiting and stick to them, without letting people in and making it complicated for us to do our job' (4)

Make women and their visitors aware of the policy before they are admitted to the ward so that they cannot say they were not aware of visiting times
'Visitors should be informed of needs of clients and reason for restricted visiting prior to admission through posters, leaflets' (13)

Controls or restrictions placed on children on the ward
'I feel that children other than clients own should not be allowed to visit' (2)
'Too many naughty children running riot (restrictions needed; it is dangerous)' (12)

Discussion

One of the key components of the NHS plan and clinical governance is to encourage involvement of service users and their families in their care at all levels. In a report by the Maternity and Neonatal Workforce Group commissioned by the Department of Health, it is reinforced that 'good maternity care starts with the wishes of the woman and her family, and aims to meet these as far as possible, whilst also ensuring the safety of both mother and baby' (Maternity Neonatal Workforce Group 2003).

This study is a step towards providing mother-friendly policies on a matter that is perhaps not apparently clinical but is of essential relevance to mothers and their families. It was carried out as part of a larger research project across the whole trust, using a slightly modified questionnaire to reflect different priorities within maternity care.

The single most significant finding from the survey was the overwhelming preference of all three groups for a combination visiting policy, where women's partners or another identified individual have open visiting, with restricted visiting for other visitors. This appears to be in line with the findings of Malcolmson et al (1999) whose participants also expressed a preference for all-day visiting for women's partners.

As part of the admission procedure to the ward it might be possible to ask each woman for the name of her designated visitor, enabling a list to be kept on the reception desk and thus relieving some of the complications for the receptionists. This policy is particularly important for maternity, as it allows parents time to bond with and gain experience of caring for their new baby.

Once a policy has been decided on, this could be included in patient information booklets, allowing women to inform their families and other potential visitors prior to admission and birth.

Another interesting suggestion by mothers that needs serious consideration is to have a separate lounge/family room away from the bed areas. This would have the benefits of reducing disturbance to women who are trying to rest during the day and providing a space, particularly for longer term inpatients, to eat meals and spend time in a more socially orientated area. This does appear to have been included in the new plans for the refurbishment of DMS, as well as quiet rooms and a waiting area for visitors.

When questioned about visitors having access during the night, more than half of visitors and all staff thought that this was not desirable. However, the exact circumstances of this were not specified and flexibility might be necessary, dependent on who the visitor was and the condition of the woman and baby.

In relation to visiting during meal times, the discrepancy between the women's and visitors' responses might be due to different perceptions of who a visitor is. Due to the design of the questionnaire, it was not possible to determine whether those who completed the visitors' questionnaire were women's partners, friends and family or an acquaintance. It might be that partners, who would not necessarily consider sitting with a woman while she was eating a meal as unusual, completed a significant number of the visitor questionnaires. For the women completing the questionnaire, however, a visitor might be perceived as being anybody and therefore not someone they would want to sit and eat in front of.

This study provides some interesting insight into the visiting preferences of the women, visitors and staff on DMS, as well as giving an evidence base on which to develop a coherent visiting policy.

Conclusion

Due to the nature of this study and the consultation of three different groups, we naturally expected some degree of diversity in responses. However, on major issues there seems to be significant harmony in the pattern of responses among our study populations: mothers, visitors and health professionals. These include the overwhelming preference for open visiting for the partner (or a known person) and restricted policy for other visitors, as well as restricting the number of visitors to four per woman. Other suggestions were also made such as the possibility of alternative areas for spending time with visitors, away from sleeping areas. These are currently being planned as part of the major refurbishment process that the hospital is undergoing.

These findings, although primarily aimed at providing evidence for local practice, might also prove beneficial for other hospitals when considering visiting policies and the needs of maternity service users.

REFERENCES

Bradley S (2001). 'The influence of nurses and parents in the evolution of open visiting in children's ward'. International History of Nursing, 6 (2): 44–51.

Carlson B, Riegel B and Thomason T (1998). 'Visitation: policy versus practice'. Dimensions of Critical Care, 17 (1): 40–47.

Clarke CM (2000). 'Children visiting family and friends on adult intensive care units: the nurses' perspective'. Journal of Advanced Nursing, 31 (2): 330–338.

Malcolmson LC, Lavender T and Walkinshaw S (1999). 'Visiting on the maternity wards: a study of the views of women and staff'. The Practising Midwife, 2 (3): 20–23.

Maternity and Neonatal Workforce Group (2003). Report to the Dept of Health Children's Taskforce from the Maternity and Neonatal Workforce Group. www.doh.gov.uk/maternitywg/

Ramsey P, Cathelyn J, Gugliotta B and Glenn LL (2000). 'Restricted versus open ICU's'. Nursing Management, 31 (1): 42–44.

The Practising Midwife 2004; 7(9): 27–30

Handle with care!

Deirdre Amos

The dangers of manual handling have been recognised since the 1960s, and have been given formal and legal recognition in the Health and Safety at Work Act (1974), supported by The Manual Handling Regulations and The Management of Health and Safety at Work Regulations of 1999. However, midwives do not always acknowledge the risks specific to them: for example, student midwives undertaking their compulsory manual handling training stated they had not done any manual handling since their placements on the gynaecological ward! This shows a lack of appreciation of the complexity of manual handling, and a lack of recognition of the many practices and procedures requiring manual handling in midwifery practice.

Hazardous manual handling situations are obvious for nurses: for example, the moving of an unconscious or paralysed patient or caring for patients attached to skeletal traction. The handling of a newborn baby as a risk factor would surprise many, but any load that is held away from the body while bending over puts strain on the spine. This position is frequently adopted when assisting with breastfeeding and when bathing a baby.

The Royal College of Midwives (RCM) states that back injury is the most common single injury for midwives and nurses, and quotes estimates of 6,000 midwives a year injuring their backs and 300 giving up midwifery as a consequence (RCM 1997). Thompson (2000) analysed questionnaires from 110 midwives on the causes of back pain, and found that 49 per cent identified assisting with breastfeeding, 33 per cent with birth positions, 7 per cent with postnatal care, and 11 per cent with no particular task (just gradual onset).

Mander (1999) identified caring for women with impaired mobility due to the use of epidural analgesia and caesarean section as additional risks. There is an increasing rate for both of these procedures (Mander 1999). Other practices that are hazardous are baby-bathing, caring for women who are high dependency or have disabilities, and handling equipment.

The insidious nature of the dangers for midwives is a risk in itself, particularly the failure to recognise that it is not a single manoeuvre or procedure that results in damage, but the cumulative effect of strain over many years (National Back Pain Association and Royal College of Nursing 1999).

Good handling techniques

Midwives must adhere to the fundamental principles of good handling techniques (Box 1.5.1), in particular avoiding twisting and bending from the waist and keeping the load close to the body. This will help to protect the large group of back muscles that support the spine. Bending the knees when lifting or moving will help to maintain the natural curves of the spine and prevent damage occurring to the intervertebral discs. Placing one knee on the bed when carrying out a manual handling manoeuvre has also been advocated to help maintain the natural curves of the spine and to get close to the load. However, some Trusts are no longer supporting this because of concern about the weight load of three people on the bed.

If damage does occur, the disc may rupture, allowing the inner part – the nucleus pulposus – to protrude and cause pressure on the spinal cord. This painful condition, known as prolapsed disc, requires orthopaedic treatment and results in the midwife being absent from work. In severe cases this could jeopardise her future working life.

Midwives must be 'back aware', not only when on duty but throughout their daily lives. Activities such as swimming, relaxation exercises and sitting in an upright position with the back well supported can be beneficial (RCM 1997). Activities in everyday life contribute to the cumulative damage to the spine, and lifting any load incorrectly – be it shopping, wet washing or children – is hazardous. Shopping should be divided into several

<table>
<tr><td>

Box 1.5.1 Principles of manual handling

- Use a slide sheet or other manual handling equipment.
- Adopt a secure base position by standing with feet a shoulder width apart, one foot slightly in front of the other.
- Bend the knees to maintain the spine's natural curves.
- Do not bend or twist from the waist.
- Keep the load close to your body.
- Raise the head to maintain the natural curves of the spine.

Source: Manual Handling Operations Regulations 1992

</td></tr>
</table>

bags, and care must be taken when transferring the shopping from the supermarket trolley to the car boot to avoid twisting and top-heavy bending. Driving for long periods without back support must be avoided (Parsons 1996). Studying can also contribute to the cumulative effect, and midwives should take frequent breaks from constantly bending over academic work or sitting for too long in front of the computer.

Births are particularly hazardous, especially if supportive equipment is not available, for example during water births. Midwives should consider the impact on themselves when planning the birth with the mother, and may need to consider adaptations. Mandelstam (2002) cites a case of a successful claim of negligence in which a midwife with a history of back problems suffered an exacerbation of back pain due to the cumulative effects of caring for women in labour. Managers were criticised for not carrying out assessment of the risks or the individual's capability.

The RCM (1997) advises bending and stooping only when absolutely necessary, frequent change of position, and using cushions and pillows to make the position more comfortable (Box 1.5.2). A mother must not be allowed to put her foot on the midwife's hip to help push: not only can it cause damage to the midwife, but it may also result in excessive hip abduction and strain on the pubis of the mother. Guidance on safer birthing positions can be found in the RCM publication Handle with Care (1997).

The Health and Safety at Work Act 1974 states that the employee has a duty to take reasonable care of the health and safety of themselves and also of any other person affected by their action at work, within their sphere of responsibility. Anyone present at the birth must be advised against practices that could be harmful, especially taking the weight of any part of the mother's body or allowing the mother to support herself by putting her arms around their neck. This can be particularly damaging since, if she falls, the mother can also drag down the person supporting her which could result in injury to either or both of the people involved.

The RCM (1997) states that a woman's partner should support her only if he/she has undertaken appropriate training at antenatal classes and has no chronic back

<table>
<tr><td>

Box 1.5.2 Principles for midwifery care positions

Although your posture and position will vary, you should always adhere to the following principles:

- Always make best use of the available equipment – eg, slide sheets and rope ladders.
- Beds and chairs should be adjusted to prevent unnecessary bending and stooping.
- Cushions and pillows can be used to make your position more comfortable when working from the floor.
- Change your position at regular intervals, where possible every few minutes.
- Bend and stoop only when it is absolutely necessary to do so – eg, examining the perineum.
- Do not hold the bend/stooped posture for a prolonged period.
- Do not allow a woman to push against your hips. It can damage your hips, and there is also a risk to the woman of excessive hip abduction and strain on the pubis.
- Place one knee on the bed. This helps to keep your back straight and to give greater stability.
- The woman's partner should support the woman only if he/she has received appropriate training at antenatal classes and does not suffer from chronic back problems.
- He/she should be made aware of the risks of providing physical support.

Source: Royal College of Midwives 1997

</td></tr>
</table>

problems. They must also be fully aware of the risks involved.

The damage that occurs from assisting with breastfeeding is cumulative, and not appreciated by many midwives. This can be reduced by remembering to maintain the natural curves of the spine as much as possible. Sitting with the mother or standing behind her to assist can be utilised – although some bending will be required, especially when initiating breastfeeding.

Putting into practice

It is not possible to eliminate the risks and dangers entirely, but the overall aim is to reduce the cumulative strain of everyday midwifery practices. The first principle is to avoid manual handling wherever possible. However, this must be linked to correct assessment. Mothers needing assistance must not be left to struggle alone because midwives fear they will injure themselves. This will result in the mother feeling neglected and alienated. A thorough assessment of the activity will ensure that mothers receive good-quality care with minimal risk to the midwife.

The mnemonic ELITE can be used to facilitate a thorough assessment (Walsh 2002):

E emphasises the need to assess the environment in which the procedure is undertaken. Any space constraints that prevent good posture must be dealt with, but poor flooring and lighting can also be hazardous.

L addresses the load to be handled and looks at factors such as: is the load bulky, difficult to grasp, unstable and extremely heavy? Tarling (1992) suggests that people are the most difficult load to manoeuvre.

I asks for the individual capability of the person doing the manual handling to be considered. If the person cannot undertake the manoeuvre on her own, she must seek assistance or utilise the correct equipment.

T stands for the task to be achieved: for example, helping a woman to move up the bed, birthing the baby or assisting with breastfeeding.

E is for equipment that must be utilised if handling is to be avoided or minimised. Midwives must be trained to use the equipment correctly.

Outside the hospital setting

If a home birth is planned, the midwife should discuss with the mother well in advance the changes that will need to be made in the home to ensure a safe and well-managed labour and birth, and also to minimise any risk to the midwife.

Working in the community can be particularly hazardous, since midwives may not have access to necessary equipment and may be working in a confined or cluttered space. Also, as a guest in the woman's home, the midwife will not have total control over the environment and will need to seek permission if she wishes to change or move anything. This always requires extra consideration and assessment.

Creating policy

Following assessment, action should be taken to reduce the risks identified. To avoid unnecessary lifting, equipment must be available. The use of rope ladders and slide sheets are particularly vital – a minimal handling policy cannot be achieved without them. Midwives working in areas where these are not available must request them from their managers. The Management of Health and Safety at Work Regulations 1992 impose a legal duty on employees to inform their employer of any shortcomings in health and safety arrangements. Once equipment is supplied to the clinical area, the midwife must use it effectively or give a sound reason for why she is not using it (Health and Safety at Work Act 1974).

As with all new equipment, it may take time for it to be used efficiently and effectively, but it can become an invaluable aid to safe practice. Slide sheets are inexpensive, especially when compared to the cost of back injury compensation payments. It should be possible to supply every woman requiring manual handling with their own slide sheet, thus eliminating any infection risks. Slide sheets can be easily laundered between clients.

Avoiding pressure sores

Correct manual handling is also essential to prevent the development of pressure sores in pregnant women and those who have just given birth. Prior (2002) identified that the incidence of pressure sores is increasing in maternity hospitals, and that legal action has resulted in significant damages being awarded. Women whose mobility is compromised following surgery, or who have an epidural in situ, are most at risk. Tissue damage can occur over bony prominences, due to friction and sheering forces as women are moved or attempt to move themselves. The use of slide sheets will eliminate both of these factors and allow easy movement of the woman.

Working together

When carrying out a manual handling procedure with one or more people, a leader must be appointed to guide the procedure and to give the relevant commands. This avoids confusion and facilitates a coordinated manoeuvre. The command should be clear, with everyone understanding when they are to act: for example, when moving a woman up the bed using a slide sheet, the command used could be: Ready? Set, Slide (National Back Pain Association 1999). The 'Ready' is posed as a question, checking that all are in position and know what they are to do. The command '1 2 3' should never be used, because there can be confusion over whether the move takes place on or after the command of '3' – thus, the lift is not coordinated (National Back Pain Association and Royal College of Nursing 1999). This could result in one person taking the weight of the whole load, leading to an acute injury.

Any mother collapsing should not be held upright but gently lowered to the floor using a manoeuvre that minimises the impact both on the midwife and on the mother. This manoeuvre should be taught to the midwife at her manual handling update session, and the midwife should be assessed as proficient since this is considered to be an advanced procedure. Once the mother's general condition has been checked and she is fit to be moved, an assessment needs to take place to decide the best method to be used. This may involve the use of a hoist. Midwives will not be familiar with hoists and should therefore ensure that a person trained to use the hoist carries out the procedure.

Legal issues

Attendance at annual manual handling updates is compulsory Trust policy, and midwives' failure to adhere to what they have been taught could result in disciplinary and legal action against that individual. Manual handling procedures are constantly reviewed and are based on the principles of neuro-muscular kinetics. The aim of these principles is to use a method of moving in a relaxed way which obtains the most from the body with the least effort. Once the midwife has been taught these manoeuvres she is legally obliged to use them. The Management of Health and Safety at Work Regulations states:

Employees must work in the way they have been trained to work, following the instructions they have been given. (Regulation 12).

Take a break

The body can be more easily damaged if the person is over-tired. The National Back Pain Association and Royal College of Nursing (1999) recommend that rest periods should be taken to give the body a chance to recover. Midwives are often called upon to work through their breaks; while this may be acceptable occasionally, it should not become normal practice. Neither should midwives routinely choose to work through their breaks in order to finish their shift early; this should be condemned by Trust management.

Conclusion

Midwives must recognise that their work entails procedures and practices that put them at high risk of strain and injury, and must incorporate correct manual handling techniques if they are to avoid injury. Constant review of practices and procedures will enable the midwife to make adaptations that will protect her from cumulative injury while still ensuring that she continues to give good-quality care.

REFERENCES

Health and Safety Executive (1974). The Health and Safety at Work Act, London: HMSO.

Health and Safety Executive (1992), revised 1998. The Manual Handling Operations Regulations, London: HMSO.

Health and Safety Executive (1992), revised 1999. The Management of Health and Safety at Work Regulations, London: HMSO.

Mandelstam M (2002). 'Wells v West Hertfordshire Health Authority 1992' in Manual Handling in Health and Social Care, London: Jessica Kingsley Publishers.

Mander R (1999). 'Manual handling and the immobile mother'. British Journal of Midwifery, 7 (8): 485–487.

National Back Pain Association and Royal College of Nursing (1999). The Guide to the Handling of Patients, Middlesex: National Back Pain Association.

Parsons (1996). 'Look after your back'. Modern Midwife, February-

Prior J (2002). 'The pressure is on: midwives and decubitus ulcers'. RCM Midwives Journal, 5 (5): 196–200.

Royal College of Midwives (1997). Handle with Care, London: RCM.

Tarling C (1992). 'Handling patients'. Nursing Times, 88 (43): 38–40.

Thompson E (2000). 'Safer birthing positions: a choice for mother and midwife'. The Column (a quarterly journal for the National Back Exchange), 12 (2): 17–22.

Walsh A (2002). Manual Handling Team Teaching Guidance, Birmingham: University of Central England.

The Practising Midwife 2005; 8(5): 15–19

Protecting the public – from me

Kirsten Baker

My friend Anna had her baby last month. Ben was born at home after a labour that Anna says 'pushed me through what I knew of myself, beyond anything I'd ever done before . . .' Holding Ben in the small hours of that Sunday morning, Anna travelled slowly back from that 'beyond' place, back to the social here-and-now world. We watched quietly as she and her partner became curious to know who their baby was. She talked to him, and to us, those of us who were gathered there to support her in her ordinary, extraordinary birth experience.

For the two of us who were there and are midwives, our job had been to enable her to go to that place; we knew that we had to create a safe place for her to do this difficult thing. Creating – and holding – that space had been, for me, messy, fraught, confronting and scary. Sadly, for midwives, this, too, is an experience that is both ordinary and extraordinary.

On Thursday Anna phoned me to say her membranes had ruptured. We waited for her contractions to start, but instead Anna had the best night's sleep she'd had for weeks! On Friday I phoned my Supervisor who suggested that I let her local hospital know. They knew of Anna's decision to have me, an out-of-area midwife and friend, to look after her. Several months previously I had notified my intention to practise, and written to the Head of Midwifery (HoM).

The reply I received was the first of many confusing and heart-sinking encounters. Despite the fact that I had not asked for one, the HoM refused to give me an honorary contract. I pointed out that I did not need one, since Anna was planning to labour and give birth at home, and that if we did go into hospital I did not propose to be her midwife. Because I am not an independent midwife I had initially wondered about dovetailing with Anna's local community midwives, and had offered to supply details and testimonials about myself to become a kind of associate of the Trust.

After my second letter, the HoM said that she was pleased that we had decided to proceed, and hoped that my friend would have the birth experience she hoped for. She required nothing further from me. This was interesting, and difficult to interpret. On the one hand it could be seen as a proper and grown-up exchange of information, and a recognition that although Anna's care was not to come under her ambit she was confident that I was a safe and competent practitioner. On the other hand, there was something of the 'washing my hands of you' to it. In either interpretation, I began to sense some odd notions of responsibility and control in our exchanges. Still, since there was clearly no possibility of working alongside the local midwives, I put this unease to one side. I found a midwife who works independently who was happy to look after Anna with me.

Supervisors' logic

The next time the Trust heard from me, therefore, was when I let them know about the ruptured membranes and the plan to wait and see until labour started. In doing so, I was of course reinforcing some of the confusion around responsibility. Why did I tell them? My Supervisor's view was that because Anna was still a client of the Trust, this was an appropriate course of action. She also pointed out that there was no reason not to tell them this clinical detail. Nothing, after all, was wrong. Where, then, did the confusion lie?

The working assumption of the Trust's Supervisors of Midwives was that Anna's primary carer (me) was potentially dangerous, dirty and stupid. In the absence of any other information, this was the logical default position. It is a sad and fragile logic, but it has been constructed and maintained through aspects of our history and culture, and it is arguably the basis for the Supervision of Midwives. The other working assumption was that expectant management – not intervening with intravenous antibiotics and expediting the labour within hours of membranes rupturing – was also dangerous, dirty and stupid.

Acting on these assumptions, as several of the Supervisors then proceeded to do, also mobilised another assumption: that they were in some way responsible for Anna and her baby. Not only did they feel the (logical) need to check with me by phone that I had warned Anna that her baby might die, and that it would be better if she came into hospital, but they also (logically) needed to check with Anna that I had done so. They needed to protect the public (this, after all, is the strapline for Supervisors) from me, and they needed to check with the public to ensure that they had done so. Obviously.

Anna's logic

Meanwhile, Anna had a different set of assumptions. Her first assumption was that she was responsible for herself and her baby. The second was that she had chosen a caregiver whom she believed to be competent. The third assumption was that had she felt at any point that obstetric intervention was required (as it had been with her first baby), she would willingly resource herself from what was available medically. The fourth assumption was that risk is something we live with. Specifically, she felt that there are risks associated with admission to hospital with ruptured membranes in terms of possible infection. She also felt that in the event of her baby being compromised by an undetected infection, she wanted to bring it into the world at home.

Different logics

All of us involved in Ben's birth were operating from within our own set of assumptions. As I attempted to construct my own, I experienced the Supervisors' and Anna's logics very differently. My starting point was simple: to facilitate a birth where Anna felt that the agency (not control – labour is too big for that) stayed with her. Whatever happened (in my view), she needed to know that her assumptions, with her and her partner as the main agents, were paramount.

This principle – an apparently uncontroversial basis on which all care should be based – was made easy for me by the fact that I found her logic fundamentally more attractive than that of the Supervisors. First, her assumption was very affirming: I had been chosen. She entrusted me to accompany her on this journey, and shared her hopes and fears with me. My role was to listen carefully; to respond with my knowledge and experience; and to create and hold a space for her, her partner and her baby. Her logic was inclusive of me – and inclusive, too, in another way: she embraced her fear and uncertainty; her

experience of risk was to encompass it rather than to deny it. Her paradigm opened her up to endless possibilities of engaging with life in a potentially new, raw and boundless way. This was how she wanted her birth to be.

Meanwhile, and in contrast to this boundlessness, the Supervisors' logic seemed to have some very clear (although paradoxical) edges around it. First, and primarily, they wanted us all to be contained within the sphere of responsibility of the local Trust. This 'wanting' may well be based on a fear that we somehow fall anyway into their sphere, which means that controlling us is critical. Containment would make us visible and accessible. This has the illusion of making any risk more manageable. By Anna choosing to stay outside this box – and as her care-givers we needed to stay with her – it became possible to dump all the notion of 'risk' with us, thereby creating an illusion of 'safety' within their confines.

What this attempt to commodify both safety and risk amounts to, in effect, is a denial of risk: by pushing it outside the box it does not have to squirm uncomfortably within their sight. What this demarcation also achieves is to make everything outside the box very scary indeed.

Curves and straight lines

Straight line thinking, exemplified by this demarcation and quantification, is a dominant model within obstetric practice. The partogram is a good example of this. Given the phallic symbolism of the upwards sloping line depicting progress in labour, small wonder that there is anxiety when the line deviates from straight. Another example is the hierarchical ladder: at one stage Anna was told she was 'under' the consultant Mr C. This unfortunate image of sexual subjugation was also a fantasy: as far as we were aware, Mr C was blissfully unaware of the story that was unfolding, and he was certainly not in Anna's house when she gave birth.

On closer examination, many of the straight lines are an illusion, and dissolve unless we create and endorse thinking (fantasies) to reiterate them. There is also a degree of internal illogic. Two examples of this include the illogic of the Trust wanting to manage my practice, but not taking any opportunity to find out anything about it. In addition to this there is the illogic of Supervisors not trusting the supervision process. If supervision works, logically I come with an inbuilt guarantee that I am competent: this is what my annual appraisal seeks to confirm. One of the many sadnesses in this story is that the supervisory system does not manage to reassure those who implement it. This fundamental mistrust is disempowering and scary for everyone.

Anna's logic was not based on straight lines. Like her increasingly curvy abdomen, and her experience of life as a woman with her hips and breasts, changing body shape, mood cycles and multi-tasking, hers was curvy and embracing. Rather than construct lines of division between herself and the existential aspects of her birth, she allowed herself to be engulfed by it: it contained her rather than she it. She was not 'under' it: she was with it, and we were with her.

Protecting Anna

Because of the mess created by this attempt to protect Anna from me, my job became more complex. I saw a need to construct some boundaries to create and hold space for her: there were aspects of what was happening that had no place there, and it was my job to try to keep them out. Some of this I did well, some less well, but what is interesting was this need to draw lines myself.

The Practising Midwife 2005; 8(8): 20–21

Responses to my actions and inactions varied as I encountered a wide range of sets of assumptions. Inevitably, to some I appear over-cautious; to others, dangerously cavalier in my approach to clinical risk. Equally, in relation to the Supervisors, I was perhaps either hopelessly naive or cynically paranoid.

As the new parents and I debriefed after what was a clinically 'good' outcome, I reflected on what had not been good about it. Clinical risk had had a part to play in the story, but actually in the end it was a small part. The much bigger players were the institutional fears and anxieties, the inappropriate structural layers of responsibility, the unhelpful pitting of midwife against midwife, and the gaping chasms of systemic illogic. It is a perilously small step from these to a culture of blame, infantilisation of women and midwives, abdication of responsibility and denial of risk. It's time to grow up.

The landscape of caring for women: a narrative study of midwifery practice

Holly Powell Kennedy, Maureen T. Shannon, Usa Chuahorm, M. Kathryn Kravetz

Our purpose was to expand knowledge on the process and outcomes of midwifery care. Narrative analysis was used to interpret stories provided by midwives to illustrate their practice and by recipients of midwifery care about their experience. A purposive sample of 14 midwives and four recipients of midwifery care was recruited as a subsample from a prior Delphi study on midwifery practice. Three broad themes were identified: 1) the midwife in relationship with the woman, 2) orchestration of an environment of care, and 3) the outcomes of care, called 'life journeys' for the woman and the midwife. The findings are discussed from the perspectives of therapeutic landscapes described in cultural geography and prior research on midwifery practice. The challenge is to confirm the associations between the processes of care identified in these narratives with both short- and long-term outcomes in the health of women and their families. These appear to go well beyond the usual perinatal measures currently used in health care research and hold implications for how care is delivered, measured, and evaluated.

Keywords: midwife, midwifery care, normal birth, power, cultural geography, therapeutic landscape

The outcomes of midwifery practice have been examined in a series of studies over the past several decades.[1–3] They have demonstrated that midwives provide safe care, achieve positive outcomes in women's and infant's health, and often use fewer interventions compared with their physician counterparts.[4] Kennedy has conducted several prior research studies to distinguish specific processes, outcomes, and experiences of midwifery care.[5,6] Although results of these studies were illuminating, further exploration was necessary to place these findings into the context of actual midwifery practice. This article presents the third stage in Kennedy's research program to develop theoretical linkages between the processes of midwifery care and outcomes for women and their families.

Background

Outcomes of midwifery care in the United States, as measured by maternal and infant morbidity and mortality, have been carefully scrutinized and are consistently excellent in both low and moderate risk populations.[1,7] The Report of the Pew Health Professions/UCSF Center for Health Professions Commission on the future of the profession notes that midwifery's many strengths and contributions have not been fully used to meet today's health care needs and that further description and outcome analyses of midwifery methods and processes are essential.[8]

The study by Thompson et al.[9] stands as seminal in the early development of midwifery theory identifying critical indicators of care. Cragin critically examined the early theoretical efforts of Lehrman, Thompson and her associates, Morten and her colleagues, and Kennedy.[5,6,9–12] She notes there is 'remarkable consistency in the identification of concepts important to the discipline, which are much broader than those derived from a medically based philosophy.' However, she emphasizes the importance of future study to refine and clarify these concepts and their contribution to midwifery knowledge and women's and family health.

Kennedy conducted two prior exploratory studies to understand the complexities of midwifery practice.[5,6] The first used phenomenology, a qualitative method that moves toward understanding a person's experience of a particular phenomenon (e.g., chronic illness, pain, or birth).[13] In this study, she examined women's experience with midwifery care.[5] The women identified the essence of the experience as one in which a relationship was built on respect, trust, and alliance. Ultimately, it was this respect that empowered the women to determine and direct their care.

Kennedy's second study used the Delphi method to gain consensus about the essential elements of midwifery practice.[6,14] This method queries a panel of experts chosen specifically for their knowledge about the issue being studied. Midwives across the country were nominated as representative of exemplary practice and adherence to a midwifery philosophy. A second panel was formed of women who had been recipients of care by those midwives. The study revealed three dimensions of practice, including therapeutics, caring, and professional.[6] Although these results moved the state of the science forward, the results came from an academic exercise and not the context of actual practice. It was essential to build on these early exploratory studies to clarify the findings and to develop a framework that could be empirically tested in clinical practice.

Methods

The research questions were 1) what processes of care and beliefs emerge as central in midwifery practice when described in actual clinical scenarios and 2) are there linkages between midwifery processes of care and short-and long-term outcomes for the woman and her family? Narrative analysis was chosen for this stage of research to best explore the context of practice. Koch[15] describes the use of narratives or stories as a valuable research method because it creates paths to solve clinical problems, provides a voice to clients and nurses, informs social policy, and addresses diversity through understanding. 'Narrative forms reveal individual's construction of past and future life events at given moments in time.'[16] Stories help the often invisible parts of our work to be seen. Narratives provide us with the opportunity to hear specific ideas, unique approaches, and thoughts about how best to provide care in the context of actual clinical scenarios.

A purposive sample of 14 midwives and 4 recipients of midwifery care were recruited to provide scenarios that described their midwifery practice or care experience. In Kennedy's prior Delphi study, panelists were asked to list specific qualities and traits, processes of care, and outcomes they believed to be most important in the practice of midwifery.[6] Many wrote vignettes as they made their list, using stories to illustrate their point. Because the current study used narrative method, we chose to recruit these storytellers. In qualitative research, this is similar to theoretical sampling in which participants are recruited specifically because of prior research findings to learn more about specific questions.[13] Three of the midwives were not in the original Delphi study but were theoretically sampled based on emerging findings. Sampling continued until no new information was emerging. This is called theoretical saturation and reflects the

point at which data collection may cease.[13] This occurred quickly with the recipients of care because their narratives were highly resonant with interview data obtained from women who participated in Kennedy's prior study on women's experience with midwifery care.[5]

The 14 midwives were an experienced group of clinicians averaging 20 years of practice (range = 6–40). Most (n = 13) were certified by the American College of Nurse-Midwives (ACNM) mechanisms; one was dual-certified through ACNM and the North American Midwives Registry, and one was not nationally certified. All were licensed to practice. They had practiced in a variety of settings throughout their careers, including hospitals, birth centers, and homes. Twelve were Caucasian, one was Latina, and one was African American, generally reflecting the demographic characteristics of U.S. nurse-midwives.[17] The recipients of midwifery care also reflected the three birth settings and one had received only gynecologic care from her midwife. All were Caucasian, which is not reflective of the general population cared for by midwives in the United States.[17] All participants for both groups were women.

The University of Rhode Island Institutional Review Board approved the study. Each participant was asked to tell one or more stories that most reflected her midwifery practice (midwives) or care experience (recipients of care). Interviews, lasting 60 to 90 minutes, were conducted by using videotape to collect the data. Informed consent was obtained from each participant before data collection with specific permission about future use of video clips in educational and professional presentations. The videotapes were transcribed, checked for accuracy, and entered into Atlas.ti software for analysis. The techniques of Geanellos[18] in story analysis were used to guide the interpretation of the data. The steps are outlined in Table 1.7.1

Table 1.7.1 Steps in narrative analysis

Steps	Analytic process
Storied experience	Presenting the storied experience of the midwives and recipients of midwifery care through the use of videotaped interviews
Reflection	Focusing on story details Deliberating, speculating, contemplating, exploring, interpreting, and discussing Coding of text using constant comparative techniques and detailed memos Attending to thoughts, feelings, assumptions, and understandings Drawing meaning and relationships
Progression	Gaining insight about practice and beliefs Linking and integrating new knowledge with old Identification of future directions for practice and research

Adapted from Geanellos.[18]

and include a presentation of the story, interpretation of its meaning, connecting it to what is currently known about practice, and identification of new knowledge.

When qualitative research methods are used, the researchers become the instrument of analysis; therefore, it is essential they are prepared and bring perspectives that will inform the process.[13] The research team was comprised of three expert midwives, including one from Thailand and two graduate midwifery students. The primary investigator was experienced in qualitative research, and two of the midwives were completing doctoral research residencies in qualitative analysis. Together, this team brought multiple perspectives, adding to the rigor during data checking, coding clarification, and interpretation.

Atlas.ti was used to assist in data management, organization of coding, tabulation of coded text, and identification of conceptual relationships within the qualitative data. An initial coding structure was created with the members of the research team using two of the narratives. The rest of the narratives were then coded, and their findings were examined for interpretive consensus in face-to-face discussions.

At the conclusion of the coding phase, the categories were compared with the prior study findings for resonance and dissonance.

The final phase of analysis was to thematically align the codes as they related to one another. This interpretative process was completed independently by two of the researchers. As the categories were aligned, the research-ers conceptually clustered them into three main themes. Considerable time was spent on this step to understand the fundamental meaning and structure of each of the themes and how they were situated in the framework. Naming them became the greatest challenge and was discussed at length with additional researchers experienced in qualitative methods.

Findings

When the results of the narrative analysis were compared with the Delphi findings, there was an overall congruence of 80% across all codes. All of the themes identified in the phenomenology study appeared in the narratives. A more complete description of the analytic comparison of the studies is reported elsewhere.[19] The congruence of the narrative analysis with the results of the prior studies is important because of the consistency of findings. However, the stories provided greater depth and description of foundational issues in practice, specifics about how the midwife enacted care, and some new findings that had not been seen in prior studies. Nineteen types of scenarios were relayed by midwives and five by the recipients during the narrative interviews and are listed in Table 1.7.2. Three overarching themes were identified: 1) the midwife in relationship with the woman; 2) orchestration of an environment of care; and 3) life journeys, or outcomes, for the woman and the midwife. Table 1.7.3 provides a listing of the codes clustered thematically with the

Table 1.7.2 Scenarios presented during the narrative interviews

Midwives (*n* = 14)		Women (*n* = 4)	
Type of scenario		Type of scenario	
Labor and birth care	14	Childbirth*	8
Low technology care	14	Gynecologic care	4
Success of the woman	13	Midwife community service	2
Advocacy for woman and/or family	11	Non-midwife childbirth experience	1
Personal introspection and growth	11	Professional presentation	1
Environment of care	10		
Defining midwifery model	10		
Relationships over time	9		
Antepartum care	8		
Intersection of lives	8		
Birth settings	8		
Feedback from woman	7		
Learning from women	7		
Frustrations in practice	5		
Changing systems	5		
Teaching midwives and others	5		
Altered consciousness during childbirth	3		
Gynecologic care	2		
Community service	1		

*Many women described more than one of their births, or their friend's births

Table 1.7.3 Thematic representation of narrative coding scheme

Processes of care			Outcomes of care
The midwife in *relationship* with the woman	*Orchestration* of an environment of care		The *life journeys* of the midwife and the woman
Founded on: • Mutuality (30) Enacted by: • Response to women's desire (30)/meeting the woman where she is (23) • Validation (29) • Participatory care (25) • Continuity (22) • Respect (22) • Intimacy (7) • Disclosure (5) Supported by: Qualities and Traits of the Midwife: • Humility/ego (16) • Integrity (14) • Realist (11) • Non-judgmental (7) • Passion for midwifery (7) • Humor (6) • Compassion (6) • Confidence (4) The Midwife's Care of Self: • Midwife relationships (7) • Personal care of self (6)	Founded on: • Advocacy (23) • Role model (9) • Conduit (7) • Accountability (5) Enacted by: Midwifery Management Process: *Gathering data* (51) • Listening to women (33) • Probing for information (21) • Home visits (11) *Assessment* (79) • Knows you/knows woman (8) • Ethical reasoning (4) *Plan* (34) • Information giving (43) • Providing options (31) • Strategy development (29) • Enlisting resources and support (24) • Consulting (15) *Implementation* (7) • Timeliness of actions (22) • Comforting care (19) • Directing (9) • Going out of way (8) • Touch (3) *Evaluation* (3) Reflection on case (76) Personal reactions (31) Follow-up (22)	Founded on: • Support of normalcy (97) • Trust in women (23) and belief in their strength (42) Enacted by: • Space-physiologic (46) • Contextual awareness (45) • Setting awareness (45) • Presence-midwife (45) • 'We'll see what happens' (40)/patience (12)/'doing nothing' (6) • Space-emotional (36) • Low technology (28) • Time (17) • Presence-other (12) • Rituals (3) Supported by: • Clinical expertise and skills (46) • Collegiality (30)/teamwork (13) • Knowledge of self and limits (16) • Intuition (15) • Cultural awareness (12) • Constant inquiry (10) • Calm (6) • Assertive (5) • Hand skills (4) • Vigilance (3)	Outcome for the Woman: • Family-centeredness (50) • Power (17)/'she did it' (10) • Trust (14) • Safety (14)/feeling safe (5) • Protection (11) • Transformation (11) • Community services (8) • Life-long memories (7) • Healing (6) • Felt cared for (5) • Satisfaction with care (3) Outcome for the Midwife: • Defining midwifery (29) • Growth as a midwife [clinical wisdom (15)/continuing to learn (18)/changing practice style (6)] • Conflict resolution (14)/changing the system (11) • Professional teaching (11) • Frustrations in practice (10) • Honor (9)/pride (4)

( ) Indicates number passages coded from the transcripts. **Founded on** indicates a philosophical belief or stance. **Enacted by** indicates processes used. **Supported by** indicates specific knowledge, skills, or personal qualities and traits of the midwife.

number of text passages assigned to them. The danger of presenting such a linear schema is that it does not fully represent the dynamic nature of practice. This is not our intent; rather, it is to simply portray how the data were conceptualized and organized.

The midwife in relationship with the woman

The first theme describes the structure of the relationship of the midwife and the woman. Mutuality emerged as foundational for the midwife's relationship with the woman. This concept suggests that the midwives regard themselves on an equal level with the woman, recognizing that women bring a knowledge base to the clinical situation as important as the midwife's. It requires being open to the woman and what she brings to the relationship, and at times, entails personal disclosure. The latter was a new finding and noted in five of the scenarios.

That the ability to be close to someone is so available and so ripe if you're only willing to take the moment and to share yourself, as much as we ask them to share with us. . . .

Respecting and responding to the woman's desires indicates the midwife regards the woman's goals even when they may differ from her personal values.

I had a hard time letting go of the fact that people don't necessarily feel like giving birth as something that should be a challenge. They say 'I want an epidural, why would anyone want to go through pain?' . . . So, I've had to give up some of that thinking-you know, [that] this is the right way; you should want to feel that pain and feel proud of yourself after you give birth. . . . Being able to support people in their choices, though they might not have been my choices.

The midwives individualized their care, identified in our coding scheme as 'meeting the woman where she is.' The actions in doing this were purposeful and geared toward knowing her as a unique person. One of the recipients of care noted how her midwife does this during her annual visits; 'She sits down, she asks you questions about the past year . . . things that are really related to your passion, what you are doing.' One of the midwives was very specific in how she personally meets the woman.

. . . my very first step is to always connect with her. That may mean squatting down where she is; it may mean pulling a chair up that puts me at eye level with her; it may be standing next to her if she's up and walking so that we have eye contact. That to me is where it begins. That somehow she sees me; she can see my eyes and my face . . . to connect with her as she is. . . .

The midwives used validation to acknowledge the woman's feelings and concerns. It was a realistic and honest reflection 'with' the woman about the current situation. One midwife described a woman in second stage with five centimeters of caput showing who suddenly said, 'I can't do this.' The midwife said her style had changed over the years in handling that situation and rather than having her push through that sense of panic at the end, she now stops and asks her why, as long as there is no physiologic reason to facilitate the birth. In this situation, the woman spent the next 45 minutes talking with the midwife and her husband about her fears of being a mother and whether she needed medication for this last stage. As soon as she decided to have some medication, she began to push and went on to deliver without it, by her choice. She later expressed delight with her birth and her baby. When asked to reflect on her change in practice, the midwife said that she had learned how validating a woman's fears often facilitated her ability to handle them.

. . . when people said, 'I can't do it,' instead of saying, 'Yes you can,' and sort of being confrontational with them, which I think initially I thought was an empowering thing to do . . . , I found [myself] saying, 'OK' - just accepting that . . . not trying to talk them out of what they are feeling about something, but just validating that their feelings are valid . . . they usually come around to grappling with it and moving ahead. . . .

We heard many stories that depicted the variety of relationships between the midwife and the woman. Although it always appeared to be professional, a personal connection, partnership, and often friendship were apparent. One of the recipients of care talked about the loss she felt in leaving the relationship at the end of the pregnancy, where she had felt so accepted and so special.

I tell you, I wasn't ready to do that. It was almost like this nervous feeling that I wouldn't see her . . . I've seen her every month and then every week. I looked forward to every visit . . . She knew me, she knew my family, she knew my profession; it was wonderful. It was like going to visit a friend every single time . . . Feeling the baby and hearing the heartbeat and her excitement was like it was her first delivery too. . . .

Kennedy's prior research had identified a number of these concepts, but the stories told in this study provided evidence specifically for how these were enacted in clinical practice. The building of the relationship between the midwife and the woman provided the foundation for the midwife to orchestrate an environment of care to meet the woman's needs and is described in the next theme.

Orchestration of an environment of care

Orchestration was chosen to describe the midwife's 'art' in creating an environment in which the woman's desires were met, where she was kept safe along the way, and where normalcy was preserved. It included an awareness of the women's context and care setting and creating space where the woman's physical and emotional needs could be met. Of the three themes, it is the most complex and suggests that the midwife maneuvers the health care system as an advocate for the woman. Preservation of 'normalcy' during pregnancy and birth was predominant, highly challenging, and is discussed more fully in a separate article devoted solely to this concept.[20]

Two important foundational concepts were advocacy and acting as a 'conduit.' Advocacy was complex and included supporting what the woman wants to have happen, aligned with what the midwife believes is safe to happen. This may be to keep interventions at bay, to cope with difficult family members, or to convince nursing staff that all is safe. Some advocacy changes policy and some occurs in closed-door sessions with consulting physicians. At times it included helping women come to grips with difficult life issues. One midwife talked of how she sometimes advocated for a woman to take charge of her life, even during labor. She described attending a birth years ago when the woman's labor began to stall,

I asked if she had any idea what was standing between her and having this baby. First she looked bewildered, . . . then she said, 'Well, I can tell you that my mother wants to come right after the baby is born and I really don't want her. I really don't want her until later. . . .' I said, 'here's a dime, go call your mother.' She marched right down there, called her mother, told her she didn't want her to come until the baby was a week old, came back, got into bed and had the baby - just about like that. Of course the activity helped, too!

One of the most intriguing foundational concepts for orchestrating care was that of working as a conduit and portrays the often invisible work of midwives. Seven of the midwives described a process where they believed they served as a channel for the woman's process. The word conduit was actually used by several and sent us to the dictionary to fully understand what they were trying to say. Conduit is derived from Latin for 'conducere,' which means to conduct, often referring to the conveyance of water.[21] When visualizing a conduit, water is flowing, but the channel conducting the water is not seen. The story in which the concept first appeared was that of a young primigravida immigrant woman. She was extremely timid and had probably been sheltered away much of her life. The midwives debated her level of risk for a birth center, but this midwife advocated for her admission to the caseload. Her labor was long and the midwife assessed that although she had an unusual pelvis, she had adequate room for birth; it would just take patience and positioning. She stayed with her throughout the labor helping her to rock, take showers, providing comfort; all the while the woman made no eye contact in her shyness. As she progressed toward full dilation, she was encouraged to just follow her body – no pressure, to just push as she felt the need. The midwife described a transformation in this young woman at the birth.

This woman, who I had never made eye contact with . . . I had never seen her smile, say a thing herself . . . all of a sudden she looked up . . . she smiled . . . she reached out, she received her baby and [en]folded it. I said to myself, here this girl was; has been kept away, and now all of sudden here she is. Done this wonderful thing . . . she was accomplished.

The midwife described her own role at this birth in the following way. 'Why I could have just faded into the woodwork because it was all her [midwife's emphasis]. I realized that I'm just a conduit . . .'

These foundational concepts imply that the midwife works to meet the woman's needs and that the woman has an experience where she is the one receiving credit for the hard work she has done. It entails a power differential that shifts control from the provider to the woman.

Another aspect of orchestrating an environment of care is exemplified in the management process, which was highly evident and underscores the majority of the clinical scenarios. This did not mean they 'managed' the birth, but rather they carefully monitored unfolding events. Critical to the assessment process was their ability to have a contextual awareness of the woman and the setting in which care takes place. This helped them create physical and emotional space for the woman that feels safe and supports her needs. The midwives believed best care was provided when the whole woman was understood in her context – specifically, what it was that she brought to the labor, birth, or health care experience.

. . . I think [you] always have to have a good ear as far as listening to people. But I think taking it a step further; listening and then trying to out what to do with all these issues that some of these people have faced in their lifetime that I have no experience with . . . listening and being able to help a woman find her strength and use her strength.

Balanced with understanding the woman's context was an awareness of the setting and environment in which midwifery care was taking place. These included professional relationships, philosophies, system policies, and those people involved with the woman. One midwife described how she negotiates the physical environment by dimming lights and 'getting the heavy medical stuff

out of sight' and then assesses the social environment of those who are attending the woman. She uses that knowledge to create a space that serves the energy and flow in the room.

Over time I had to learn or become more aware of the social environment. Where was the strong, confident energy coming from in the room? Where was the black hole of fear? Where are the hope and excitement and encouragement? I began to feel that those things could be translated into real awareness . . . To be able to walk into a room and know what is serving and what is not . . . That's a feeling, I don't have a lot of science about that. It's a feeling. I come in, I read the tempo, the dance of the labor and who's in sync and who's out of step. [Then] just very subtly, and in a low key way redirect it, or repace it; and hopefully bring it to place where the mom is getting what she needs.

Much of the orchestration we saw in the stories is probably not seen by the women it served. We heard many battles as midwives fought to change hospital policies and restrictive protocols, go out on limbs to create a plan of care that met a woman's unusual needs, and to build communities and safe places for women. As a process, orchestration appeared to be directly linked with outcomes and are described in the following theme.

Life journeys for the woman and the midwife

We chose to call the third major theme 'life journeys' to reflect the effects of midwifery care as short- and long-term outcomes for the woman and the midwife. We selected this term because the narratives often portrayed effects beyond the common indicators used in women's health care. We were struck by the depth of the sense of accomplishment and emotion that went with the stories. The midwives described transformative experiences in which women achieved victories and strength. They also described their own growth, learning, and at times humility. This theme drew on the earlier foundational concepts, including a trust in the woman's strength and a belief that she would make the right decisions for herself. It required accountability to reflect, to continue to learn, to change when needed, and to revolutionize systems to improve care for women. There was a clear sense of outcome and journey for the midwife. This had not been seen in the prior studies and represents a new finding. We have chosen several stories to portray these life journeys.

A sense of achievement and healing was described by one of the recipients of midwifery care as she told about her births.

I also had a lot of doubt about myself and my capability of having a natural birth and all of that . . . I very much felt like a failure after that first birth [in a hospital]. So I went into it not sure that I could do it at all . . . I just kept putting one foot in front of the other, and I think that she [the midwife] sort of sensed that because at one point at the very end she said,

'I think you're holding back or something.' Then I told her I was just very afraid that I couldn't do a natural birth, and I would be at home with no way to change that situation. I just wasn't sure I could do it. She reassured me that I could . . . [She went on to give birth at home] . . . But that was a really healing thing for me because he [the baby] was able to go right to my stomach. He was able to nurse immediately and he didn't cry.

One midwife described her care of a woman and her family over many births (including grandchildren) throughout her career. Both the woman and the midwife grew and learned from one another.

When given the opportunity at every moment, she engaged sharing . . . it affirmed to her that someone was listening and that whatever she had to say was incredibly important to her. That had not been her previous experience in her births prior to the fourth baby. So while I was learning from her in a unique way over those years, she was gaining more and more empowerment about her right as a woman to be heard, and that was beginning to carry over into other aspects of her children's health care with pediatricians and emergency room visits . . . I think she was learning through the relationship that we had over time that not only was it her right, but she should demand to be listened to and was becoming a very strong woman.

In completing our description of the theme of life journeys, we have chosen one story that provides a sense of understanding of the potential for short- and long-term outcomes and effects of care. The midwife cared for a young woman many years ago, facilitating her family's presence in a hospital setting not particularly conducive to family birth. Other than that, she did not recall a great deal about the birth. Sixteen years later, a young man walked into her clinic with his aunt and requested to see her.

After so many years I had forgotten this lady. His mom had developed breast cancer and she had died. One of the things she had asked was to come find me and go over the story about how he was born. So we sat in my office and cried and told him the story of how he was born. It's amazing to me that someone should remember you so many years later.

As the midwife recounted this story, she became emotional about the impact this had on the woman and her family, and on herself. The researchers hearing the story had a glimmer of the midwife's skill as she 'midwifed' the young man and his aunt in their grief and loss, and marveled at the mother's wisdom in sending him back to his birthroots for solace. The midwife's emotion in the telling of the story was, in part, the realization of how little is known about the potential impact of a clinician's actions on a person's life memories. It also helped us to identify that life journeys and outcomes are also experienced by the midwife.

These three overarching themes provide us with a sense of the complex and intricate nature of midwifery practice and its short- and long-term effects. Figure 1.7.1 portrays these conceptually to reflect the multifaceted processes and interconnectedness of midwifery care 'with women for a lifetime.'

Discussion

These stories have provided a robust portrayal of midwifery practice. The first research question asked what processes of care and beliefs were central to midwifery practice. Two of the three themes identify essential processes of midwifery practice. The mutual relationship between the midwife and the woman provided the foundation for the midwife to orchestrate care to meet the woman's needs. The second research question asked what linkages there might be between care processes and short- and long-term outcomes for the woman and her family. We believe the identification of the third theme – life journeys – demonstrates there are specific outcomes related to how care is provided and can be measured. Story after story reflected women's sense of safety, accomplishment, power, and at times, transformation.

Figure 1.7.1 Conceptualization of the midwifery model of care. The figure portrays the connection of midwife and woman and what each brings to the care experience. An environment of care is created that reflects the input from both (open lines) and results in outcomes or 'life journeys' for each.

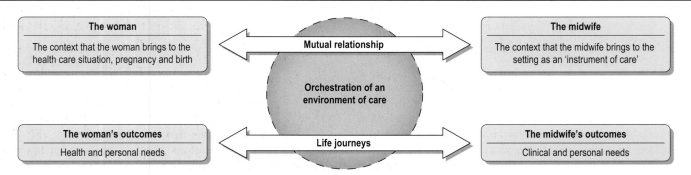

The themes are multidimensional and complex. Gesler and Kearns[22] use 'cultural geography' to examine the concepts of place and space and their relationship to health and health behaviors. They describe a 'therapeutic landscape' as one that incorporates the environment, social constructs, and beliefs about health and healing properties. That framework aligns with the themes we identified from the narratives. The relationship between the midwife and the woman could be described as the bedrock of the landscape. Orchestration of an environment of care might be seen as navigating the terrain with the woman. Finally, the 'life journeys' could be seen as the horizon, or the future.

Mutuality emerged as foundational in the first theme, implying a relationship of equality between the midwife and the woman. We would propose that the narratives in this study reveal an 'engaged presence' in which the midwives gather astute observations, but we believe the woman's knowledge and a subjective stance make it possible to more fully understand the situation. For example, the midwife who asked the woman 'what is standing between you and having this baby?' had clinically observed a stalled labor, but also knew the answer for its protraction may lie with the woman. This is a different position from the objective 'clinical gaze' of modern medicine described by Foucault.[23] This application of shared knowledge and engagement may be key in understanding how midwives achieve positive outcomes. As many of the stories portray, establishing a relationship with a woman and discovering her world and worries may alter a labor, create a lifelong memory, or help her find her inner strength. Melender and Lauri found this in their work with women's fears surrounding pregnancy and birth.[24] Rather than protecting a woman from her fears, they emphasize the importance of giving her the opportunity to deal with them.

The second major theme was the orchestration of an environment of care to meet the woman's needs. We believe this theme is the most complex and little acknowledged in today's health care arena. Metaphorically, we likened this to an orchestra, in which the conductor (midwife) must know the musicians (woman/family), score (fundamental knowledge), technical supports (staff), and acoustics (health care setting/policies). The midwife draws on the strengths of all, blending and highlighting as needed, but in the end it is the musicians who perform and make the real music. In this respect, it moves beyond the notion of navigation, 'to manage, steer or control,'[25] to the ability to combine various elements harmoniously.[26] In the prior Delphi study, the midwives believed that it was important to 'create a respectful setting.'[6] The findings from this study clarified the intricate ways in which they did this. We saw repeatedly in the stories the midwife assess and orchestrate the environment by creating emotional and physical space to help the woman achieve her desires. Emotional space gave a woman time to talk through her fears, or to work through a painful memory. Physical space sometimes just meant the removal of scary medical equipment; regardless, the space felt safe to the woman. These concepts are also seen in Abel and Kearns' study exploring geographic perspectives of birth places.[27] Using narratives, they found that women who gave birth at home believed they had more control, continuity with their provider, and familiarity with their surroundings.

The last theme portrayed the outcomes, or what we chose to call 'life journeys,' for the woman and the midwife. In the past Delphi study, the highest ranked identified outcome was 'optimal health of the woman and/or infant in the given situation.'[6] Neither this nor the other identified outcomes in that study conveyed the potential for lifelong memories and effects of the pregnancy, labor, birth, and care experiences that were evident in this analysis. Simkin has done significant research in describing long-term birth memories for women.[28,29] She found that women with the highest satisfaction with their birth experience believed they had accomplished something important, were in control, and that these were related to their self-confidence and self-esteem. Their memories of the birth were vividly accurate 15 to 20 years after the birth, and negative experiences were rarely shared with the provider.

The ethical schema of care described by Thompson and her colleagues[9] was also evident in the findings. Compassionate care requires a concern and respect for the woman. Perhaps the most profound messages were also the subtlest in the realistic approaches the midwives used in caring for women. They did not shy away from the hard questions as they strived to understand someone whose life and desires might be very different from theirs. It takes courage to ask a question for which you may not have an answer, but the asking sends a message of respect, care, and a commitment to work together toward a solution. The concept of competence, or clinical expertise as we conceptualized it, was seen in the midwives' ability to assess the situation and orchestrate the environment as needed. It was often dazzling and deft. Those are powerful adjectives, but so were the stories and complex maneuvers orchestrated by the midwife to achieve specific and challenging goals with the woman.

The findings of these narratives are similar to van der Hulst and van Teijlingen's[30] use of stories to describe four aspects of midwives work from the Netherlands, Canada, and the United Kingdom: 1) obstetric technical care (procedures), 2) risk selection for midwifery appropriate clients, 3) social environment (harmonization with the woman's personal situation), and 4) relational care (provider–client trust based on connection). The resonance of their findings with this study suggests that these dimensions are central to midwifery and may be the differentiating factors from the practice of obstetrics.

Several limitations should be noted with the samples in this study as well as in Kennedy's prior research. All of the recipients of care who participated in the studies are assumed to have been satisfied with their care; therefore, the perceptions of women who were dissatisfied were not heard. There was also a lack of ethnic diversity among the participants in the studies. The perceptions of ethnically diverse women and midwives are essential to understand what they have to say about midwifery care. Finally, sampling only 'exemplary midwives' is problematic by creating the question, what is 'non-exemplary?' Future research should focus on all kinds of midwives in all kinds of settings to remove this artificial dichotomy and continue to refine the core elements central to the model of care.

These findings have moved ahead with conceptualization of a model of care reflecting processes of care and effects and outcomes less apparent in prior research. It provides a platform to begin to examine in clinical practice settings and to move toward theory testing. Empirical study should be directed to elucidate the association of relationship between the midwife and woman, specific care processes, and the effect of those on outcomes. Specific questions to consider might include how women perceive their relationship with the midwife and how does that influence her decision making, satisfaction with care, and perception of control during her care experience. How does the belief in normalcy and trust in the woman to give birth translate into the use of technology and its association with perinatal outcomes? Besides the usual perinatal morbidity and mortality indicators, what are other outcomes that should be examined in relationship to a model of care? These could include maternal role adaptation, self-esteem, childbirth self-efficacy, anxiety, postpartum depression, health care behaviors, and breastfeeding, among many others.

Conclusions

It is critical that the immediate and long-term effects of midwifery practice be recognized. We are facing monumental challenges in health care today. Our current health care system is struggling to balance rising costs with an ever-increasing reliance on, and demand for, technological innovation. Midwifery care has been demonstrated over and over to be excellent and associated with positive maternal-infant outcomes. This prompts the troubling question: if midwives have such good outcomes, why then are they not the primary provider of women's health care in the United States? The answers are likely complex but must be explored. It may lie in the often-invisible nature of their work. The midwives in this study were negotiators, not dictators. They believed that power rested with the women and not necessarily in themselves. This does not mean to imply that they were weak or compliant; in fact, they were often the opposite. Yet, their consistent approach in being a background, rather than a foreground presence may prevent them from being seen as a substantial force for change in our delivery of health care for women in the United States. In addition, emphasis on presence and relationship, rather than routine use of technology, may be misaligned with an institutional and consumer fascination with machines as the solution to achieve optimal birth outcomes. In this study, the midwife represented the 'instrument' of care. It was the midwife's ability to communicate, engaged presence, and clinical judgment that presided, not the technology that was used. Consequently, strategies must be developed to document midwifery care and outcomes in ways that are understood from public health, consumer, marketing, and economic perspectives. Their invisibility as a strategy to help women realize their own strength is admirable, but they must work to increase their public visibility if they are going to continue to make a difference in the lives of women.

Acknowledgements

This study was partially funded by the University of Rhode Island Foundation. The authors thank the women and midwives who freely shared their stories and thoughts with us during the study; Debra Erickson-Owens, CNM, MS, and Emily MacDonald, CNM, MS, for their assistance with initial data collection and analysis; and Drs. Kathryn A. Lee, Teresa Juarbe, Paulina Van, Leslie Cragin, and Jeanne DeJoseph for their endless reviews of this manuscript.

REFERENCES

1. Raisler J. Midwifery care research: What questions are being asked? What lessons have been learned? J Midwifery Womens Health 2000;45:20–36.
2. MacDorman MF, Singh GK. Midwifery care, social and medical risk factors, and birth outcomes in the USA. J Epidemiol Community Health 1998;52:310–317.
3. Oakley D, Murray ME, Murtland T, Hayashi R, Anderson F, Mayes F, Rooks J. Comparisons of outcomes of maternity care by obstetricians and certified nurse-midwives. Obstet Gynecol 1995;88:823–829.
4. Harvey S, Jarrell J, Brant R, Stainton C, Rach D. A randomized controlled trial of midwifery care. Birth 1996;23:128–135.

5. Kennedy HP. The essence of nurse-midwifery care. The woman's story. J Nurse Midwifery 1995;40:410–417.

6. Kennedy HP. A model of exemplary midwifery practice: Results of a Delphi study. J Midwifery Womens Health 2000;45: 4–19.

7. Cragin L. Outcomes in moderate risk women: comparison of midwifery and obstetrical care [unpublished doctoral dissertation]. San Francisco: University of California, 2002.

8. Dower CM, Miller JE, O'Neil EH, and the Taskforce on Midwifery. Charting a course for the 21st century: the future of midwifery. San Francisco, CA: Pew Health Professions Commission and the UCSF Center for the Health Professions, 1999.

9. Thompson JE, Oakley D, Burke M, Jay S, Conklin M. Theory building in nurse midwifery: The care process. J Nurse Midwifery 1989;34:120–30.

10. Lehrman EJ. A theoretical framework for nurse-midwifery practice [unpublished doctoral dissertation]. Tucson: University of Arizona, 1988.

11. Morten A, Kohl M, O'Mahoney P, Pelosi K. Certified nurse-midwifery care of the postpartum client: A descriptive study. J Nurse Midwifery 1991;36:276–88.

12. Cragin L. The theoretical basis for nurse-midwifery practice. J Midwifery Womens Health (in press).

13. Speziale HJS, Carpenter DR. Qualitative research in nursing. Advancing the humanistic perspective, 3rd ed. Philadelphia: Lippincott Williams & Wilkins, 2003.

14. Keeney S, Hasson F, McKenna HP. A critical review of the Delphi technique as a research methodology for nursing. Int J Nurs Stud 2001;38:195–200.

15. Koch T. Story telling: Is it really research? J Adv Nurs 1998; 28:1182–1190.

16. Sandelowski M. Telling stories: Narrative approaches in qualitative research. J Nurs Scholarship 1991;23:161–166.

17. Rooks JP. Midwifery and childbirth in America. Philadelphia: Temple University Press, 1997.

18. Geanellos R. Storytelling: A teaching-learning technique. Contemp Nurse 1996;5:28–35.

19. Kennedy HP. Enhancing Delphi research: methods and results. J Adv Nurs (in press).

20. Kennedy HP. Keeping birth normal: research findings on midwifery practice. J Obstet Gynecol Neo Nurs (in press).

21. Oxford English Dictionary (electronic version). Query: Conducere. [cited February 4, 2003]. Available from: *http://www.oed. com*.

22. Gesler WM, Kearns RA. Culture/place/health. New York: Routledge, 2002.

23. Foucault M. The birth of the clinic. An archaeology of medical perception. New York: Pantheon Books, 1973.

24. Melender H-L, Lauri S. Fears associated with pregnancy and childbirth-experiences of women who have recently given birth. Midwifery 1999;15:177–182.

25. Oxford English Dictionary (electronic version). Query: Orchestrate. [cited August 7, 2003]. Available at: *http://www.oed.com*.

26. Oxford English Dictionary (electronic version). Query: navigate. [cited August 7, 2003]. Available from: *http://www.oed.com*.

27. Abel S, Kearns RA. Birth places: A geographic perspective on planned home birth in New Zealand. Soc Sci Med 1991;33: 825–834.

28. Simkin P. Just another day in a woman's life? Women's long-term perceptions of their first birth experience. Part I. Birth 1991;18: 203–210.

29. Simkin P. Just another day in a woman's life? Nature and consistency of women's long-term memories of their first birth experiences. Part II. Birth 1992;19:64–81.

30. van der Hulst L, van Teijlingen ER. Telling stories of midwives. In: Devries R, Benoit C, van Teijlingen ER, Wrede S, editors. Birth by design. New York: Routledge, 2001:166–179.

Journal of Midwifery & Women's Health 2004; 49(1): 14–23

(Reprinted with permission from Journal of Midwifery & Women's Health)

Midwives: praise and beyond

Mavis Kirkham

Some months ago, all midwives in the Doncaster and Bassetlaw Hospitals NHS Trust were sent a questionnaire entitled 'Influence your future'. The questionnaire asked midwives what parts of their job were particularly satisfying and how this satisfaction could be extended; and what parts of their job were particularly frustrating and stressful and how this could be overcome. From the responses, it was clear that relationships with clients and colleagues were crucially important. Being appreciated and respected was stated as important by many midwives. Positive feedback from clients, colleagues and management was particularly satisfying.

A worrying number of midwives reported that they felt 'not appreciated', 'not valued' or 'not respected', and the language used demonstrated the distress of some. A few wrote of the 'culture of blame' which we know to be widespread in NHS midwifery (Kirkham 1999). A considerable number expressed a need for positive feedback, using phrases such as 'give praise more freely' or 'give praise where praise is due'; and described a need for 'more appreciation for each other'.

Is praise a good thing?

In considering what to do about this aspect of the survey findings, we were helped by the thoughts of Mary Smale, an NCT breastfeeding counsellor who is central to our work in Doncaster on peer support for breastfeeding (Kirkham 2000, Curtis et al 2001). In discussing praise in clinical care, Mary has stimulated my thoughts greatly by moving beyond the immediate response that praise is necessarily a good thing. She maintains that those who praise us can also blame us, and that the giving of praise therefore carries the potential for being an exercise of power over another, rather than being empowering for the person receiving the praise. From this viewpoint, it is clearly important that midwives and mothers are helped to develop skills of self-validation, rather than being

dependent on others for praise and encouragement. These views are highly thought-provoking, and so we decided to invite Mary to run workshops for midwives in Doncaster and Bassetlaw.

The first event, entitled 'Receiving and giving positive feedback', was attended by 12 midwives from a range of posts in Doncaster and Bassetlaw. We sat in a circle of comfortable chairs and wondered what to expect. Mary opened by describing the aim of the session as 'time for refreshment', which would clearly extend beyond the tea and biscuits we were enjoying! Rather than asking us to share personal revelations while we felt a bit nervous, Mary gave us each a small form on which to write our name and answers to four questions:

- Families and other workers sometimes thank me for . . .
- What I like mothers, fathers and others to say to me is . . .
- One of the best bits of feedback I ever got was . . .
- It felt good because . . .

We then shared our thoughts in the circle, and all contributed with enthusiasm. The ice was certainly broken. We told stories of good feedback from clients, of being thanked, sometimes of events a long time ago. Only one midwife recounted words of appreciation from a colleague, and that colleague was outside midwifery.

In response to careful questioning, we started to examine our need for appreciation and the very different aspects of midwifery we might be thanked for from 'just being there' to very hard, complex work. We explored the paradox of excellent midwifery being enabling for clients but largely invisible – so unlikely to be praised. We were challenged to examine whether we were thanked for the right things.

Only when we were all very much engaged with the subject did Mary suggest we pause to create our ground rules for the session.

How it feels to be blamed

After discussing praise, Mary asked us to examine what it feels like to be blamed. We all had experiences to contribute, and produced a very long and alarming list of feelings and responses, many of which had long-term consequences. After examining this list, Mary referred to the work of Carl Rogers, which two of us knew from doing counselling courses. She used this to examine issues of praise, blame and power: 'Anyone who gives praise also has the power to blame'. She then challenged us as to what we actually want from people. She did not quite ban the word 'praise', but encouraged us to be more precise. We wrote our wants on yellow petals, which we put together to create a wonderfully dense flower (see Fig. 1.8.1). The repeated petal was 'respect'.

Mary then divided the room with two ropes. One represented 'high challenge' to 'low challenge', the other, 'high support' to 'low support'. We were then asked to stand in the area that represented our work situation. Most of us huddled in 'high challenge/high support', with some in 'high challenge/low support'. We were helped to examine what this feels like in the long term and in the short term, and the support needs generated by 'high challenge' work. We examined natural places to go for this support, and turned to each other.

With carefully designed exercises, we examined what women want of us and the consequences of going on supporting and encouraging women if we ourselves are

Figure 1.8.1 Midwives' 'wants' were written on yellow petals, put together to create a wonderfully dense flower. The repeated petal was 'respect'.

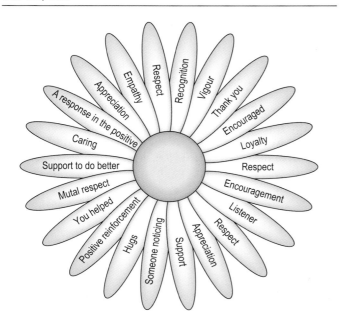

unsupported. We discussed our fears and not wanting people to think that we can't cope.

Mary highlighted our powerful metaphors of 'bursting at the seams' and 'leaking', with friends being called on 'to mop up'. She made the analogy with birth as an out-of-control state, lactating women leaking and midwives often holding back their tears. We shared useful references ranging from the nursing text Behind the Screens (Lawler 1991) to The Vagina Monologues. With laughter and real reflection, we observed that 'we joke about the deepest things'.

When feedback is useful

We examined what it feels like to get the feedback we want. We spoke of where we put such feedback and the literal meaning of encouragement: 'in the heart'. We found ourselves far more likely to write down and reflect on negative experiences than positive ones. We acknowledged our tendency to home in on the negative, and found that negative feedback is often precise whereas praise is often general. Mary facilitated us in looking at what kind of feedback is most useful. We identified really useful feedback as specific, realistic, speaking of actions (not the person) and offering alternatives. In a skilful exercise, we practised using the headings we had generated.

We all described something we had achieved that we had not thought we could do. That created a real buzz, and led to a discussion on knowing our boundaries.

Skills: better than 'quite good'

Mary then set us exercises in naming our own skills. We could cope with being 'quite good' but found being called 'excellent' very uncomfortable. We acknowledged, however, that women want their midwives to be better than 'quite good'!

Most of the rest of the session was taken up with highly relevant exercises in active listening, highlighting key skills in offering validation and how we could develop these skills. We were then asked to complete two written questions:

- I am going to try out with others . . .
- I am going to try out by myself . . .

I resolved to try out with others specific, owned feedback and to try out by myself writing down and keeping the good things in my practice. We each kept our resolves on paper.

We wrote down our feedback. Mary shared hers: she was nervous at undertaking a new form of workshop but 'glad that we would play'. I enjoyed and learnt from such active play with a facilitator who made us all feel safe and appreciated. Relationships within the group were certainly enhanced.

The written feedback was very positive. The participating midwives felt comfortable and cared for within the group and able to share personal experiences and views. In this safe setting we could question our own responses to colleagues and make practical plans to be more supportive. It was helpful to see into our similar concerns and anxieties. A number of participants described gaining insights as well as skills. The exercises enabled us to focus on developing specific skills which we had already decided were needed. The quality of facilitation was noted and appreciated.

The session was deeply educational in that Mary facilitated us in drawing out and owning the key issues. The exercises kept us moving physically, emotionally and intellectually. The balance of work as individuals, in pairs or in the whole group ensured that we were constantly engaged but never felt exposed. It was a really invigorating morning, and an example of positive response to midwives' identified needs.

Mary will conduct a similar session in Bassetlaw soon. We then plan to cascade these workshops for midwives who have not yet attended. Mary will act as guide and mentor to those who facilitate future workshops.

This session really enabled us to address our needs for validation and support. These have long been recognised in midwifery. One workshop cannot, in itself, solve long-standing needs, but it enabled us to make a start in examining our requirements and learning skills for mutual support and validation.

Acknowledgements

I would like to thank Vivienne Knight, Head of Midwifery, Doncaster and Bassetlaw Hospitals NHS Trust, for commissioning the workshops, and Mary Smale for designing and running them.

REFERENCES

Curtis P, Stapleton H, Kirkham M and Smale M (2001). 'Evaluation of the Breastfriends Doncaster 2000 Initiative'. WICH, University of Sheffield.

Kirkham M (1999). 'The culture of midwifery in the NHS in England'. Journal of Advanced Nursing, 30 (3): 732–739.

Kirkham M (2000). 'Breastfriends Doncaster 2000'. The Practising Midwife, 3 (7): 20–21.

Lawler J (1991). Behind the Screens: Nursing, Somology and the Problem of the Body, London: Churchill Livingstone.

The Practising Midwife 2004; 7(4): 18–20

Topics for further reflection

Several of the articles in this section relate to ideology, an area that has been discussed a great deal in relation to birth over the past few decades. The differences between the midwifery model and the medical model have been discussed at length, and the past few years have seen both an increase in the research around the midwifery model and a deepening of the level of debate in this area; both of which are reflected in the articles in this section.

- Do you feel that this debate in general or any particular article that you have read have impacted upon your personal ideological standpoint in relation to birth and, if so, how?

In her article about the situation that she and a woman she cared for experienced around expediting labour after membrane rupture, Kirsten Baker makes some fascinating points about how different people – and groups – work from different sets of assumptions.

- Where do you stand in relation to the different positions that Kirsten describes? Do you feel particularly strongly (whether in agreement or disagreement) about any specific parts of this article? If so, why do you think that this might be the case?

Another area that has been explored in more depth in recent years relates to midwives ways of thinking, being, knowing and practising, and some of the articles in this section also touch upon those areas.

- Mary Nolan describes two kind of thinkers in her article; holistic thinkers and analytical thinkers. Do your preferred ways of thinking fall into one of these categories, and do you think this affects the way you talk to women? How do you adapt your approach when working with women who think in different ways from you?
- The research carried out by Holly Powell Kennedy and her colleagues offers many interesting insights into the practice of the midwives they studied. Do the findings of this study resonate with the way you practice? What is the most significant aspect of this study for you?

Finally, tensions often arise where there exist differences in perspective, or where there is a gap between the ideal and the reality, or between the needs of different groups.

- Do you feel that there exists a gap between the theory of manual handling (or health and safety in general) and the reality of what happens in practice? If so, how do you manage that?
- What is your perspective on the subject of visiting policies in hospital maternity wards? Do you agree with some, or all, of the responses shared? Do you feel that the policies in your local hospital are woman-centred? How can we work towards developing policies which are women-centred while recognising that women may have different needs from each other and that midwives and other staff have their own needs and preferences as well?

Focus on . . .

The Birthing Environment

SECTION CONTENTS

How women choose where to give birth

Tina Lavender, Jean Chapple

The need to assess women's views on childbirth issues is contained in a vision of a maternity service that offers both safety and satisfaction (Department of Health 1992). However, although maternity services are generally rated highly, there is a variation in what women want and receive (Audit Commission 1997). An earlier survey found that women who choose home birth do so to avoid unnecessary intervention, to be on familiar territory, because they feared hospital setting, to have a continuing relationship with a midwife or because they had given birth at home previously (National Birthday Trust 1997). The reasons for giving birth in hospital were safety or previous hospital birth. However, recent findings suggest that women's needs are not always being met in many hospital units (Newburn 2003), yet despite this the majority of women continue to give birth in hospitals.

There is overwhelming evidence that safe and effective maternity services based on a philosophy of normality can be provided by appropriate use of midwifery-led care and appropriate referral for women who are low risk (Zander and Chamberlain 1999). It can therefore be argued that if neither mother nor baby is at risk, then the woman should be the only person who decides where she gives birth. This is supported by a large prospective study of 625 women in Holland, which found a relationship between interventions and planned birth site (van der Hulst et al 2004). Women intending to have a home birth experienced fewer interventions compared with those who opted for a hospital birth. Home-like settings, established in or near conventional wards, are also associated with benefits (Hodnett et al 2005), including reduced intervention and increased maternal satisfaction. Furthermore, a structured review of midwife-led birth centres found that, of the five studies included, all reported a benefit for women intending to give birth in a free-standing, midwife-led unit (Walsh and Downe 2004). It is unsurprising, therefore, that maternity providers are increasingly exploring alternatives to large obstetric units.

There is, however, a lack of research that looks at birth settings in relation to both women's and midwives' views. We therefore remain unclear as to what factors are currently influencing women's decisions.

The project

This project was commissioned by the Department of Health (UK) to inform the Children's National Service Framework (Department of Health 2004). This Framework provides new national standards across the National Health Service and social services for children.

The project's aim was to identify models of maternity care which provide a service that is consistently safe, equitable, sustainable, meets the needs of the current and future population and offers choice in relation to the type of service that women can access. The overall project included observational visits of different maternity sites, focus group interviews with midwives (Lavender and Chapple 2004) and a survey of women's views. This article reports on women's views in the antenatal period.

Methods

We carried out a survey of pregnant women in 12 maternity units in England between January and March 2002, following approval from Local Research Ethics Committees, Research and Development Managers and/or Audit Co-ordinators.

A purposive sampling strategy was adopted to ensure the inclusion of units that serve women from various socio-economic/ethnic backgrounds, from different areas of England (urban and rural). The strategy ensured that units were included that offered different birth settings (home, free-standing unit, midwife-led unit (MLU), obstetric unit) and varied in size (from 50 births to 6,000 births).

A five-day snapshot of women's views in the antenatal period were sought in an attempt to gain the views of a representative sample in a short timeframe. Questionnaires were administered by local midwives and administrative staff and returned to post boxes in the clinical areas. In some units interpreters were made available to assist women from ethnic minority groups to complete the questionnaire.

The questionnaire

The questionnaire was specifically designed but incorporated a number of questions from previous local audits (Lavender et al 1999, Saunders et al 2000). It was descriptive in design and included open and closed questions. The main body of the questionnaire incorporated a series of statements which women were asked to agree or disagree with. Positive and negative statements were included to prevent respondents answering uniformly, without consideration of the statement. Content validity was achieved through review of the literature, our own experience and informal discussions with key stakeholders. Stakeholders included clinical midwives, obstetricians, consumers, consumer representatives and researchers. A pilot study confirmed readability and acceptability to women.

Analysis

Pre-coded quantitative data was entered onto SPSS (version 10.1). Double entry of random data sets was carried out to ensure data accuracy. We computed means and standard deviations for continuous baseline variables and frequencies and percentages to describe the categorical data. Comparisons were made according to parity, Jarman Underprivileged Area Scores (UPA) (Jarman 1983), age and ethnicity. Significance was calculated with the chi-squared test for categorical data.

Open responses were included to provide some rationale for the structured answers provided. Thus, emerging theoretical themes were compared and analysed with existing literature and related directly to the responses to the structured questions. Responses were independently analysed by two researchers to minimise the potential for interpretation bias.

Results

Of the 14 units invited to participate, 12 were able to do so within the allocated time frame; two units had lengthy ethical procedures. In total, 2,902 questionnaires were distributed to participating units and 2,071 (71 per cent) returned. The response rate between units varied from 59 per cent to 85 per cent.

Demographic and baseline details

Half of the questionnaires were returned from district general hospitals (n = 1,053: 51 per cent), the remainder being returned from university hospitals incorporating midwife-led units (n = 781: 38 per cent) and free-standing birth centres (n = 231: 11 per cent). The mean age of women was 29 (SD 7) and gestation on completion of the questionnaire was 29 weeks (SD 9). Just over half of the women were multigravid (1,125: 54 per cent), the majority having given birth to one child previously (n = 946: 46 per cent). Most were 'white-European' (n = 1744: 84 per cent), and English was the first language (n = 1867; 90 per cent) of the majority. There was a wide variation in UPA scores, the median score being 4 and range –37 (affluent) to 68 (underprivileged).

Choice of birth setting

When asked, 'Were you given a choice of places where you can give birth?,' only 932 (45 per cent) of women said 'yes.' These women were asked to record in a free text space what these choices were; this varied, as can be seen in Table 2.1.1.

In 202 cases women stated that they were not offered a choice of birth setting due to 'medical conditions.'

Only 158 (7.6 per cent) women ever considered giving birth at home, of which 107 (67.7 per cent) stated they had changed their mind as the pregnancy progressed. The main reasons for women changing their minds included 'safer in hospital,' 'medical reason' and 'family pressure.' Pressure from midwives and obstetricians was also noted. Women suggested that this occurred covertly and overtly. One woman, for example said:

'I told the doctor at the hospital [that] I was going to have my baby at home and he said "you are being foolish putting your baby at risk".'

Table 2.1.1 Birth setting choices offered in current pregnancy

	N	(%)
Home or hospital	316	(34)
Choice of hospitals	246	(26)
Hospital or birth centre	72	(8)
Midwife-led unit or obstetric unit	66	(7)
Home, midwife-led unit or obstetric unit	62	(7)
Place not specified	63	(7)
Hospital, birth centre or home	41	(4)
Birth centre or MLU	59	(6)
Home	7	(1)

N = 932

Another said:

'I could tell by the way she [midwife] went silent that she didn't approve so I gave in . . . I got the impression that nobody wanted me to have a home birth and the nurse [midwife] seemed pleased when I changed my mind.'

Women clearly did not believe home birth to be a real option. One woman said:

'The midwife said I could request a home birth but because of staff shortages there may not be a midwife available anyway, so I didn't see the point.'

Factors which women considered important in determining where they wished to give birth are summarised in Table 2.1.2. Women in this survey used the free text spaces to provide the rationale for the structured responses in Table 2.1.2. The following quotes represent some of the most frequently recurring issues.

Statement 1: It is not important for me to have my baby in the same place as I receive my antenatal care

Although almost a third of women wished to have antenatal care in the same place that they were to give birth, the remainder were either indifferent or disagreed. Women who disagreed tended to be those who had received some of their antenatal care at home. Comments

such as 'I felt much more relaxed when the midwife came to see me in my house' were frequently used.

Statement 2: It is important that my antenatal appointments are at a location close to where I live

The majority of women wanted their antenatal care to be provided locally. Some expressed that it would be unreasonable to travel any distance:

'It would be too inconvenient to travel for antenatal care, especially when you're working and/or have got other kids.' (Free-standing unit)

Some women stipulated the maximum amount of time to arrive at the antenatal clinic that they believed to be reasonable:

'When you are pregnant you don't want to be getting on and off buses. You want to be there in no more than 15 minutes otherwise you're fit for nothing when you arrive.' (District General Hospital)

Statement 3: I would be willing to travel if it meant I would receive higher quality care for my baby and me around the time of giving birth

The locality of a birth centre did not appear to be a major issue to a large number of women (n = 1,407: 68 per cent). This was confirmed by the fact that a number of women

Table 2.1.2 Statements to support structured responses

	Strongly disagree		Disagree		Neither agree nor disagree		Agree		Strongly agree		Missing	
	N	(%)	N	(%)	N	(%)	N	(%)	N	(%)	N	(%)
1. It is not important for me to have my baby in the same place as I receive my antenatal care	178	(9)	622	(30)	620	(30)	429	(21)	140	(7)	88	(4)
2. It is important that my antenatal appointments are at a location close to where I live	25	(1)	145	(7)	353	(17)	1029	(50)	460	(22)	65	(3)
3. I would be willing to travel if it meant I would receive higher quality care for my baby and me around the time of birth	53	(3)	165	(8)	384	(19)	971	(47)	436	(21)	68	(3)
4. It is important to me that a midwife helps me to give birth to my baby even if complications develop	42	(2)	110	(5)	426	(21)	957	(46)	472	(23)	70	(3)
5. I would feel unsafe if a specially trained doctor was not immediately available when I am in labour	57	(3)	293	(14)	369	(18)	803	(39)	483	(23)	72	(4)
6. It is not important to me that a midwife I know helps me to give birth to my baby	161	(8)	520	(25)	663	(32)	527	(25)	132	(6)	74	(4)
7. It is important to me to that a special care baby unit is in the same place that I give birth	18	(1)	153	(7)	312	(15)	790	(38)	735	(35)	69	(3)
8. It is important to me to be able to have an epidural at any time of day or night	71	(3)	261	(13)	612	(30)	626	(30)	412	(20)	93	(5)
9. It is important to me that a pool is available for my labour/birth	96	(5)	425	(21)	962	(46)	364	(18)	147	(7)	82	(4)
10. I want to be looked after by midwives and not have doctors involved	177	(9)	612	(30)	789	(38)	314	(15)	106	(5)	79	(3.8)
11. I would not want to transfer to a hospital a few miles away if my baby or I develop a problem	395	(19)	635	(30.6)	373	(18)	373	(18)	209	(10.1)	86	(4.2)

N = 2,071

had booked to give birth in a unit that was out of their area:

'I had heard so much about this unit. I was told how personal it was and would have travelled any distance to get here' (Free-standing unit)

However, others had travelled in an attempt to distance themselves from what they perceived to be poor intrapartum care:

'This isn't my nearest hospital. I had to pass my local hospital to get here but it was worth it. My experience of labour was much better this time. You just want the best for you and the baby . . .' (Obstetric unit)

Statement 4: It is important to me that a midwife helps me to give birth to my baby even if complications develop

Women clearly wanted the support of a midwife during labour to 'be there,' 'offer support,' 'assist the doctor' and 'offer advice.' However, women appeared unclear as to the full range of skills possessed by a midwife. Furthermore, some women rated a midwife's technological skills by the place where the midwife worked. For example, one woman said:

'Community midwives are not good enough to work in a hospital . . . They are great for giving baby advice, though.' (Obstetric unit without MLU)

Another said:

'Midwives working in the busy hospitals are better equipped than those who do not; I would have more confidence in them.' (District general hospital)

Some women who had previously experienced a birth in a free-standing unit or at home did not support this notion. Their views were expressed in terms of 'confident midwives who knew exactly what to do at the right time.'

Statement 5: I would feel unsafe if a specially trained doctor were not immediately available when I am in labour

Women believed that a doctor was necessary to 'identify risks' and act appropriately in emergency situations. Again, many comments related to the midwives' role, which suggested that some women were not aware that midwives are competent at dealing with emergency situations:

'Midwives work for the doctors so [the doctors] must be around when you give birth. What if you develop a problem?' (Obstetric unit with MLU)

Furthermore, many women said: 'I would not feel as important if a doctor did not see me during labour.' This was particularly true of women from ethnic minority groups.

Statement 6: It is not important that a midwife I know helps me to give birth to my baby

Many women stated that knowing their midwife was unimportant or they were ambivalent:

'It is more important that the midwife is kind and caring. You could have a real dragon and be glad to get rid of her!' (Obstetric unit with MLU)

However, those women who stated that they did know their midwife saw this as a positive experience:

'The midwife saw me throughout my pregnancy and will be there at the birth. She also delivered my last baby which makes it all that more special.' (Free-standing unit)

Statement 7: It is important to me to that a special care baby unit is in the same place that I give birth

A large number of the open responses centred on issues of safety. For example, one woman said:

'Although I don't think my baby will have a problem it is nice to know that the special care baby unit is there if I need it.' (Large teaching hospital)

Women who had experience of a free-standing unit or home birth did not project the same anxieties:

'I'm not worried about having a special care baby unit. I have had a home birth before and know the midwives can deal with problems. The chances of anything going wrong are so small anyway.' (Free-standing unit)

Statement 8: It is important to me to be able to have an epidural at any time of day or night

Approximately half of the respondents said they wished an epidural to be available but this did not necessarily mean that they were intending on having one; rather, 'it's nice to know an epidural is there, just in case.' Those in midwife-led units (within same building as obstetric units) were concerned that if they needed an epidural they wouldn't be given priority:

'I want to go to the midwife-led unit as I've heard it's really relaxed but my mate went there and had to wait ages for an epidural because the doctor was doing one on the main delivery suite.' (Obstetric unit with MLU)

Statement 9: It is important to me that a pool is available for my labour/delivery

The majority of women were undecided as to whether pool availability was important to them. Some who had experienced labour/birth in a pool wrote of the benefits of such a birth in terms of 'excellent pain relief' and 'relaxing way to labour.'

Statement 10: I want to be looked after by midwives and not have doctors involved

A minority of women stated that they wanted midwifery care only. Some said: 'Why do I have to choose either a doctor or a midwife; why can't I have both?' Women also appeared to perceive the midwife's role as a 'doctor's assistant' as opposed to an autonomous practitioner:

'Although midwives are kind and caring you feel more confident if you know that a doctor is around, just in case there's an emergency.' (District general hospital)

Statement 11: I would not want to transfer to a hospital a few miles away if my baby or I develop a problem

Half of the women questioned said that they would transfer to another hospital if a problem developed. However, some women stated that they would not consider a free-standing birth centre, MLU or home birth because of the potential to transfer.

'I am going to X unit because I know that everything is there if I need it. I don't see the point in going to a small hospital when you could get transferred anyway.' (Large teaching hospital)

Yet those women who had previously been transferred in the intrapartum period maintained that '[they] would rather have started off in the stand-alone unit and been transferred than never have been there in the first place.'

Comparisons of baseline variables

There were no differences in women's views according to age or under privileged area score. Primigravid women were more likely to say that they were willing to travel for intrapartum care (agree plus strongly agree) (684/946 vs. 723/1121, × 2 14.04, p < 0.01) and it was important to have a pool available (299/946 vs. 211/1121, × 2 30.04, p < 0.01) when compared to multigravidae. Women from ethnic minority groups were more likely to say that they wanted antenatal care close to where they live when compared to the white European group (245/303 vs. 1244/1744, × 2 11.3, p < 0.01). Women from ethnic minority groups were more likely to feel unsafe if a doctor was not immediately available (235/303 vs. 1051/1744, × 2 32.3, p < 0.01) and wanted a SCBU in the place where they give birth (255/303 vs. 1270/1744, × 2 16.8, p < 0.01).

Discussion

This survey provides insight into views of women from different geographical locations who have been exposed to different models of maternity care and have different birth setting options. Unlike many surveys, the quantitative findings are contextualised using the qualitative responses.

Not all women were offered a full array of birth setting options, either because these options were not available or perhaps the information was not communicated to them. All units, however, should be able to offer a home birth service. Few women stated that they would ever consider having a home birth. The reasons provided by women for not choosing home birth centred on safety issues; however, disappointingly, responses also suggest that women did not always believe it to be a real choice. These findings are similar to those of Madi and Crow

(2003) who also found that women lacked information regarding available services and demonstrated midwives' reluctance to initiate discussions regarding home birth.

The survey demonstrated that women's decisions are based on multiple factors. Although women were not requested to rank the items that they felt were most important, clearly they felt more strongly about some issues than others. The majority wanted antenatal care to be provided locally (72 per cent) but were prepared to travel for intrapartum care (68 per cent). This has implications for trusts when developing operational strategies.

Women also stated that they wanted to give birth in a unit that had doctors readily available (62 per cent) and a special care baby unit on site (73 per cent), but they also wanted midwifery support (69 per cent). The open responses indicate that women opting for obstetric units felt reassured by the access to what they believe to be appropriate personnel and equipment in case of an emergency situation. However, importantly, this survey discovered that women might be unaware of the fact that midwives have the ability to work autonomously, identify risk and deal with obstetric emergencies. This could be because the traditional image of a midwife prevails or, alternatively, women may be accurately reporting what they see and experience. Nevertheless, some women were concerned that the care they may receive at home, in a free-standing unit or a midwife-led unit may be inferior to that in an obstetric unit. This appeared to be compounded by a belief that obstetricians were more able than midwives. There is a huge drive for childbirth to be viewed as a normal life event (RCM 2004), however to achieve this philosophy women must understand the roles of professionals. Given the reduction in junior doctors' working hours under the New Deal (Department of Health 1991) and the European Working Time Directive (Council of the European Communities 1993), and a reduction in the GP involvement in intrapartum care (Weigers 2003) women's acceptance of the midwife as lead professional is imperative for the implementation of future government strategies.

Only a third of women believed it to be important to know the midwife who helps them to give birth. It is unclear, however, from this study as to whether those who did know their midwife were more satisfied than those who did not. Continuity of care was highlighted as being important in the Changing Childbirth document (Department of Health 1993). However, a more recent review of continuity of care found women valued consistent care as opposed to continuity per se (Green et al 2000). While acknowledging that national policies advocate the continuity of care model, there is no evidence to suggest that women are really more satisfied with care from only one person. It is suggested that a limited number of carers with good co-ordination of care could be the norm (Clement and Elliot 1999).

Study limitations

This survey only had the ability to retrieve a minimal amount of information on previous maternity experience – yet this is likely to have influenced women's views. Women did not have access to all birth settings; responses may have reflected only what women knew was available, as it is difficult to comment on an unfamiliar concept of care (van Teijlingen et al 2003). Furthermore, the relatively small number of women from ethnic minority groups meant that it was not possible to explore each individual's ethnicity. Examining these women as a single cohort did not allow for consideration of cultural variations.

The response rate from some units was disappointing, and women who failed to respond may have had different views. However, opinions were similar irrespective of demography (age, parity, ethnicity, and level of deprivation). Furthermore, the study was not able to capture the views of women who chose not to attend for antenatal care, or who were receiving care from an independent midwife; such views would have made an important contribution. The duration of the project also meant that it was not feasible to follow a single cohort of women through their whole maternity experience.

One could argue that the closed questions set the agenda for women's open responses. However, women commented on issues that had not been directly asked in the closed questions – for example, the skills possessed by a midwife.

Implications for research

Further work should include primary qualitative research to obtain a deeper understanding of the rationale for women's views of birth setting in relation to locality; an exploration of the views of GPs, obstetricians, paediatricians and anaesthetists towards different birth settings; and evaluative work to explore the hypothesis that women's perceptions of a midwife's role influences her birth place decisions.

Implications for practice

In the 1970s a concerted effort took place to convince women that hospital was the best place to give birth (Peel 1970). It is perhaps therefore unsurprising that now, in the 21st century, many women continue to believe this to be the case, and indeed for some women it is. However, midwives need to ensure that women are fully informed of all birth options available to them, and resist the urge to overtly or covertly influence decision-making. Furthermore, midwives should inform women of their skills and qualifications and reinforce this during practice by projecting themselves as confident practitioners.

There was no evidence in this survey that women associated different professionals with the different spectrums of the childbirth continuum. Instead, they appeared to see obstetricians caring for all women and midwives assisting them to do this. Highlighting the fact that midwives are not only experts in normal birth, but are also skilled at identifying complications and dealing with emergencies, may be one way to convince women of the safety of a variety of birth settings.

Acknowledgements

We thank the Department of Health for funding the project, the women who participated, the individual units that facilitated the administration of questionnaires and the Liverpool Midwifery Research Department for assisting with data management.

REFERENCES

Audit Commission (1997). First Class Delivery: Improving Maternity Services in England and Wales, Abingdon: Audit Commission Publications.

Clement S and Elliott S (1999). 'Psychological health before, during and after childbirth'. In: G Marsh and M Renfrew (eds.) Community-based Maternity Care. Oxford University Press, Oxford.

Council of the European Communities (1993). 'Council Directive of 23rd November 1993 concerning certain aspects of the organisation of working time (93/104/EC)'. Off J Eur Comm; L307: 18–24.

Department of Health. NHS Management Executive (1991). Junior Doctors: The New Deal. London: Department of Health.

Department of Health (1992). Maternity Services. Government response to the second report from the health committee, session 1991–2. London: HMSO; 2018.

Department of Health (1993). Changing childbirth, Part 1: Report of the Expert Maternity Group. London: HMSO.

Department of Health (2004). The National Service Framework for Children, Young People and Maternity Services. London: Department of Health. www.publications.doh.gov.uk/nsf/children

Green J, Renfrew M and Curtis P (2000). 'Continuity of carer: what matters to women'. Midwifery; 16 (3): 186–196.

Hodnett ED, Downe S, Edwards N and Walsh D (2005). 'Home-like versus conventional institutional settings for birth'. The Cochrane Database of Systematic Reviews, No.1, CD000012.

Jarman B (1983). 'Identification of underprivileged areas'. British Medical Journal, 286: 1705–1708.

Lavender T and Chapple J (2004). 'An exploration of midwives views of the current system of maternity care in England'. Midwifery, 20: 324–334.

Lavender T, Warnock T and Nolan J (1999). Midwifery Led Audit. Liverpool Women's Hospital. Unpublished report.

Madi BC and Crow R (2003). 'A qualitative study of information about available options for childbirth venue and pregnant women's preference for a place of delivery'. Midwifery, 19, 328–336.

National Birthday Trust (1997). 'National Birthday Trust's 1994 Home Births Survey'. In: G Chamberlain, Wraight A, Crowley P (eds) Home Births. Pergamon Press: Carnford.

Newburn M (2003). 'Culture, control and the birth environment'. The Practising Midwife, 6: 20–25.

Peel Report (1970). Domiciliary Midwifery and Maternity Bed Needs. Report of the standing Maternity and Midwifery Advisory Committee (Chairman Sir John Peel). London: HMSO.

Royal College of Midwives (2004). Campaign for Normal Birth www.rcmnormalbirth.net/

Saunders D, Boulton M, Chapple J et al (2000). Evaluation of the Edgware Birth Centre Report, Middlesex: North Thames Perinatal Public Health.

van der Hulst LAM, van Teijlingen ER, Bonsel GJ et al (2004). 'Does a pregnant woman's intended place of birth influence her attitudes toward and occurrence of obstetric interventions?' Birth, 31: 28–33.

van Teijlingen ER, Hundley V, Rennie AM et al (2003). 'Maternity satisfaction studies and their limitations: what is, must still be best'. Birth, 30: 75–82.

Walsh D and Downe S (2004). 'Midwife-led birth centers: a structured review'. Birth, 31: 222–229.

Weigers TA (2003). 'General practitioners and their role in maternity care'. Health Policy, 66 (1): 51–59 (review).

Zander L and Chamberlain G (1999). 'Place of birth'. British Medical Journal, 318: 721–723.

The Practising Midwife 2005; 8(7): 10–15

Home birth: a social process, not a medical crisis

Sheila Kitzinger

The creation of the NHS was a brave and splendid revolution. As a child, I remember my mother's excitement. She had been a midwife and had also worked in one of England's first family planning clinics. She used to talk about the distress surrounding pregnancy and birth for many impoverished women who were unable to have any control over their reproductive lives. They saved money in a tin on the kitchen shelf so that their children could get medical care, but could not afford it themselves. Together with the improved nutrition that came about as the result of food rationing during and after the Second World War, the NHS changed the health of a nation. Government policy on birth initiated in 1993 (UKCC 1998: 27–28) seemed to herald another revolution, and for the first time promised woman-centred care.

But the changes made have not matched the fine talk. The system is fettered by fortress-like management structures and insensitive, defensive attitudes. We may have reached the stage where legal action is necessary. Barbara Hewson, the barrister who appealed against court-enforced caesarean sections, and won a landmark case, considers that home birth is a question of human rights. Kafka said: 'Every revolution evaporates and leaves behind it only the slime of a new bureaucracy.' I believe that the birth revolution has to be continually recreated if we are to improve the quality of childbirth for women and their babies everywhere.

Why do some women want home birth?

Women rarely feel they need to justify the choice of a hospital birth. Those who opt for hospital tend to think of it as the normal way to have a baby. If asked why they are going into hospital they may say that it is safer for the baby and themselves, they can get an epidural there, and that since expertise and equipment is based at the hospital, they will have speedy access to skills and technology. Some say that birth is messy and this is why they prefer

it to take place in hospital. Some say that their male partners insist that hospital is best, and that the men could not cope with home birth.

A large proportion of women who have given birth previously in hospital seek a home birth because the hospital birth was distressing. They hope that it will avoid a style of birth in which they are confronted by strangers, denied information and choice, treated like a 'lump of meat', and feel completely out of control. One woman, who questioned the need for induction of labour, described how the obstetric registrar told her: 'When I go to the garage, I do not tell the mechanic how to fix my car.'

A study reveals that women in Sweden who choose to give birth at home or a birth centre want to feel in control and think that this is much more likely at home or in a midwife-run birth centre. They want to make their own decisions, manage without pharmacological pain relief, have a known midwife, and give birth naturally. They see birth as a social, rather than a medical, event. The authors of this study conclude that: 'If women had free choice of place of birth the home birth rate in Sweden would be 10 times higher and the 20 largest hospitals would need to have birth centers' (Hildingsson et al 2003).

Women who call me often talk about why they seek a home birth. Their main concerns are described below.

To handle birth without drugs

One reason is that the women do not want to be dosed to the eyeballs with drugs. All anaesthetic and analgesic drugs cross the placenta to the fetus. I have heard an obstetric anaesthetist describe the placenta as 'a sump for drugs.' Drug transfer is flow-dependent. Fetal plasma has a lower pH than maternal plasma, so the drug concentrates in the fetus. Pethidine is a weak analgesic but a strong respiratory depressant. After a single dose there is a higher concentration in the fetus than in the mother, and it can be detected in the newborn baby for 62 hours.

An epidural can bring blessed relief from pain and does not produce respiratory depression. When given by an experienced anaesthetist it is usually safe. But epidurals often have side-effects for the mother and the baby: 15 per cent of mothers and babies develop fever during labour. The baby may be taken to the special-care nursery for investigation and tests to discover if it has septicaemia. The mother's blood pressure may drop suddenly when the epidural is given, and this reduces the amount of oxygen passing through the placenta to the baby. So other drugs have to be available to raise the mother's blood pressure again.

Delivery may be by forceps or ventouse because the tone of the pelvic floor muscles is lost, the head gets stuck in the wrong position, and the mother cannot push the baby out. The vaginal operative delivery rate is four times higher in women who have epidurals than in those who do not, and the caesarean rate is twice as high (Findley and Chamberlain 1999, Goer 1999, MacArthur and Weeks 1995, Thorp et al 1993).

To give birth without intervention

Each intervention in childbirth has a knock-on effect that can be positive or negative. It may help to support the physiology of normal labour, or disrupt it so that there is a cascade of further interventions. There is evidence that induction of labour leads to other interventions, including greater need for pain-killing drugs. One study showed that induction more than doubles the likelihood that delivery will be by caesarean section (Seyb et al 1999). Continuous fetal monitoring is also associated with other interventions, including instrumental delivery and caesarean section (Haverkamp et al 1976, Renou et al 1976, Thacker and Stroup 2000, Vintzileos et al 1993).

The problem is that fetal distress is often diagnosed when it is not present (Ecker et al 2001). In UK hospitals the trend is towards routine admission cardiotocography for 20 minutes. This has the effect of classifying a large group of women as having abnormalities when, in fact, labour is normal and the baby is fine. In one study, 32 per cent of print-outs were defined as unsatisfactory, and the women went on to have continuous CTG (Impey et al 2003).

Labour can be disturbed by midwifery interventions, too, some of which have been made for many years without any analysis of their effect. As one midwife teacher expresses it: 'Decades of repetitive performance of asking a woman to get on a bed, or asking her to push, have had the effect of making such interventions invisible' (Anderson 2002).

Amniotomy, for example, is often used routinely, and injections of pethidine are part of normal midwifery practice. In the USA, multiple interventions are the norm. The First National Survey of Women's Child-bearing Experiences reveals that 93 per cent of women had continuous electronic fetal monitoring, 86 per cent an intravenous drip, 74 per cent of those who gave birth vaginally were expected to lie on their backs while pushing the baby out, 67 per cent had artificial oxytocin to start or to stimulate uterine contractions, 63 per cent had epidurals, 58 per cent had a hand inserted into the uterus after birth, 55 per cent had their membranes artificially ruptured, 52 per cent had a catheter in the bladder, and 52 per cent had suturing to repair an episiotomy or tear. Less than 1 per cent of women gave birth without such interventions, and they nearly all came from the less than 1 per cent home births in the sample (Declercq et al 2002).

To enable the baby to have a smooth and gentle introduction to the world

Newborn babies can see and hear. They look around and fix their eyes on the nearest interesting face. They startle if they hear loud noises, and turn towards the sound of the mother's voice, because they heard it when inside her body. All this is delayed if the baby is crying so much that other stimuli are shut out, or is so drugged that he or she cannot respond to anything. At birth, babies often cry for about five minutes. A very heavily drugged baby feels floppy and may only whimper, or may not cry at all.

A distressed baby may cry until it is exhausted. In general, babies who have received analgesic drugs from their mothers cry longer than babies of mothers who have received no drugs (Belsey et al 1981, Ransjo-Arvidson et al 2001, Sepkoski et al 1992).

A newborn baby who has not been dosed with medication in the maternal bloodstream is in an ideal neurophysiological state to start out on the exciting task of getting to know its mother and to breastfeed (Ransjo-Arvidson et al 2001). Given time, and in a relaxed environment, a baby will spontaneously creep up towards the breast (Belsey et al 1981) and then start to root, turning its head from side to side, mouth open and searching for the nipple. It uses its hands as well as its mouth. Immediately after birth the hands are relaxed, but after a few minutes they start to explore. The baby sucks its fingers and strokes and massages the breast, licks it and, in its own time, latches on and sucks (Matthiesen et al 2001).

This process usually takes about an hour, during which time the baby should not be disturbed or taken away. There is no hurry to weigh, bath or dress a newborn. It is much easier to create a birth setting in which babies can behave spontaneously, and mothers can behave more spontaneously, too, at home than in hospital. The mother responds to the baby's stimulation with a rush of oxytocin, which causes the uterus to contract and expel the placenta and makes her nipples erect, ready for feeding. She is excited, and touches the baby, first with her finger tips, then with the whole palm, and enfolds the baby in the crook of her arm. She cannot take her eyes off her baby, who stares and searches her face, fascinated by her eyes and mouth, and the movements as she smiles and speaks. A new relationship is unfolding. Two people are getting to know each other.

To have a midwife they know

Women seeking a home birth do not just want a 'named midwife' or 'continuity of care' offered by a team of midwives whose faces and names they struggle to recognise. They want a midwife whom they come to know during pregnancy, and who by the time the baby is due has become a close friend. There is a world of difference between knowing your midwife's name and phone number or meeting a large group of midwives, any two of whom might attend you in labour, and having a special relationship with someone you like and trust, and who really knows you.

It is reasonable to be cared for by two to four midwives working together, but not to have to confront a group the size of a football team. Unfortunately, when women are booked for a home birth they are often told that they will be cared for by a team of midwives, or that someone might come out from hospital when labour starts whom they have never before met, and that even this cannot be guaranteed: if the labour ward is short staffed, home birth is impossible and they must come in. This leaves many pregnant women feeling very unsure of what is going to happen. They are up against an administrative structure that is rigid and implacable. However reassuring the individuals they meet, they cannot fight the system. So what may have been the priority reason that leads a woman to choose home birth – personal, sensitive, woman-to-woman care – her choice is denied her.

If she is seeking a personal relationship with the midwife, it is sensible to try to find a midwife who has responsibility for her own caseload. This system operates in only a few areas within the NHS. It is what independent midwives offer. But, because these work outside the NHS, they have to be paid for.

To be free to move around

The medical management of childbirth that was introduced in the 20th century confined women to bed, because this was the easiest place for a doctor to keep an eye on them, and they could maintain their modesty by being covered in bedding. Whereas prior to this time it was taken for granted that women in labour were upright, moved around, and used a rope from the rafters, window ledges and a table or chair to get into comfortable positions, once a doctor was in charge, even in home births,

the requirements of medical supervision, together with modesty, dictated that a woman should be in bed and under the covers. In her own home a woman can move freely, supporting herself in any position she chooses, using furniture with which she is familiar. She does not need special equipment to stand, squat or kneel.

Movement is almost invariably restricted in hospital, since the mother is harpooned to electronic equipment, and perhaps an intravenous drip. There is no question of this happening in the environment of home. She can squat in front of a chair, the children's toy box, be on all fours on the floor, or in the bath or on the bed, lean against the kitchen units or a window ledge, rock her pelvis, knees spread, against the dining room table or a desk, or over a hammock and do a gentle belly dance with strong, flexible support – any of these, and more.

In hospital, birth tends to be much more static, especially once the second stage is reached. The main participants are positioned as if in a tableau and according to their status in the hierarchy. The senior obstetrician or midwife in charge stands at the end of the delivery table or bed between the woman's legs. Others are grouped around, with her partner up at her head. She may look down and see a man's face between her legs. He may be a total stranger.

To avoid hospital cross-infection

Streptococcus B is the main cause of neonatal sepsis. Mothers and babies are especially at risk when interventions take place that entail early artificial rupture of the membranes; frequent pelvic examinations; insertion of foreign bodies, such as catheters and other instruments, into the vagina; and the crowding of women together under insanitary conditions, with midwives caring for several women simultaneously.

Home birth is the setting for a social, rather than a medical, model of birth. Other reasons for choosing home birth are to do with human values. Birth and the events surrounding it have traditionally been a domestic ritual and female celebration. In the Christian calendar women organise making pancakes on Shrove Tuesday, hot cross buns at Easter, and family get-togethers at Christmas, so in the past women planned and choreographed what was to happen during birth and the lying-in, and cooked special dishes to keep up the labouring woman's strength, and to celebrate after the birth.

Childbirth took place in women's space, not a male-dominated institution. At all levels of society women gathered, bringing their charms, herbs and 'simples' to support the mother. Even when a doctor attended, but birth still took place at home, it was expected that other women would be present to help. Doctors complained that they could do nothing without the women's agreement. It was the move from home to hospital that finally got rid of the group of women companions.

At home, birth is a social process, rather than a medical crisis. It is an intimate and domestic event, and the parameters of time are quite different from those of hospital births. The medical model defines childbirth in terms of three stages: the first stage in which the cervix dilates to 10cm, the second stage in which the baby is expelled, and the third stage in which the other products of conception (placenta and membranes) are expelled. Birth is segmented into specific periods of time, and the time taken for each phase is noted on a record sheet. A holistic view of birth time does not mean that the midwife is neglectful of, or casual about, the passage of time or the efficiency of uterine function, but that she assesses it in terms of the woman's personality, her behaviour and relationships and the setting in which the birth is taking place.

With the switch to hospital, birth became a medical drama, unfolding as if on a stage or at an altar. The lighting is often harsh and inflexible, and the mother may be under the full glare of fluorescent lights, more suited to a fast-food joint or fish and chip shop. Imagine being told to make love in the setting of the hospital delivery room typical of almost anywhere in the world today. There is a hard, narrow bed in the centre of the room, a trolley with metal instruments, and a pervasive odour of antiseptics. A clock is on the wall opposite the delivery table and there is a spyhole window in the door, which opens and closes as complete strangers pop in and out to have a look or to relay a piece of information about what is happening in another room down the corridor.

Or try enjoying a meal in a laboratory surrounded by steel instruments while harpooned to electronic equipment. Specialists in gastroenterology watch and time you, rate your performance, write up detailed notes, and exhort you to try harder and swallow faster.

Our bodies tend to function more effectively when we are in a familiar environment that we ourselves can control, and in which we can relax and behave spontaneously. The challenge to hospitals is to create an environment in which this is possible for all women, whether low or high risk.

Acknowledgement

This article is reproduced from: Kitzinger S (2005) The Politics of Birth, Edinburgh: Books for Midwives, pages 99–122.

REFERENCES

Anderson A (2002). 'Peeling back the layers: a new look at midwifery interventions'. MIDIRS Midwifery Digest, 12(2): 208.

Belsey E M, Rosenblatt D B, Lieberman B A et al (1981). 'The influence of maternal analgesia on neonatal behaviour'. I. Pethidine. British Journal of Obstetrics and Gynaecology, 188: 398–406.

Declercq E R, Sakala C, Corry M P et al (2002). Listening to Mothers: Report of the First National US Survey of Women's Childbearing Experiences'. Conducted for the Maternity Center Association by Harris Interactive, Rochester, NY.

Ecker J L, Chen K T, Cohen A P et al (2001). 'Increased risk of cesarean delivery with advancing maternal age: indications and associated factors in nulliparous women'. American Journal of Obstetrics and Gynecology, 185 (4): 883–887.

Findley I and Chamberlain G (1999). 'ABC of labour care: relief of pain'. BMJ, 318 (7188): 927–930.

Goer H (1999). The Thinking Woman's Guide to a Better Birth, New York: Penguin Putman.

Haverkamp A D, Thompson H E, McFee J G et al (1976). 'The evaluation of continuous fetal heart rate monitoring in high-risk pregnancy'. American Journal of Obstetrics and Gynecology, 125 (3): 310–317.

Hildingsson I, Waldenstrom U and Radestad I (2003). 'Swedish women's interest in home birth and in-hospital birth center care'. Birth, 30 (1): 11–22.

Impey L, Reynolds M, MacQuillan K et al (2003). 'Admission cardiotocography: a randomised controlled trial'. Lancet, 361 (9356): 465–470.

MacArthur C and Weeks S (1995). 'Epidural anaesthesia and low back pain after delivery: a prospective cohort study'. BMJ, 311 (7016): 1336–1339.

Matthiesen A S, Ransjo-Arvidson A B, Nissen E et al (2001). 'Postpartum maternal oxytocin release by newborns: effects of infant hand massage and sucking'. Birth, 28 (1):13–19.

Ransjo-Arvidson A B, Matthiesen A S, Lilja G et al (2001). 'Maternal analgesia during labor disturbs newborn behavior: effects on breastfeeding, temperature and crying'. Birth, 28 (1): 5–12.

Renou P, Chang A, Anderson I et al (1976). 'Controlled trial of fetal intensive care'. American Journal of Obstetrics and Gynecology, 126 (4): 470–476.

Sepkoski C M, Lester B M, Ostheimer G W et al (1992). 'The effects of maternal epidural anesthesia on neonatal behavior during the first month'. Developments in Medicine and Child Neurology, 34 (12): 1072–1080.

Seyb S T, Berka R J, Socol M L et al (1999). 'Risk of cesarean delivery with elective induction of labor at term in nulliparous women'. Obstetrics and Gynaecology, 94 (4): 600–607.

Thacker S B and Stroup D F (2000). 'Continuous electronic heart rate monitoring for fetal assessment during labor'. Cochrane Library, Issue 2, Oxford: Update Software.

Thorp J A, Hu D A, Albin R M et al (1993). 'The effect of intrapartum epidural analgesia on nulliparous labor: a randomized, controlled, prospective trial'. American Journal of Obstetrics and Gynecology, 169 (4): 851–858.

United Kingdom Central Council (1998). Midwives' Rules and Code of Practice, London: UKCC.

Vintzileos A M, Antsaklis A, Varvarigos I et al (1993). 'A randomised trial of intrapartum electronic fetal heart rate monitoring versus intermittent auscultation'. Obstetrics and Gynecology, 81 (6): 899–907.

Home birth: safe as houses?

Jeanette Kinsey

After our second daughter was born in a planned home birth, I decided to look into the research regarding the safety of home birth. I was spurred on by the fact that my family had been quite concerned at our decision to birth at home. I am a midwife trained and practising in this country; the results of the research have been published in Sweden, my home country, but I would like to share it with readers of The Practising Midwife as well. I also want to share the, for me, very positive experience of birthing at home.

The case for home births

In the UK, 2 per cent of women have a planned home birth, although this figure varies depending on where you live (DoH 2003). The regional differences are considerable. In Sweden, the home birth rate is as low as 0.1 per cent (Madison 2002). In both countries, research shows that more women would choose to birth at home if this were available. The main difference between the UK and Sweden is that here you are legally entitled to choose where you give birth, and home birth should be an option for any woman who has been assessed as low risk. This is supported through the Changing Childbirth report (DoH 1993), and the home birth rate has increased from 1 per cent to 2 per cent since this report came out.

In 2002, the Royal College of Midwives (RCM 2002) published a position paper that again stressed the woman's choice and stated that home births should be available as standard, integral to the entire service. Further, a Cochrane review (Olsen and Jewell 2000) recommended that all women assessed as low risk should be offered the option of considering a planned home birth.

In Sweden, this service is not provided by the country's national health service. Instead, the woman who wishes to have a home birth has to contact an independent midwife herself and pay for her services, thus leading to a low home birth rate.

The safety of planned home birth remains a controversial issue and is the subject of much debate. Hospital births are often seen as a safer alternative. There are, however, several pieces of research indicating that home birth is as safe as, if not safer than, a hospital birth. Some of these will be presented here.

Fewer instrumental deliveries

In research conducted by the National Birthday Trust Fund (Chamberlain et al 1997), nearly 6,000 women who planned a home birth at 37 weeks were matched with women who planned to birth in hospital. It was found that the rate of instrumental and caesarean section deliveries were halved in the group that planned a home birth. Women who gave birth at home had a lower rate of episiotomies, of postpartum haemorrhage and less use of pharmacological pain relief.

The babies born at home had higher Apgar scores, and fewer needed any resuscitation. There were five cases of stillbirths or neonatal deaths among babies planned to be born at home. One neonatal death occurred at home, two babies were stillborn, and two neonatal deaths occurred in hospital after transfer before or during labour. There were four cases of stillbirth and one neonatal death in the hospital birth group. About 16 per cent of women were transferred to hospital in late pregnancy or labour, most of them primigravidae.

It would seem that a woman who is well assessed prior to a home birth does not put herself or her baby at any greater risk than a woman with a similar pregnancy who plans to birth in hospital (Chamberlain 1999). A study performed in the USA (Murphy and Fullerton 1998) supports this statement as long as care is provided by qualified staff and within a system that promotes transfer to hospital should this be necessary.

Olsen (1997) also concludes in his study that home birth is an acceptable alternative for selected pregnant women, and leads to a reduction in medical interventions. This study comprised more than 24,000 low-risk pregnant women and analysed mortality and morbidity, including Apgar score, perineal tears and medical interventions.

In British Columbia, Canada, it was not until 1998 that women could choose to give birth at home, with a qualified midwife in attendance. With the aim of evaluating the safety of home birth, a study was performed between 1998 and 1999 that comprised 862 births. It found that women who gave birth at home with a midwife in attendance had fewer interventions during labour compared with women who birthed in hospital, and there was no higher risk for mother and baby associated with home births (Janssen et al 2002).

Training essential

However, there are studies from both UK and Australia showing that although home birth is a safe option for women without any complications, it is not suitable for women in high-risk categories (Bastian et al 1998, Zander and Chamberlain 1998). Midwives attending a home birth must be trained to recognise problems early in order to facilitate early transfer to hospital if required. They also need regular updating in the resuscitation of the newborn, and it is crucial that they have the appropriate equipment available for resuscitation.

I believe that the type of environment in which the woman finds herself is closely linked with the debate on the safety of home birth. There are several other authors supporting this, stressing the influence of the environment on the progress of labour (Anderson 2002, Newburn 2003, Wickham 1999). Home birth needs less medical augmentation of labour, as the woman is more relaxed in her own home. Labour would thus seem more likely to progress normally and lead to the safe arrival of her baby.

Our story

After the birth of our first daughter in hospital, I knew I would like to give birth at home the next time. I had nothing against birthing in hospital the first time, as I knew that it was necessary. I had growth scans performed in the third trimester, and as growth was tailing off the decision was made that I ought to be induced at 39 weeks' gestation. It was a devastating decision for me at the time. However, I was found to be 3cm dilated and an ARM could be performed.

After a walk around the hospital, contractions started. Mobility was maintained throughout labour by standing up and using a rocking chair, although a CTG was used to monitor the baby at times. My husband, Tony,

massaged my back with massage oil through most of the labour, which I found very helpful. I remember thinking that I wished every woman in labour could experience the same. I also think that it made my husband feel part of the process to a greater extent. In the latter part of the labour I used Entonox, which was a very welcome relief at that point. After a five-hour labour, Elisa was born, weighing 5lb 9oz (2.520kg).

This experience gave me a confidence in my own body. I have seen so many women go through the birth process and many times have marvelled at their capability and strength to give birth to their babies. I now know that this strength only comes to the woman during this process, but the people surrounding the woman have to listen to her in order for her to be able to keep her strength and concentration.

I feel that this can best be achieved in a home-like environment.

So when I was pregnant again at the end of 2002, Tony and I discussed the possibility of a home birth. We decided that if all was well at the end of the pregnancy, this was what we would like. Again I was referred for ultrasound scans to monitor the growth of the fetus. This baby was larger and the growth did not tail off, so the consultant gave me his blessing for a home birth. I had a good pregnancy and felt ready, confident and very excited about having a home birth. In the back of my mind I was also prepared that all might not go to plan, and a transfer to hospital might be necessary. But I did not let this overshadow the excitement.

I was 40+3 when I felt a gush of water at 6pm – the membranes had ruptured. I had experienced strong Braxton Hicks contraction for days previously, but on this day the baby had felt exceptionally low in my pelvis. There were some tightenings following the membranes rupturing, 1:5, but not very strong. I called the midwife to inform her what was happening so that she could arrange cover at the midwife-led unit. Midwife Jane came to see me, listened to the fetal heart and brought me a birthing ball. I wanted to send her back to the unit, but as I laboured fairly quickly the first time she didn't want to leave me without performing a vaginal examination – 4cm, thick cervix, was the verdict. The tightenings seemed to be further apart, and she left.

With our babysitter Cathy present, Tony and I went for a long walk around the village. As we were walking back I felt something move sharply inside me and after that the contractions started coming thick and fast. I managed to read my three-year-old a short bedtime story at 11pm. She was excited at having Cathy there but went to sleep. Contractions were now coming 1:2 and very strong. If I was to have a hospital birth, this would have been the point to set off – I would not have liked to sit in a car to go anywhere at all!

Midwife Jill, whom I had never met, was summoned and soon arrived. The fact that I had not met her did not matter to me. At this point I was ready to go upstairs to the bedroom where the birth was planned to take place. I knelt on the floor resting over the birthing ball. Cathy, who is a qualified massage therapist (well-chosen babysitter!) massaged my back with lavender oil. She worked fantastically with me. Together with her and my husband's help, I managed to breathe through the powerful contractions and no further pain relief was needed. We continued like this through the contractions while listening to music by Eva Cassidy until the urge to push suddenly took over at 01.05. It was all very calm. At 01:08 Annie was born, with her hand in front of her head.

As everything had progressed well, I now decided to have a physiological third stage. The baby started suckling as soon as she reached the breast, and after a few contractions the placenta was birthed. An intact perineum with some grazes was found on inspection and I was very pleased. I moved from the floor up to the bed while Annie was weighed – 6lb 10oz (3.070 kg). Annie fed again, and the midwives (the second midwife, Shirley, who was my mentor during my community placement, had arrived at some point but I was too concentrated really to take notice) packed their bags.

After the helpers left, all three of us soon went to sleep. By morning we were awake and ready to show Elisa (who had slept all night) the new addition to the family. When she looked into the Moses basket where earlier she had put her dolls, she exclaimed, 'A baby!.' That was a fantastic moment, and it was so nice that we hadn't needed to leave her.

Conclusion

In conclusion, I would suggest that while home birth is not ideal, or recommended, for all pregnant women, more women should have the opportunity to plan a home birth. I think that a lot of women would benefit physically, psychologically and emotionally from going through the satisfying process of planning for the birth, and have the feeling of being more in control of the situation, the pain and their body.

REFERENCES

Anderson T (2002). 'Out of the laboratory: back to the darkened room'. MIDIRS Midwifery Digest, 12 (1): 65–69.

Bastian H, Kierse M J N C and Lancaster P A L (1998). 'Perinatal death associated with planned home births in Australia: population based study'. BMJ, 317 (7155): 384–388.

Chamberlain G (1999). 'Birth at home: a report of the national survey of home births in the UK by the National Birthday Trust'. The Practising Midwife, 2 (7): 35–39.

Chamberlain G, Wraight A and Crowley P (1997). Home Births: the Report of the 1994 Confidential Enquiry by the National Birthday Trust Fund, Carnforth Parthenon Publishing Group.

Department of Health (1993). Changing Childbirth: report of the Expert Maternity Group, London: HMSO.

Department of Health (2003). NHS Maternity Statistics, England: 2001–2002, London: Office of National Statistics.

Janssen P A, Lee S K, Ryan E M et al (2002). 'Outcomes of planned home births versus planned hospital births after regulation of midwifery in British Columbia'. Canadian Medical Association Journal, 166 (3): 315–323.

Madison C (2002). Personal communication, Jan.

Murphy P A and Fullerton J (1998). 'Outcomes of intended home birth in nurse-midwifery practice: a prospective study'. Obstetrics and Gynecology, 92 (3): 461–470.

Newburn M (2003). 'Culture, control and the birth environment'. The Practising Midwife, 6 (8): 20–25.

Olsen O (1997). 'Meta-analysis of the safety of home birth'. Birth, 24 (1): 4–13.

Olsen O and Jewell M D (2000). 'Home versus hospital birth (Cochrane Review)'. The Cochrane Library, Oxford: Update Software, issue 2, 2003.

Royal College of Midwives (2002). Position Paper 25: Homebirth, London: RCM. Published in RCM Midwives' Journal, 5 (1): 26–29.

Wickham S (1999). 'Home birth: what are the issues?'. Midwifery Today, summer, s16–18.

Zander L and Chamberlain G (1998). 'Place of birth'. BMJ, 318: 721–723.

The Practising Midwife 2005; 8(7): 27–29

The influence of maternity units' intrapartum intervention rates and midwives' risk perception for women suitable for midwifery-led care

Marianne M. P. Mead, Diana Kornbrot

Summary

Objective: to test the hypothesis that midwives working in higher intervention units would have a higher perception of risk for the intrapartum care of women suitable for midwifery-led care than midwives working in lower intervention units.

Methods: an initial retrospective analysis of the computerised records of 9887 healthy Caucasian women in spontaneous labour enabled the categorisation of 11 units as either 'lower intrapartum intervention' or 'higher intrapartum intervention' units. A survey of the midwives involved in intrapartum care in these 11 units, using standardised scenario questionnaires, was used to investigate midwives' options for intrapartum interventions, their perceptions of intrapartum risk and the accuracy of these perceptions in the light of actual maternity outcomes.

Findings: midwives working in maternity units that had a higher level of intervention generally perceived intrapartum risks to be higher than midwives working in lower intervention units. However, midwives generally underestimated the ability of women to progress normally and overestimated the advantages of technological interventions, in particular epidural analgesia.

Conclusions: variations in intrapartum care cannot be solely explained by the characteristics of the women. The influence of the workplace culture plays a significant role in shaping midwives' perceptions of risk, but it seems even more likely that the medicalisation of childbirth has had an influence on midwives' appreciation of intrapartum risks. Intervention rates for low-risk births are often higher than recommended by research. The level of interventions varies across hospitals and higher rates are associated with higher perception of risk by midwives. Attention needs to be given to the influence the workplace plays in shaping midwives' perception of risk; and to the effect of organisational culture on intervention rates.

Introduction

Maternity services have experienced major and often conflicting changes in the industrialised world since the second world war. The epidemiological findings published in Birth Counts (Macfarlane and Mugford, 2000) show a progressive decrease in perinatal mortality (stillbirths at 28 weeks gestation and deaths in the first week of life)in England and Wales: from 57.7/1000 in 1940, to 45.2/1000 by 1945, 38.5/1000 in 1948 and finally to 6.8/1000 in 1998. The recent changes of the definition of stillbirth from 24 weeks gestation shows that the perinatal mortality rate in 1998 was 6.8/1000 (Macfarlane and Mugford, 2000). Maternal mortality also saw a significant decrease in the same years from 224/100 000 total births in 1940, to 147/ 100 000 in 1945, 86/100 000 in 1948 and finally to 7.3/100 000 in 1998 (Macfarlane and Mugford, 2000). Improvements in the general health of the population (Tew, 1995) as well as the availability of antibiotics, anaesthesia and blood transfusion have contributed to making pregnancy and labour much safer for both mothers and babies. Yet this higher level of safety has been associated with the development of a strong biological model of care, including a shift towards hospital care (Tew, 1995), supported in the UK by various governments' recommendations (Ministry of Health, 1956, 1959;

Standing Maternity and Midwifery Advisory Committee (Chairman J. Peel), 1970). This medicalisation of childbirth was associated with a rise in intrapartum interventions, e.g. induction of labour (Rayburn and Zhang, 2002), electronic fetal monitoring (Martin, 1998) and epidural analgesia (Chamberlain et al., 1993; Government Statistical Service, 2002; Harris and Chapple, 2000), and a rise in abnormal deliveries (Macfarlane and Mugford, 2000; Government Statistical Service, 2002). Some practices have been challenged: the rate of episiotomies fell from 51% for all deliveries in 1975 to 23% for the year 1989–1990 and stood at 14% for the year 2000–2001 in England (Government Statistical Service, 2002); the rate of induction of labour reached 41% in the early 1970s (Edozien, 1999), but went down to 16.8% in 1992–1993, to rise again to 21–22% in the years 1998–2001 (Government Statistical Service, 2002). Elective caesarean sections have on the other hand increased from 4.5% in 1980 to 9.8% in 2000–2001 (Government Statistical Service, 2002), but the overall rate of caesarean section has risen from 8.5% in 1975 to 17.5 in 1997 (Macfarlane and Mugford, 2000). The increased use of interventions has been associated with a reduction in the rate of deliveries undertaken by midwives: from 75.6% in 1989–1990 to 66.2% in 2000–2001 (Government Statistical Service, 2002).

The demands of some women's organisations and pressure groups eventually led to changes in attitudes, culminating in the UK in the publication of the report Changing Childbirth (Department of Health, 1993). At a more international level, Care in Normal Birth: A Practical Guide was making simple recommendations for an increased use of midwifery skills and a reduced use of technologies such as electronic fetal monitoring and epidural (WHO, 1996; Goddard, 2001).

Despite recommendations and guidelines suggesting a reduction in its application, the use of electronic fetal monitoring is widespread in the UK: only 5% of women suitable for midwifery-led care did not have any form of electronic fetal monitoring in a survey of 92 hospitals (Williams et al., 1998). The use of regional analgesia is rising – from 17% in 1989–1990 to 32% in 2000–2001 (Government Statistical Service, 2002). The rise in caesarean sections has been linked with higher levels of intervention (Thorp et al., 1989; Goffinet et al., 1997; Lieberman et al., 1999), although some studies have questioned the link between epidural and caesarean section (Howell, 2000). The rise has also been influenced by cultural changes and fear of litigation (Nozton et al., 1994; Penn and Ghaem-Maghami, 2001).

An exaggerated or underestimated perception of risk can affect judgment (Slovic et al., 1982). No studies dealing specifically with obstetric events or midwifery behaviour could be found in the literature, but the literature on perception of risk and associated behaviour suggests that

risk appreciation is often inaccurate (Johnson et al., 2002; Windschitl, 2002) and that practitioners are often excessively optimistic about the accuracy of their diagnosis (Ermenc, 1999). However, there is evidence that the medico-legal context in which midwives and obstetricians now practise may affect their perception of risk and lead them to practise defensively (Symon, 1998, 2000a; Young, 1999), even though the concept itself may be difficult to define (Symon, 2000b). Furthermore, even though clinical guidelines are being developed (National Institute for Clinical Excellence, 1999), question marks remain about their use: they must be interpreted and applied in the context on individual care, and that 'under common law, minimum acceptable standards of clinical care derive from responsible customary practice, not from guidelines' (Hurwitz, 1999, p. 661) but 'if clinicians implement faulty guidelines it is they, rather than the authors of such guidelines, who are likely to increase their liability in negligence' (Hurwitz, 1999, p. 661).

Midwives are the main intrapartum care providers for healthy women in the UK and make key decisions with women about what may constitute their optimal care. It is likely that customary practice and the environment in which they work may influence the care they give and the recommendations they make. Therefore, this study was undertaken to test the hypothesis that midwives working in higher intervention units have a higher perception of risk for the intrapartum care of women suitable for midwifery-led care than midwives working in lower intervention units.

Objectives

- To compare the level of intrapartum intervention for women suitable for midwifery-led care in 11 maternity units using one computerised data collection programme in order to categorise them as either lower intervention or higher intervention units;
- to describe midwives' perception of risk for women suitable for midwifery-led care and test the hypothesis that midwives' perception of risk will be higher in higher intervention units;
- to compare the accuracy of midwives' perception of the probability of outcomes to the actual labour outcomes.

Methods

A retrospective comparison of the intrapartum intervention rates of women suitable for midwifery-led care in 11 maternity units led to the dichotomous classification of each unit as either 'lower intrapartum intervention' or 'higher intrapartum intervention' units (Mead and Kornbrot, 2004). The midwives' perception of risk during the first and second stages of labour was explored through questionnaires, using standardised scenarios and closed questions, and the responses from the midwives working in either 'lower intrapartum intervention' or 'higher intrapartum intervention' units were compared.

The questionnaire was designed to include areas of interest for the admission procedure and the first and second stages of labour. The scenarios were developed on the basis of the information that could be retrieved from the St. Mary's Maternity Information System (SMMIS) database, so that a comparison could be established between the midwives' perception of risk and the actual outcomes associated with specific interventions. The SMMIS data only include factual data and the question-naires therefore only ask midwives what care they would provide, but did not ask them to justify that care. The particular intrapartum interventions were also identified in the guide for care in normal birth (Wagman, 1991; World Health Organization, 1996). Previous evaluations of the SMMIS database had established its reliability (Cleary et al., 1994).

The standardised scenario presented the situation of a woman who would be suitable for midwifery-led care:

X, 24 years old, primigravida, 39+ weeks gestational age, no previous medical history, a normal singleton pregnancy, in spontaneous labour, arrives at the delivery suite. Her contractions started three hours ago, are now regular and moderately strong at a rate of two to three per ten minutes. She has had a show and her membranes are intact.

Midwives were presented with four situations of increasing intervention to assess their perception of risk to the mother and the fetus: labour progresses (1) without intervention, (2) with an ARM, (3) with an epidural sited, and (4) with an ARM, continuous CTG and an epidural.

Midwives were asked the same questions for each of the four situations: how likely is labour to be completed within 6, 12, 18 or more than 18 hours (the answers for labour completed within 6 hours and between 7 and 12 hours were totalled to identify labours completed within 12 hours); how likely is continuous electronic monitoring to be used at delivery; how likely is normal fetal oxygen-ation, slight or severe fetal hypoxia; how likely is meco-nium stained liquor; how likely is the mother to have a normal delivery, a forceps or ventouse extraction, or an emergency caesarean section.

A pilot study of the questionnaire was undertaken in a unit which was not involved in the main study. It demonstrated difficulties with the understanding of the concept of probabilities. This supported the findings of previous studies on the use of probabilities or base rates which had demonstrated that estimations of probabilities on a range of 0 to 1 was more difficult for individuals to handle than estimations of probabilities of a particular

outcome for 100 people of similar characteristics (Tversky and Koehler, 1994; Doherty and Krebs, 1997; Kleiter et al., 1997; Macchi et al., 1999). Questions such as 'On a scale of 0 to 100, how likely is Mrs X to have a normal delivery, or a forceps delivery/vacuum extraction or caesarean section?' were replaced by:

If 100 women were similar to Mrs X,

how many would complete
labour within six hours? . . . . /100
between seven and 12 hours? . . . ./100
between 13 and 18 hours? . . . ./100
after 18 hours?. . . . . /100
(The total of these four answers should be 100.)

Midwives were also asked to supply personal informa-tion on their initial and present midwifery academic level, the length of their present employment, the number of contracted hours, average annual deliveries, experience of litigation and previous observation of the, then, UKCC Professional Conduct Committee hearing.

SPSS for Windows was used for the statistical analysis. The SMMIS data had been made available in text format and transferred onto an SPSS data file. Differences between categorical variables were analysed using the chi-square test and differences between continuous vari-ables were analysed by ANOVA. The differences between the SMMIS data and the midwives' responses were explored using descriptive statistics.

Ethical approval was granted by a Multi-centre Research Ethics Committee (MREC) as well as the Local-Research Ethics Committees (LREC) of the 11 units involved in the study.

Sample

Following an initial comparison of four neighbouring maternity units (Mead et al., 2000), it was envisaged that the three highest and the three lowest caesarean section rates units submitting their data centrally would be selected for this study, but three of the 12 units that regu-larly returned their data were teaching hospitals. Since it was possible that the practice in these units may vary substantially from that of district general hospitals the decision was made to use all units. One unit involved in other research studies declined to participate. One hospi-tal, officially classified as a district general hospital, had a strong history of research and was used for the training of medical students and was classified as a teaching hospital for the purpose of this research. Eleven units, seven Dis-trict General and four teaching hospitals, all situated in London and Hertfordshire, reporting 35 367 cases for the year 1998, were therefore included in the study. Only the cases of nulliparous Caucasian women (4909 deliveries) who could be identified as suitable for midwifery-led care were used because the standardised scenario clearly identified a nulliparous woman suitable for midwifery care.

Eight hundred and twenty-eight midwives identified by their manager as having cared for women during the intrapartum period in these 11 units during 1998 were sent a personally addressed envelope at work, including an information sheet, the questionnaire and a self-addressed return envelope. The information sheet informed the potential respondents that answering the questionnaire was entirely voluntary and anonymous, and completion of the questionnaire would imply consent to take part in the study.

Despite MREC and LREC approval, further demands were made by different midwifery managers. In some units no record of the names of the midwives was allowed because this was perceived to be the only way to protect the anonymity of the respondents. Unfortunately this also meant that no reminders could be sent to individuals. The absence of funding also meant that self-addressed stamped envelopes could not be provided.

Findings

Two hundred and forty-nine midwives returned their questionnaire, a response rate of 30.1%, ranging in the units from 10% to 55%. The response rate was highest in the five units linked to the midwifery education department for the clinical experience of student midwives. The number of respondents varied between six and 37, median 23, per unit. One hundred and thirty-seven midwives (55%) worked in the five 'lower intrapartum intervention' units and 112 (45%) in the six 'higher intrapartum intervention' units. The majority of the midwives qualified at certificate level (154/224 – 69%), 20% (45/224) at diploma level and 10% (25/224) at degree level; the differences between 'lower intrapartum intervention' and 'higher intrapartum intervention' units were not significant ($\kappa^2 = 5.552$; df = 2, $p = 0.062$). The present educational level was higher, but not significantly so, in 'higher intrapartum intervention' units, with only 32% (31/97) of midwives still at certificate level compared to 50% (57/115) in 'lower intrapartum intervention' units, and 35% (34/97) of midwives at degree level, compared to 21% (24/115) in 'lower intrapartum intervention' units ($\kappa^2 = 7.996$; df = 2; $p = 0.018$).

There was no difference in the rate of day or night duty worked by midwives working in either type of units, but midwives in 'higher intrapartum intervention' units were more likely to work predominantly in hospital, rather than in both hospital and community, or predominantly in the community: 56 of 102 midwives (55%) in 'higher intrapartum intervention' units worked mostly in hospital compared to 56 of 103 (46%) in 'lower intrapartum intervention' units. Only 13 (13%) midwives in the 'higher

intrapartum intervention' units worked mostly in the community. This compared to 34 (28%) in the 'lower intrapartum intervention' units ($\kappa^2 = 7.448$; df = 2; $p = 0.024$). This increased rate of midwives working in hospital also meant that a higher proportion of midwives working in 'higher intrapartum intervention' units undertook more than 20, or more than 50 deliveries a year: 78 of the 103 midwives (76%) working in the 'higher intrapartum intervention' units versus 69 out of 125 (55%), and 40 out of 103 midwives (39%) working in 'higher intrapartum intervention' units versus 25 out of 125 (20.0%) respectively. These differences were significant ($\kappa^2 = 10.389$; df = 1; $p = 0.001$ and $\kappa^2 = 9.829$; df = 1; $p = 0.002$; respectively).

Only 24 (11%) midwives reported ever having been directly involved in obstetric litigation and only 43 (19%) midwives had ever attended a UKCC professional conduct committee hearing as an observer. The differences between the unit categories were not significant.

There were no significant differences in the length of time midwives had been qualified (13.02 versus 11.36 years – $F (1, 218) = 1.861$, $p = 0.174$) or the weekly contracted hours (30.07 versus 31.32 hours per week – $F (1, 212) = 0.159$, $p = 0.283$) but midwives in 'lower intrapartum intervention' units had been with their present employer for significantly longer than their counterparts in 'higher intrapartum intervention' units (10.33 years versus 7.85 years – $F (1, 216) = 16.985$, $p = 0.009$). However, an overall mean of nearly eight years with the present employer does suggest a certain degree of familiarity with the accepted practices of their unit.

These very summary findings identified that midwives in 'higher intrapartum intervention' units had achieved a slightly higher overall level of academic qualification, and were more likely to work mainly in hospital and undertake a greater annual number of deliveries.

Analysis of SMMIS data for 1998

At the end of 1999, the 1998 computerised data of the 11 maternity units were made available. The data were systematically reduced to retain only the data of Caucasian women suitable for midwifery-led care. This followed the practice adopted for the previous comparison of the intrapartum care of four neighbouring units (Mead et al., 2000). A total of 10 822 non-Caucasian women (31% of the initial total) were excluded. The following criteria of exclusion were applied: previous medical history, present pregnancy complications, gestational age below 37 or above 42 weeks, fetal abnormalities and stillbirths, grand multiparae, previous perinatal or neonatal mortality, presentations other than cephalic, elective caesarean sections and induction of labour. Only the cases of women 'booked' at the hospital they were intended to deliver at were kept in the analysis. These exclusion criteria meant that a further 14 658 (41%) women were removed on the basis that they may not have been suitable for midwifery-led care. Nine thousand, eight hundred and eighty-seven women, 60% of the Caucasian women, remained in the analysis at the end of the data reduction.

At various points during the data reduction, comparisons of the potential differences in the background of the women or in the management of specific conditions (breech, previous caesarean section, onset of labour and home births) were investigated. The data of the 9887, including 4909 nulliparous women suitable for midwifery-led care were then examined for differences in the rates of augmentation, use of electronic fetal monitoring and epidural analgesia, as well as methods of delivery.

Specific criteria were used for the development of separate primiparous and multiparous intrapartum scores (Mead and Kornbrot, 2004). The rate of each of the interventions was calculated for each of the 11 units and each unit was awarded a ranked score between 1 and 11 for each intervention, the lowest score indicating the lowest rate of intervention. The sum of these ranked scores was then calculated to achieve each unit's overall intrapartum scores, calculated separately for primiparae or multiparae. The two-tailed Pearson correlation coefficient of each unit's score of primi-and multiparae was significant ($r = 0:703$; $p = 0:016$), indicating a strong similarity between the intrapartum interventions for primiparae and multiparae in these 11 units. As the standardised scenarios involved primiparae, the score of the primiparae was used to explore the potential link between level of intrapartum intervention and midwives' perception of risk.

The ranked scores enabled units to be categorised as either 'lower intrapartum intervention' (five units) or 'higher intrapartum intervention' units (six units). The four teaching hospitals were identified as belonging to the 'higher intrapartum intervention' group. However one Teaching hospital had a lower overall score than two District General hospitals.

Midwives' perception of risk

The areas of interest for the admission procedure were general maternal observation, palpation, anticipated birth weight, possibility of fetal hypoxia and meconium stained liquor (see Table 2.4.1). Except for the difference in the perception of the risk of meconium stained liquor on admission (9.84% versus 13.55% – $F = 5.014$, df = 1,241, $p = 0:026$) there were no significant differences in the perception of risk by midwives from 'lower intrapartum intervention' and 'higher intrapartum intervention' units. Midwives' perception of the potential birth weight corresponded with reality. However, there were some notable differences. Only 1% of women were recorded on the

Table 2.4.1 Admission observations (%)

Questionnaire	SMMIS variable	SMMIS $n = 4909$	'Lower' $n = 137$	'Higher' $n = 112$
Temperature >37.5°C	Pyrexia	1	7	8
Pulse 60–100 bpm	N/A[a]		94	92
Diastolic <90 mmHg	N/A		87	86
Proteinuria	N/A		11	11
Ketonuria	N/A		17	15
Cephalic presentation[b]	Presentation at delivery	97	94	93
Breech presentation	Presentation at delivery	3	5	5
Transverse lie	None identified		1	2
Engaged head	N/A		82	80
Birth weight 3–4 kg	Birth weight	75	75	75
Birth weight <3 kg	Birth weight	14	15	15
Birth weight >4 kg	Birth weight	11	10	11
CTG – normal	N/A on admission		82	82
CTG – slightly abn.	N/A on admission		13	13
CTG – very abn.	N/A on admission		4	5
Meconium[c]	Mec. in labour	20	10	14

[a]N/A – not available

[b]Fetal presentation – SMMIS $n = 6274$ (data reduction at onset of labour stage for nulliparae)

[c]Level of significance between 'lower' and 'higher' intervention units – $p = 0.026$

database as having been pyrexial during the whole of labour, but midwives' perception of the probability of pyrexia varied between 7.41% and 8.49%. The proportion of breech presentation at term on the database was 2.8%, but midwives' perceived this to be either 4.84% or 5.37%. Information was not available on SMMIS for the quality of admission CTGs.

Where labour was identified as progressing without any intervention, the SMMIS data identified 95% of nulliparous women delivered within 12 hours, but midwives perceived this to be the case for 68% in 'lower intrapartum intervention' units and 63% in 'higher intrapartum intervention' units (Table 2.4.2). The differences between the 'higher intrapartum intervention' and the 'lower intrapartum intervention' units were not significant. There were no differences between the perception of the risk of intra-uterine fetal hypoxia. Midwives identified that 82% or 83% of women would not have had any fetal hypoxia in labour. That corresponded with a rate of 87% of nulliparous women who either had no CTG or had a CTG diagnosed as 'normal'. There were, therefore, no differences between units and between perception of risk and reality for fetal hypoxia during labour. The SMMIS data identified that 42% of these women had an epidural in the absence of any other intrapartum interventions. This compared with a perception of 46% and 61% between the 'lower intrapartum intervention' units and the 'higher intrapartum intervention' units. These differences were highly significant ($F\ 1,239 = 38.421$, $p < 0.001$). However, these differences also reflect the proportion of epidurals used for nulliparous women in the two categories of maternity units. In reality, 87% of the nulliparous women who progressed without intervention had a normal delivery. This compared to a perception of 72% and 65% between the different units, a significant difference between units ($F\ 1,234 = 13.365$, $p < 0.001$). The differences in the perception of operative vaginal deliveries were also significant between the units: 16.4% versus 22.3% ($F\ 1,234 = 20.252$, $p < 0.001$). This compared to an actual rate of 12%. The perception of the rate of caesarean sections did not differ between the two categories of units (12% versus 12%), but this was remarkably higher than the actual rate of 1% for nulliparous women in spontaneous labour who progressed without intervention (see Table 2.4.2).

Where the questions dealt with the situation 'labour progresses with an ARM', midwives again underestimated the proportion of nulliparous women who would deliver within 12 hours, 88% versus 76% and 68% respectively for 'lower intrapartum intervention' and 'higher intrapartum intervention' units (Table 2.4.3). The differences between the units were significant ($F\ 1,227 = 5.822$, $p = 0.017$). The differences in the proportion of normal CTG did not vary between the categories of units and

Table 2.4.2 Actual and perceived outcomes if labour progresses without intervention (%)

Questionnaires	SMMIS variable	SMMIS $n = 801$	'Lower' $n = 137$	'Higher' $n = 112$
Delivery <12 h	Length first stage	95	68	63
No hypoxia	CTG no/normal	87	82	82
Epidural*	Pain relief	42	46	61
Normal delivery*	Delivery	87	72	65
Forceps/ventouse	Delivery	12	16	22
Caesarean	Delivery	1	12	12

Level of significance between 'lower' and 'higher' intervention units:
*$p < 0.001$

Table 2.4.3 Actual and perceived outcomes if labour progresses with an ARM (%)

Questionnaires	SMMIS variable	SMMIS $n = 588$	'Lower' $n = 137$	'Higher' $n = 112$
Delivery <12 h*	Length first stage	88	76	68
No hypoxia	CTG no/normal	80	78	79
Epidural**	Pain relief	52	50	65
Normal delivery***	Delivery	84	71	64
Forceps/ventouse	Delivery	14	17	23
Caesarean	Delivery	2	12	13

Level of significance between 'lower' and 'higher' intervention units:
*$p = 0.017$
**$p = 0.001$
***$p = 0.035$

with reality. Just over half the women (52%) who had had an ARM also used an epidural, but there were differences in the perception of epidural use – 50% versus 66% in the different categories of units. These differences were significant ($F\ 1,232 = 33.588$, $p < 0.001$), but may again reflect practice in the different units. Eighty-three per cent of nulliparous women who had an ARM in the absence of other interventions had a normal delivery, but this rate was perceived to be significantly different in the two unit categories – 71% and 64% ($F\ 1,231 = 16.148$, $p < 0.001$). Similar levels of differences were found when looking at the risk of operative vaginal delivery – 17% versus 23% ($F\ 1,231 = 25.072$, $p < 0.001$), but the differences in the risk perception for caesarean section were not significant. However, the actual caesarean section rate was 2%, but estimated to be 12% and 13% in the 'lower intrapartum intervention' and the 'higher intrapartum intervention' units respectively (see Table 2.4.3).

Where the situation was 'labour progresses with an epidural', there were no significant differences in the midwives' perception of risk for the length of labour, fetal hypoxia or caesarean section between 'lower intrapartum intervention' and 'higher intrapartum intervention' units

(Table 2.4.4). However, the differences between actual data and perception of risk were important. Seventy-one per cent of the nulliparous women who had had an epidural delivered within 12 hours, but midwives estimated this chance at 59% and 55% respectively. Midwives were also more optimistic about the rate of normal CTG – around 77% in both categories of units, compared to an actual rate of 63%. The perception of the delivery outcomes demonstrated differences between the units for normal deliveries (57% versus 51%, F 1,232 = 6.549, $p = 0:011$) and for operative vaginal deliveries (29% versus 34%, F 1,232 = 6.701, p = 0:010), but the midwives' perception for normal deliveries was substantially higher than reality since only 42% of nulliparous women who were initially suitable for midwifery-led care had a normal delivery when an epidural was used (see Table 2.4.4).

Discussion and conclusions

The aim of this study was to identify whether there were differences in perception of risk between midwives working in 'lower intrapartum intervention' and 'higher intrapartum intervention' units (Mead and Kornbrot, 2004), and whether these risk perceptions matched reality. An initial study of actual intrapartum interventions and outcomes for 4909 nulliparous women suitable for midwifery-led care enabled the categorisation of the units involved into the two intervention categories, and the subsequent comparisons of risk perception according to unit categorisation.

The management and organisation of the midwives' survey used to test the hypothesis linking intervention rates and risk perception was complex, partially because of the complexities of MREC and LREC submissions (Lux et al., 2000; Tully et al., 2000), but also because of further requests made by managers who wanted added assurance that the anonymity of the midwives would be guaranteed. The absence of funding further complicated

the task. These difficulties and the complexities of the questionnaire may account for the poor response rate. However, a total of 249 midwives responded and this number allowed the comparison of risk perception between midwives working in 'higher intrapartum intervention' and 'lower intrapartum intervention' units.

The analysis of the scenarios supported the initial hypothesis that midwives from 'lower' intervention units have a lower perception of risk than midwives working in 'higher' intervention units, but only for some aspects of intrapartum care: length of the first stage of labour, use of epidural analgesia, normal delivery. However, midwives generally underestimated the ability of women to deliver within 12 hours, irrespective of their unit's intrapartum intervention score category. In the clinical situations 'no intervention' or 'ARM', midwives overestimated the risk of abnormal deliveries, but their appreciation of the risk of fetal hypoxia did not deviate significantly from the reality (see Tables 2.4.2 and 2.4.3). However, in the clinical situation 'epidural', midwives strongly underestimated the level of fetal hypoxia and the associated rise in abnormal deliveries (see Table 2.4.4).

This study clearly showed that there was a relationship between practice and midwives' perception of risk. Midwives working in 'higher intrapartum intervention' units generally had a higher perception of risk than their colleagues working in lower intervention units. However, irrespective of these differences, midwives generally underestimated the ability of women suitable for midwifery-led care to progress normally from spontaneous labour to delivery. Midwives generally overestimated the advantages of interventions such as epidural analgesia.

The aim of this study was to examine midwives' perception of risk given some specific and common intrapartum situations rather than the actual interaction between midwives and women suitable for midwifery-led care. Questions have been raised about the limitations of alternative methods of investigation that provide only a limited reflection of the reality compared to the real world in which events happen and are not controlled by either a laboratory environment or conveniently neat questions (Fischhoff, 1996). The approach used in this study was justified on several counts. Firstly, the use of standardised scenarios enabled the control of potential extraneous variables that would have been inherent to the examination of real-life situations. Secondly, the survey enabled the recruitment of a larger number of midwives than would have been possible in an observational study, and this enabled the statistical comparison of midwives working in units classified as either 'lower' or 'higher' intervention maternity units. Thirdly, although the use of secondary and retrospective data forced the reliance on a previously defined database program and prevented the collection of information that may have been useful to

Table 2.4.4 Actual and perceived outcomes if labour progresses with an epidural (%)

Questionnaires	SMMIS variable	SMMIS $n = 2171$	'Lower' $n = 137$	'Higher' $n = 112$
Delivery <12 h	Length first stage	71	59	54
No hypoxia	CTG no/normal	63	78	77
Normal delivery*	Delivery	42	57	51
Forceps/ventouse**	Delivery	38	29	34
Caesarean	Delivery	20	14	15

Level of significance between 'lower' and 'higher' intervention units:

*$p = 0.011$

**$p = 0.01$

assess the underlying reported reasons for interventions, e.g. augmentation of labour or emergency caesarean section, the SMMIS database had previously been assessed as reliable (Cleary et al., 1994) and the availability of large databases enabled the comparison of the intrapartum practice available for women suitable for midwifery-led care in several units. The overall degree of control fell short of what would be expected in experimental studies, but this retrospective approach did have the major advantage of not having any influence on the intrapartum treatment of the women suitable for midwifery-led care.

The findings suggest that midwives' perception of risk are strongly influenced by the environment in which they work. Another part of the research which included this study examined the midwives' perception of their own and their colleagues' intrapartum practice using the same standardised scenario (Mead, 2003). This revealed marked variations in practice between units, but also demonstrated some potential discomfort in midwives' practice because they generally reported their practice to be more evidence based than that of their colleagues. This was also true when midwives were asked what their unit policy would recommend. The rate of practices that midwives would opt for was often different than the rate of policies identified as recommended by their unit policies (Mead, 2003). This would suggest that implicit or explicit clinical guidelines or philosophies may exercise an influence on practice, but may also act as a deterrent for the development of new forms of practice based on evidence (Kirkham and Stapleton, 2000).

The findings also suggest that although the perception of risk is higher in higher intervention units, the level of error of perception is important and this may affect the intrapartum care and interventions midwives advise as adequate for women suitable for midwifery-led care. On the other hand, the information available to midwives to answer the questions dealing with common clinical situations suggests that more information ought to be extracted from routinely collected computerised maternity data to enable midwives to calculate specific probabilities of events. Annual reports, though useful, tend to project overall information rather than details of the outcomes of pregnancies suitable for midwifery-led care (Harris and Chapple, 1998, 2000). The information that could be systematically gathered from the analysis of the computerised data relating to the intrapartum care of women suitable for midwifery-led care could help provide a more comprehensive account of events during the intrapartum period and the outcomes that could be expected.

If midwives' perception of risk is at odds with reality, irrespective of the level of intrapartum intervention, it is likely that the information provided to women will be biased towards labour being presented as more risky than it actually is. This may in turn lead women to adopt attitudes towards labour that favour a more, rather than a less interventionist approach.

Reports such as the confidential enquiries into maternal deaths (Department of Health et al., 1991; Department of Health, 1994, 1996, 1998) or perinatal mortality (Confidential Enquiry into Stillbirths and Deaths in Infancy, 1997, 1998, 1999, 2000), together with regular units' perinatal mortality or morbidity meetings may also encourage an abnormally high perception of risk.

The findings of this study suggest that further research involving a systematic approach aimed at reducing the degree of erroneous risk perception by midwives may be helpful if a lower degree of intrapartum intervention, and a corresponding higher rate of normal intrapartum outcomes, are to be achieved. It would also be useful to know if medical practitioners, GPs as well as obstetricians, have similar misperceptions of intrapartum risks for women suitable for midwifery-led care. Should these findings be confirmed for other health professionals, approaches could be devised to improve the quality of risk assessment and in turn the provision of intrapartum care more suited to individual women's needs. This may in turn be instrumental in reducing the rate of unnecessary routine intrapartum interventions and their potential consequences.

Acknowledgements

This study was undertaken as part of a PhD programme of work.

REFERENCES

Chamberlain, G., Wraight, A., Steer, P., 1993. Pain and its Relief in Childbirth – The Results of a National Survey Conducted by the National Birthday Trust. Churchill Livingstone, London.

Cleary, R., Beard, R., Coles, J., et al., 1994. The quality of routinely collected maternity data. British Journal of Obstetrics and Gynaecology 101 (12), 1042–1047.

Confidential Enquiry into Stillbirths and Deaths in Infancy, 1997. 4th Annual Report, Maternal and Child Health Research Consortium, London.

Confidential Enquiry into Stillbirths and Deaths in Infancy, 1998. 5th Annual Report, Maternal and Child Health Research Consortium, London.

Confidential Enquiry into Stillbirths and Deaths in Infancy, 1999. 6th Annual Report, Maternal and Child Health Research Consortium, London.

Confidential Enquiry into Stillbirths and Deaths in Infancy, 2000. 7th Annual Report, Maternal and Child Health Research Consortium, London.

Department of Health, 1993. Changing childbirth: report of the expert maternity group. HMSO, London.

Department of Health, 1994. Report on confidential enquiries into maternal deaths in the United Kingdom 1988–1990. HMSO, London.

Department of Health, 1996. Report on confidential enquiries into maternal deaths in the United Kingdom 1991–1993. HMSO, London.

Department of Health, 1998. Report on confidential enquiries into maternal deaths in the United Kingdom 1994–1996. HMSO, London.

Department of Health, Welsh Office, Scottish Home and Health Department et al., 1991. Report on Confidential Enquiries into Maternal Deaths in the United Kingdom 1985–1987. HMSO, London.

Doherty, G., Krebs, M., 1997. Do subjects understand base rates? Organizational Behavior and Human Decision Processes 72 (1), 25–61.

Edozien, L., 1999. What do maternity statistics tell us about induction of labour? Journal of Obstetrics and Gynaecology 19 (4), 343–344.

Ermenc, B., 1999. Discrepancies between clinical and postmortem diagnoses of causes of death. Medicine, Science and the Law 39 (4), 287–292.

Fischhoff, B., 1996. The real world: what good is it? Organizational Behaviour and Human Decision Processes 65 (3), 232–238.

Goddard, R., 2001. Electronic fetal monitoring. Is not necessary for low risk labours. British Medical Journal 322 (7300), 1436–1437.

Goffinet, F., Fraser, W., Marcoux, S., et al., 1997. Early amniotomy increases the frequency of fetal heart rate abnormalities. British Journal of Obstetrics and Gynaecology 104 (5), 548–553.

Government Statistical Service, 2002. NHS Maternity statistics, England: 1998–99 to 2000–01, Bulletin 2002/11, London.

Harris, J., Chapple, J., 1998. SMMIS in North Thames (West) F Annual Maternity Figures 1996. Department of Epidemiology and Public Health, Imperial College School of Medicine, London.

Harris, J., Chapple, J., 2000. SMMIS in North Thames (West) F Annual Maternity Figures 1998. Department of Epidemiology and Public Health, Imperial College School of Medicine, London.

Howell, C., 2000. Epidural versus non-epidural analgesia for pain relief in labour (CochraneReview). Update Software, Oxford.

Hurwitz, B., 1999. Legal and political considerations of clinical practice guidelines. British Medical Journal 318 (7184), 661–664.

Johnson, R., McCaul, K., Klein, W., 2002. Risk involvement and risk perception among adolescents and young adults. Journal of Behavioral Medicine 25 (1), 67–82.

Kirkham, M., Stapleton, H., 2000. Midwives' support needs as childbirth changes. Journal of Advanced Nursing 32 (2), 465–472.

Kleiter, G., Krebs, M., Doherty, M., et al., 1997. Do subjects understand base rates? Organizational Behavior and Human Decision Processes 72 (1), 25–61.

Lieberman, E., Lang, J., Frigoletto, F., et al., 1999. Epidurals and cesareans: the jury is still out. Birth 26 (3), 196–198.

Lux, A., Edwards, S., Osborne, J., 2000. Responses of local research ethics committees to a study with approval from a multi-centre ethics committee. British Medical Journal 320 (7243), 1282–1283.

Macchi, L., Osherson, D., Krantz, D., 1999. A note on super-additive probability judgment. Psychological Review 106 (1), 210–214.

Macfarlane, A., Mugford, M., 2000. Birth Counts, Statistics of Pregnancy & Childbirth, Vol. 2 – Tables. The Stationary Office, London.

Martin, C., 1998. Electronic fetal monitoring: a brief summary of its development, problems and prospects. European Journal of Obstetrics & Gynecology and Reproductive Biology 78 (2), 133–140.

Mead, M., 2003. Intrapartum care of women suitable for midwifery led care–midwives' perception of their own and their colleagues' practice. Evidence-based Midwifery 1 (1), 4–11.

Mead, M., Kornbrot, D., 2004. An intrapartum intervention scoring system for the comparison of maternity units' intrapartum care of nulliparous women suitable for midwifery-led care. Midwifery 20 (1), 15–26.

Mead, M., O'Connor, R., Kornbrot, D., 2000. A comparison of intrapartum care in four maternity units. British Journal of Midwifery 8 (11), 709–715.

Ministry of Health, 1959. Report of the Maternity Services Committee (Chairman Lord Cranbrook). HMSO, London.

Ministry of Health CCG, 1956. Report of the Committee of Enquiry into the Cost of the National Health Service. HMSO, London.

National Institute for Clinical Excellence, 1999. A Guide to Our Work. NICE, London.

Nozton, F., Cnattingius, S., Bergsjo, P., et al., 1994. Cesarean section delivery in the 1980s: international comparison by indication. American Journal of Obstetrics and Gynecology 170 (2), 495–504.

Penn, Z., Ghaem-Maghami, S., 2001. Indications for caesarean sections. Best practice & research. Clinical Obstetrics and Gynaecology 15 (1), 1–15.

Rayburn, W., Zhang, J., 2002. Rising rates of labor induction: present concerns and future strategies. Obstetrics & Gynecology 100 (1), 164–167.

Slovic, P., Fishhoff, B., Lichtenstein, S., 1982. Facts versus fears: understanding perceived risk. In: Tversky, A. (Ed.), Judgment Under Uncertainty: Heuristics and Biases. Cambridge University Press, Cambridge.

Standing Maternity and Midwifery Advisory Committee (Chairman J. Peel), 1970. Domiciliary Midwifery and Maternity Bed Needs. HMSO, London.

Symon, A., 1998. Litigation: The Views of Midwives and Obstetricians. Hochland & Hochland Ltd, Hale, Cheshire.

Symon, A., 2000a. Litigation and defensive clinical practice: quantifying the problem. Midwifery 16 (1), 8–14.

Symon, A., 2000b. Litigation and changes in professional behaviour: qualifying the problem. Midwifery 16 (1), 15–21.

Tew, M., 1995. Safer Childbirth? A Critical History of Maternity Care. Chapman & Hall, London.

Thorp, J., Parisi, V., Boylan, P., et al., 1989. The effect of continuous epidural analgesia on cesarean section for dystocia in nulliparous women. American Journal of Obstetrics and Gynecology 161 (3), 670–675.

Tully, J., Ninnis, N., Booy, R., et al., 2000. The new system of review by multi-centre research ethics committees: prospective study. British Medical Journal 320 (7243), 1279–1282.

Tversky, A., Koehler, D., 1994. Support theory: a nonextensional representation of subjective probability. Psychological Review 101 (4), 547–567.

Wagman, H., 1991. Obstetric practice and fear of litigation – letter. The Lancet 338 (8773), 1019.

Williams, F., du V Florey, C., Ogston, S., et al., 1998. UK study of intrapartum care for low risk primigravidas: a survey of interventions. Journal of Epidemiology and Community Health 52 (8), 494–500.

Windschitl, P., 2002. Judging the accuracy of a likelihood judgment: the case of smoking risk. Journal of Behavioral Medicine 15 (1), 19–35.

WHO (World Health Organization), 1996. Care in Normal Birth: A Practical Guide. WHO, Geneva.

Young, D., 1999. Whither cesareans in the new millenium? Birth 26 (2), 67–70.

Birth centres: a success story

Denis Walsh

Introduction

Stephen Ladyman, until last month the Parliamentary Under Secretary of State for the Community, wrote recently that the National Service Framework (NSF) for Children, Young People and Maternity Services encompassed 'local options for midwife-led care including midwife-led units in the community or on a hospital site' (Ladyman 2005: 68). By so doing, he opened up the possibility of the expansion of free-standing birth centres (FSBCs): there are more than 60 in England, and an increasing number in Wales and Scotland. FSBCs are becoming a serious alternative to large hospital provision, and their re-emergence as a model of care has sparked a lot of interest in their evidence base.

In this article I want to discuss some of that evidence, in particular the findings from ethnography of an FSBC in the Midlands (Walsh 2004). Rather than detailing these findings, I will draw out some of the critical success factors from the narrative of the centre over the past 15 years. These may hold some relevance for other birth centres, both free-standing and integrated, and even larger maternity units.

Setting and method

The birth centre studied was in the Midlands, and catered for around 300 women a year. It was sited within a small district hospital, with the nearest consultant maternity unit 15 miles away. The centre was staffed by midwives and maternity care assistants (MCAs) who provided a 24-hour service. There were three birth rooms and capacity for five postnatal women.

The aim of the study was to explore the culture, beliefs, values, customs and practices around the birth process. After gaining ethics approval for the study, participant observation was undertaken over a nine-month period and included all hours of the day and all days of the week.

In addition, an opportunistic sample of 30 women were interviewed approximately three months after giving birth at the centre. A purposive sample of 10 midwives and five MCAs (midwifery care assistants), representing a breadth of clinical experience, were also interviewed.

Critical success factor 1: empowerment through struggle

It seems that most FSBCs have a history of struggle related to recurrent threat of closure. This is in itself interesting because no such pressure appears to be paralleled in large maternity units, which seem more likely to be expanded than retracted. It probably tells us something about the respective power of each. Large facilities are 'a given', and have a kind of self-validating dynamic, underpinned by professional power and the technocratic birth model (Davis-Floyd 2001). Small birth centres are vulnerable to the centralising tendency of health care services and to the relative lack of clout of birth centre stakeholders, commonly midwives, service users and some general practitioners. When they succeed in overturning bureaucratic and professional power, their victories are especially noteworthy.

The birth centre staff in this study, along with many others, achieved this end through their commitment to the cause and their skilful managing of the anti-closure campaign, something they grew into as the months passed. In the end they were astute managers of the local media, using radio and television to support their cause. They were already adept fundraisers, conducting an ongoing programme throughout the year, and used the money in this case to support their campaign.

Networking with women users and with local and national politicians had become second nature to them, but most striking was their self-belief and confidence. 'We were in their faces [health service bureaucrats] all the time,' commented one of the midwives. Notably absent from their actions were the 'doing good by stealth' and passive aggression tactics that Kirkham (1999) observed in midwives in her midwifery supervision study.

This sense of empowerment is beautifully captured in the following extract from a staff interview, undertaken after they had secured the future of the birth centre:

I really wouldn't mind having a go at anything. That's not how I was a few years ago! But now it's another dimension! We've really grown here. I feel much more responsible. I don't want to sound arrogant, but I am important, I am doing things, I am making a difference. I go home and I'm thinking about what we can do, where we can go . . . (Midwife, Transcript No. 38, p13)

There is no doubt that fighting a successful campaign can politicise birth centre staff in ways that are rarely seen in acute maternity care settings, so that they become powerful advocates for the birth centre model. In this study, the staff forged strong alliances with women users, and were not intimidated by medical and bureaucratic power. Of course, some birth centre struggles are lost, and the risk of that is always in the background. When they succeed, however, their flow-on effects not only secure the future of the model but have a profound impact on the ethos and operation of the birth centre, as the following discussion outlines.

In this sense, the experience of struggle, though challenging and demanding for those involved, can have positive effects on the solidarity and empowerment of birth centre staff and women users. For the birth centre stakeholders, it has cemented a belief in the sustainability and longevity of the model. In addition, it provides something else of immense value, for their story is much more than an isolated, one-off occurrence, successful only because of the unique context. It happened to real midwives in a setting that was once a traditional general practitioner unit and was turned around to become a contemporary birth centre. It is, therefore, a source of inspiration and encouragement to anyone who has dreamed of more humane maternity care.

Critical success factor 2: autonomy and self-regulation

Another striking feature of the birth centre study was the independence of its internal operation and hands-off attitude of the external community manager. She trusted the staff to self-manage and self-regulate. The clinical leader, based on site, espoused a consultative and enabling leadership ethic that resulted in all staff assuming accountability and ownership for the birth centre. This was evident from the remarkable attention to birth environment and decor. The staff were constantly making-over the interior to hone its ambience for optimum birthing. Much of this work was done very pragmatically, eschewing bureaucratic and institutional mechanisms so that processes resembled how one might approach home decorating.

Another amusing anecdote captured the sense of this. A woman and her partner were visiting the birth centre with a view to booking to have their baby there. An MCA was explaining to them how the staff had raised all this money and decorated the rooms themselves. In fact, one of the staff was painting a ceiling as the couple walked around. She was wearing an old pair of knickers on her head to protect her hair!

After a while, the partner said, 'I don't think you should tell me how you beat the system to get all this done because I'm the Chief Executive of the Trust that owns this building. I've heard about what you have achieved here!' Before they left, the couple donated some money to the trust fund.

Clinical governance and risk management have ushered in an era of intense monitoring in the NHS (Walsh 2003). Extensive organisational standards and clinical guidelines now dominate service provision, and this is denounced by some authors as an oppressive 'evaluation imperative' that is as much about control, regulation and avoidance of litigation as it is to do with best practice and evidence-based care (Strathern 2000). The birth centre presents a counter-balance to these trends by trusting the local staff to self-manage and self-regulate. Their commitment to and ownership of the facility drives them to pursue excellence, and mimics what Brown and Crawford (2003) found in autonomous, community-based mental health teams – a 'clinical governance of the soul'. This is an internal and shared dynamic that motivates the staff to put the women before organisational need. It is ethically and value rooted, a self-imposed discipline to offer optimum care, facilitated by sleek organisational processes. It changes the low-trust/high-control approach typical of bureaucracies to high trust/low control.

The critical success factors here were the marrying of power devolution with enabling leadership and non-bureaucratic, non-institutional ways of working. This cocktail of ingredients has real possibilities for application in other birth settings.

Critical success factor 3: building community and social capital

A sense of fulfilment and enjoyment was palpable among birth centre staff. The very first staff interview revealed this in a startling response to the question: what's it like working here?

Working is like having your favourite chocolate bar. You really want it, you get to have it and you still want some more. It's lovely. (Midwife, Transcript No. 31, p1)

This contentment was articulated many times in subsequent interviews, and over time a number of factors emerged that clearly contributed to it.

Ninety per cent of the staff were part time, and were very willing to be flexible about working patterns. These were deregulated, both in planned off-duty (a variety of shift patterns to suit individual staff needs) and in unplanned day-to-day flexibility where the demands of home and family life were clearly valued. Reciprocal covering of the beginning and end of shifts in response to need was endemic and worked extremely well in addressing work/life balance issues. This extended to reciprocal childcare arrangements and a blurring of work/home boundaries that was as refreshing as it was unusual in my experience. The following story was related to me by one of the MCAs:

> The very young children of one of the midwives found it hard to settle at night if their mother was on a late shift. Her husband used to bring them into the unit around seven and she would go through a bed-time routine with them before he would return them home. (Field note, No. 9, p4)

A staff social life away from work was well established. Monthly outings were regular throughout the year, with all the staff getting to some of them. These served as 'destressers' for work, and cemented relationships among staff – so much so that the pattern continued after staff retired. They also contributed towards their collective memory, and photograph albums in the centre recalled these occasions. Support through personal crises was another marker of the communitarian ethos, prompting one of the staff to comment at the end of an interview: 'I love this place. It has been really good to me.'

In capturing the essence of these dimensions of birth centre life, the theory of social capital seems to fit well. Social capital is about the networks, relationships, values and informal sanctions that shape social interactions in different settings. Markers of social capital include participation, volunteerism, non-reciprocal giving and trust, all manifest in the life of the birth centre (Aldridge et al 2002).

High levels of social capital are said to contribute to individual and collective wellbeing, and those settings that exhibit it are sought after by Western governments wanting to realise its value (Portes 1998). The significance of social capital to the health service is certain to increase. At the birth centre, it has clearly contributed to staff fulfilment and therefore will impact on staff recruitment and retention and probably even on sick leave levels.

Conclusion

The selection of these critical success factors is not exhaustive, and represents my reading and interpretation of this ethnographic study. Others may see different subtleties at work, equally explanatory of this remarkable birth setting. I have written a lot more elsewhere about some of the fruits of these effects in relation to the distinguishing features of labour and postnatal care (Walsh 2005a), the altered sense of time/temporality (Walsh 2005b), the rejection of the assembly-line motif for labour care (Walsh 2005c) and the challenging intersection of risk and normality in this context (Walsh 2005d).

Modelling the best of birth centres' ways of doing and being is an effective way of learning for similar settings. There is an accruing bank of knowledge out there now as birth centres traverse various stages in their life cycle. They are still a relatively new model in their present incarnation, though surely the lessons of success are as old as midwifery itself. I would like to be bold and suggest that birth centres can inform acute obstetrics in modelling a compassionate and humane service that always privileges relationships over technocracy and organisational need.

REFERENCES

Aldridge S, Halpern D and Fitzpatrick S (2002). Social Capital: a Discussion Paper, London: Performance and Innovation Unit.
Brown B and Crawford P (2003). 'The clinical governance of the soul: "deep management" and the self-regulating subject in integrated community mental health teams'. Social Science & Medicine, 56: 67–81.
Davis-Floyd R (2001). 'The technocratic, humanistic and holistic paradigms of childbirth'. International Journal of Gynaecology & Obstetrics, 75: S5–S23.
Kirkham M (1999). 'The culture of midwifery in the National Health Service in England'. Journal of Advanced Nursing, 30: 732–739.
Ladyman S (2005). 'Improving postnatal care for every woman'. Editorial. British Journal of Midwifery, 13 (2): 68–69.
Portes A (1998). 'Social capital: its origins and application in modern sociology'. Annual Review of Sociology, 24, 1–24.
Strathern M (2000). 'The tyranny of transparency'. British Educational Research Journal, 26 (3): 309–321.

Walsh D (2003). 'The risk discourse and its effects on maternity care'. Health Care Risk Report, 9 (10): 11–13.
Walsh D (2004). 'Becoming Mother': an Ethnography of a Free-Standing Birth Centre, unpublished PhD thesis, University of Central Lancashire.
Walsh D (2005a). ' "Nesting" and "matrescence": distinctive features of a free-standing birth centre'. Submitted to Social Science & Medicine, March 2005.
Walsh D (2005b). 'Temporality in a birth centre', C McCourt (ed), Childbirth, Midwifery and Concepts of Time, awaiting publication.
Walsh D (2005c). 'Subverting assembly-line birth: childbirth in a free-standing birth centre'. Submitted to Social Science & Medicine, March 2005.
Walsh D (2005d). 'Risk and normality in maternity care'. In: A Symon (ed), Risk and Choice in Childbirth, awaiting publication.

Defining and developing the birth centre

Mary Stewart

The recent publication of the National Service Framework (NSF) for Children, Young People and Maternity Services (Department of Health 2004) stated that maternity care providers should ensure that women have the option of giving birth in a midwife-led unit. This seems like a ringing endorsement of birth centres, but what exactly are we talking about when we use that term? It seems such a straightforward question, but the truth, in fact, is rather more complicated. I was recently involved in a structured review into birth centre outcomes (Stewart et al 2004). The process of review was fascinating and educational on several levels, and I thought it would be helpful to summarise the recommendations that we made as a result.

Definitions

Our key recommendation was that a standard baseline definition of the term 'birth centre' needs to be developed and implemented. Arguing over terminology can seem to be a case of splitting hairs, but in the case of birth centres it really is fundamentally important that this definition is agreed and used. Having such a definition is really important because it would make it more possible to understand what's happening, so that you can make a fair comparison of centres that are like each other rather than lumping disparate birth locations together. When we looked at the research around birth centres we found that definitions differ quite markedly.

It became clear to us when we wanted to find out what evidence there was around outcomes for women who had planned to give birth in a birth centre and outcomes for their babies that definitions differ quite markedly. Even the use of terminology such as 'freestanding' or 'alongside' can become complicated. For example, if a birth centre is on the same geographic site as an obstetric unit, but is in a separate building, should it be referred to as alongside or freestanding? When assessing the research

evidence, is it possible to compare the findings from a unit that is two miles from the nearest obstetric unit, with one where the distance is 30 miles or more?

Until we get to grips with these difficulties, it is impossible to make any real sense of the large amounts of data that have been gathered in different birth centres around the UK. Without wishing to be facetious, I have even begun to wonder whether there is a need to copyright the term, in order to protect its meaning. I have recently seen advertisements in the midwifery press that refer to the labour ward in an obstetric unit as a birth centre, which seems to make a mockery of everything that birth centres should represent. As Sara Wickham (2003: 23) pointed out a couple of years ago 'it depends on whether one sees "birth center" as simply another term for a place where babies are born, or as a concept which is intensely political, grounded in the normalcy of birth and autonomous midwifery and needing careful valuing by those who value this.'

Options

The birth centre review suggested that women who use birth centres are more likely to be Caucasian, and better educated than women who give birth in hospital. This was not a surprising finding and seems be a variant of the inverse care law, first described by Julian Tudor Hart (1971) who argued that the people who need most often get the least. Although the finding is not surprising, there is little evidence available to explain why this is so, and this led us to make our second recommendation, that further research is needed to evaluate what influences women in making decisions about where to have their babies. If women are making active, informed choices to give birth in hospital, then we need to respect and support that choice. However, research done by Madi and Crow (2003), which focused on home birth, points to the influence of the midwife. Their work indicates that some midwives seem to offer women the whole range of choices of place of birth, whereas other midwives withhold information, and do not suggest any alternative to birth in hospital.

Outcomes

A recent and welcome debate in midwifery, led in particular by Soo Downe (Downe 2004) and the Royal College of Midwives (RCM 2004) has been around the promotion and protection of normal birth. It would be nice to assume that birth centres increase the likelihood of normal birth but, as with all assumptions, such a belief may be misplaced. Our review showed that, at the moment, there is no reliable evidence to demonstrate that birth centres are sure to improve outcomes for women or their babies, nor that there is reliable evidence that birth centres cause harm. However, this lack of certainty about the direction of effect should not be interpreted as meaning that we don't need to put effort into asking important questions about safety and effectiveness. It is clear that the current evidence base comes from research of relatively low quality, carried out using a range of methods and definitions. This makes it inappropriate to pool results and compare findings.

Most of the research we reviewed included outcomes for type of birth, eg, spontaneous, instrumental or caesarean section, and the findings suggest that women who plan to have their baby in a birth centre seem more likely to have a spontaneous vaginal birth. However, there is a need for more robust evidence to demonstrate whether or not this is really the case. I was also surprised and disappointed to find that only two of the papers we reviewed included data on breastfeeding rates among women who give birth in a birth centre. So, our third recommendation was that a large-scale randomised controlled trial is needed to evaluate a range of outcomes for women who plan to give birth in a birth centre, including rate of spontaneous vaginal birth, and infant feeding.

It is important to know the outcomes such as mode of birth for women who have their baby in a birth centre. It is just as important to evaluate the much rarer maternal and neonatal outcomes of mortality and major morbidity. We found few studies which considered these important but infrequent outcomes. Several of the papers had gathered data over a long period of time. Indeed, one (Moster et al 2001) had collected data over a 29-year period. While such studies provide useful information it is hard to draw firm conclusions as clinical practice will have changed over time, and it is hard to know what effect this may have had on the findings. We recommended that a standard system of data collection should be developed in NHS trusts to record and evaluate these rare outcomes, in order to compare findings in a meaningful way. It would also be possible to do this on an international level

so that findings could also be compared among different developed countries. Such systems of data collection would, in turn, help women to make fully informed choices about where they wish to have their baby.

Concepts of care

The previous two recommendations focus on physical outcomes for women and their babies, and these are hugely important. However, it is just as important to know how women feel about the care they receive. Our review showed, perhaps unsurprisingly, that women who gave birth in a birth centre were generally highly satisfied with the care they received and commented on the respect, perceived control and support they experienced. However, the findings were not conclusive. There was also evidence from one study (Watts et al 2003) that women who have to be transferred from a birth centre to hospital during labour may find the experience very traumatic. It is impossible to know what these trends mean. We recommended that valid and reliable measures for evaluating data on psychosocial outcomes should be developed and implemented. These outcome measures could then be used to carry out a national survey to explore the psychosocial outcomes of women who use birth centres. We also recommended that such a national survey should include the in-depth experiences of women who need to be transferred from birth centre care.

Improving data collection

As part of the process of data collection for this review, I wrote to all heads of midwifery and supervisors of midwives in the UK, asking if they had any relevant information that may have been gathered in their Trust, including the results of locally published, unpublished or ongoing studies. We were grateful to colleagues who sent fascinating data that had been gathered from both freestanding and alongside birth centres. However, there was no consistency in the method of data collection, nor in the types of data that had been collected. This meant that it was impossible to compare results between Trusts. This felt like a missed opportunity and so our final recommendation was that a standardised system of data collection should be developed and implemented in order to record the reasons why women are transferred from birth centre care, and other outcomes such as levels of postpartum haemorrhage, Apgar scores and other measures of neonatal wellbeing.

Conclusion

Implementation of the NSF for children, young people and maternity services provides a wonderful opportunity for midwives to carry out research that explores outcomes for women and their babies who receive birth centre care. Every cell in my body tells me that birth centres can provide a space where normal birth is the norm and where midwifery care flourishes. I also know that in these days of limited resources this is not enough: passion and belief need to be supported by evidence. However, I feel excited by the opportunities we are being offered. I hope that when another review of birth centres is carried out in the future, the authors will be able to comment on a wide range of high quality research that clearly demonstrates how and why birth centres work. Women, their families and communities deserve our commitment to asking questions about such vital issues.

Acknowledgements

I am deeply grateful to Rona McCandlish for her patient guidance and support during the birth centre review. I also thank Peter Brocklehurst and Jane Henderson for their advice and contributions. Thanks, too, to Jane Sandall and Mary Newburn for their thoughtful and helpful comments.

REFERENCES

Department of Health (2004). National Service Framework for Children, Young People and Maternity Services, London: DH Publications.

Downe S (2004). Normal childbirth: Evidence and Debate, Edinburgh: Churchill Livingstone.

Hart JT (1971). 'The inverse care law'. Lancet, i: 405–412.

Madi BC and Crow R (2003). 'A qualitative study of information about available options for childbirth venue and pregnant women's preference for lace of delivery'. Midwifery, 19: 328–336.

Moster D, Terje L and Markestad T (2001). 'Neonatal mortality rates in communities with small maternity units compared with those having larger units'. British Journal of Obstetrics and Gynaecology, 108: 904–909.

Royal College of Midwives (2004). http://www.rcm.org.uk/data/info_centre/data/virtual_institute.htm

Stewart M, McCandlish R, Henderson J and Brocklehurst P (2004). Review of Evidence About Clinical, Psychosocial and Economic Outcomes for Women with Straightforward Pregnancies who Plan to Give Birth in a Midwife-led Birth Centre, and Outcomes for Their Babies, Oxford: National Perinatal Epidemiology Unit.

Watts K, Fraser DM and Munir F (2003). 'The impact of the establishment of a midwife managed unit on women in a rural setting in England'. Midwifery, 19: 106–112

Wickham S (2003). 'A compromise for change'. The Practising Midwife, 6 (11): 23.

Improving the birthing environment

Anne Haines, Linda Kimber

Part 1 comprises an article that describes how environmental changes in a busy consultant unit encouraged normal birth and Part 2 is an article that concludes this report.

PART 1

This article discusses the process of environmental changes within a consultant unit reinforced by the preparations to undertake a feasibility study. The environmental issues were an important facet of the study that aimed to explore the benefits of the Linda Kimber Massage Programme in pregnancy, labour and childbirth. This feasibility study was conducted in preparation for a pilot randomised controlled trial which began in December 2004.

The environmental changes supported women and their babies by normalising their birth experience and encouraged a continuation of the maternal-infant interactions following birth. Our experience is that this is possible within a busy consultant unit with a birth rate of 1,500 per year.

Background

During recent years, the use of pharmacological analgesia in labour has risen (ENB 1999), and there are concerns about the increase in epidural anaesthesia and obstetric interventions (Howell 2000).

With this in mind, it was decided to explore an existing massage programme in use on the unit to identify any trends that might reverse the process.

The feasibility study required cooperation and shared learning among the midwives, medical staff and the researchers, as well as required consistency with the environment in which women laboured and birthed their babies.

Part of the model of care for the study related to environmental issues and their importance in the promotion and support of the biological process of normal labour (McNabb 2003). The massage techniques were incorporated within this model (see Figure 2.7.1).

Regardless of birthing method, babies were greeted with immediate skin contact with their mother. The only time this was to be interrupted was if the baby required resuscitation or ongoing special care. With these principles in place, midwives were engaged and the process of discussion and eventual implementation began.

Implementation

The study acted as a catalyst and accelerator of these changes already identified as a need within the unit.

The main elements underpinning this model of care reflected the views of Anderson (2003) when she described the concept of 'normal birth' as:

- a physiological process
- non-intervention
- supportive environment
- empowerment.

The locale in which we were implementing this change was a busy consultant unit with much movement, chatter and clinical activity. Odent (2004: 19) warns, 'Don't stimulate the neocortex of a labouring woman.'

With this in mind, healthy debate and a pleasant working environment were encouraged. However, we discouraged the continuation of bustle and buzz within the birthing room. During labour, women are hypersensitive to disruption, disturbance and a sense of being observed, as it upsets the normal hormonal responses and can affect progress in labour (Odent 2004: 21). Dim lighting was introduced to help create a place of safety where the woman could 'let go' in birth, feeling secure and private (Norton 1998).

The massage techniques were taught to couples in preparation for childbirth: they were encouraged to

Figure 2.7.1 Model of care.

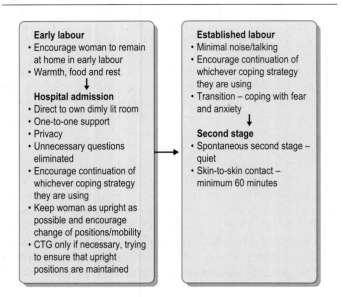

practise a method by which they could be still, calm and regain control between contractions, making the most of this well-earned break. This was taught under the umbrella of 'going to a safe place', and these words were reinforced by the midwife or partner if needed. This became an automatic response for the woman following each contraction. A deliberate effort was made to avoid unnecessary questions and to develop an observational method of care. Partners were made aware of the need for stillness and quiet in supporting the labour process.

We acknowledged when designing the model of care that women varied in their requirement for privacy. Naakteborgen (1989) discusses this need, likening it to other mammalian species. The analogies include species such as the domestic cat, which requires absolute solitude to birth its offspring, in contrast to elephants which birth protected by group members. Likewise, some women display a preference for solitude during labour, while others are happy to have helpers present (Buckley 2004).

Implementing this complex model within a consultant unit needed careful and diplomatic review by the multi-disciplinary team. This took time, but was integral to its success.

A series of regular meetings was held with the midwives and medical staff, not only to inform them of the study methodology but also of the required model of care needed to effect the environmental changes. The Linda Kimber Massage Programme and the biological process of labour and childbirth were reinforced.

This was a shift from the existing model familiar within this multi-disciplinary arena. Agreement was sought as

the model of care was reliant on the cooperation of all staff involved in the care of the women.

The methodology relied on the implementation of this model providing staff with a legitimate opportunity to use and assess it, supported by the researchers and their peer group.

Each element in the model of care was considered:

1. Warmth and privacy

The temperature within the room was regulated to the woman's requirements – this most often resulted in a warm environment in which the mother would feel safe and comfortable, removing her clothing if she wished. A quiet, calm atmosphere within the room was achieved to allow the woman to 'change her level of consciousness, reverting to the primitive brain which controls the instincts of birth' (Gaskin 2003: 241), and therefore complement the biological process of labour without distraction. Up-lighters were already in the birthing rooms to support dim lighting.

We improved the look of the rooms by adding duvets to the beds and curtains to screen off equipment such as lithotomy poles. Curtains also screened the doors, adding to the privacy. These were all simple, cost-effective initiatives. The 2003 NCT conference, 'Creating a Better Birth Environment', reiterated the importance of privacy and a homely, non-clinical room as factors that are more likely to improve normal birth.

2. Mobility and upright positions

The room needed reorganisation to encourage free movement and the use of alternative positions. The bed needed less focus within the room, increasing the floor space; floor mats, beanbags and balls were provided. Midwives assisted women and the birthing partners to alter the room to meet their individual needs. This encouraged familiarity with their surroundings and a sense of belonging within an institution. Page (1995) discusses the need to create an environment in which women feel comfortable to follow their instinct to move into the positions they prefer.

Given the choice, most women will adopt upright positions in labour to relieve painful contractions and assist their baby to assume optimal position for descent through the birth canal. Only recently has this regained importance, contradicting claims made by authors such as Silverton (1993) that 'most women prefer to remain semi-recumbent upon the delivery bed.' This claim is more likely to be as a result of professional choice than that of the woman.

Listening to and observing women in normal labour has helped this swing back to more traditional positions for childbirth.

Michel Odent (1994) suggests that it is during the second stage of labour that women become active and assume more upright positions – using more restful stances during the first stage of labour. It is clear from the literature that no one way is right for all, and the most effective way to support women is to facilitate their choices on an individual basis. Women are likely to be restless and change positions frequently during labour and need a variety of options available to them. Most commonly, left to their own instincts, women will adopt more traditional positions for childbirth such as all fours or squatting (Gaskin 2003: 228).

3. Communication

Communication among the professionals was essential throughout the change process. Once the rooms were reorganised and the environment made more conducive, the biological process of natural childbirth was considered in more detail. At this time we were extremely fortunate to have the knowledge and passion of Mary McNabb, a research midwife with an interest in neuro-endocrinology, who inspired the midwives with her explanation of the biological process of childbirth (McNabb 2004). Supported by research papers, this created an increased understanding of the processes and explained how midwives can support rather than potentially inhibit them. A challenging journey, but a general belief in the normality of childbirth began to return (Edwards 2003).

At times there was pressure from the medical staff to intervene during labour, some more proactively than others. The consultants leading the obstetric teams displayed a wide range of ways to manage different situations; some allowed more negotiation and individualised care than others. Some of the medical staff had difficulty adjusting their clinical practice when presented with women labouring in altered positions – for example, using mats and beanbags or birth balls. The response was variable; some cooperated fully and understood when the woman chose to remain on the mat for examinations, while others were worried by women naked in the rooms and were put off by the low lights. These individual responses could be explained by previous working experiences and possible cultural influences.

4. One-to-one support

Klaus et al (1986) discuss how constant human support can benefit women in labour and improve perinatal outcomes. In their study the support was provided by doulas – their constant presence was thought to reduce anxiety, thus enhancing the biological process of childbirth. In most cultures, normal birth practice would include the provision of continuous social support by women. This practice is often missing within Western cultures where women are more likely to birth their babies within large institutions and are often left alone for periods (Klaus et al 1986).

In an effort to enhance women's birth experiences, an important element of our model of care was that one-to-one support by the midwife should be considered normal practice. This not only supported the woman, but helped direct the birth partner into a more effective and supportive role.

The midwife's role was to observe the process and encourage and support, only intervening if needed. Staying in the room for periods formed part of the philosophy; the aim was to allow a non-invasive assessment of the woman's progress in labour without her feeling rushed or overly observed (Odent 2003: 21). The one-to-one support provided a coping strategy to allow couples to work effectively together, and have their needs identified and met.

5. Fetal heart monitoring

Mobility and upright positions, although limited, were encouraged and made possible even when continuous external fetal heart monitoring was indicated.

Women with a complex pregnancy will often require this type of monitoring during labour, whereas for those with straightforward pregnancies monitoring of the fetal heart can be kept to a minimum by intermittent auscultation.

Although continual use of technology in this way may be considered intrusive and an invasion of the woman's privacy in so much as she feels observed (Odent 2003: 21), a careful balance between maintaining a safe but non-controlling environment is desirable. Berg and Dahlberg (1998) report that women who experience obstetrically complicated childbirth will most often refer to the support and being recognised as a 'genuine participant' as far more significant than the length of their labour or the use of technical interventions.

Midwives helped the couples assume positions for labour, accommodating the monitoring equipment as discreetly as possible in order to support free movement. Some midwives perceived a lack of control of the labour process and preferred the woman in one place, often the bed. This attitude took time and support to overcome – help was needed to absorb this new initiative and soon fundraising was under way to obtain a mobile fetal telemetry system.

PART 2

The authors conclude their report on how 'normal' birth was encouraged in a busy consultant unit.

Second stage

Another important element of the model of care implemented during the study was to encourage spontaneous pushing rather than directed pushing during second stage.

Hansen et al (2002) conducted a randomised controlled trial (RCT) considering active management versus spontaneous second stage. They concluded that when passive descent of the presenting part was allowed to occur there were fewer fetal heart decelerations than when active pushing was commenced immediately at full dilatation.

Passive management of the second stage relies on maternal pulses of oxytocin and pressure of the presenting part on the pelvic floor, creating waves of involuntary expulsive behaviour from the woman (see Figure 2.7.2). This management allows for a latent phase in the second stage of labour followed by a shorter active phase, allowing rest and recovery both for the women and her baby prior to the birth itself. Women control their breathing throughout the contraction, improving fetal and maternal oxygenation. Studies have shown that the practice of breath-holding and sustained and directed pushing seems to compromise maternal-fetal gas exchange (Aldrich et al 1995, Thomson 1995).

During second stage and at the time of birth we continued to provide a quiet, calm and dimly lit environment. If an instrumental delivery was indicated, we requested that the environment that the couple had created was respected, and that the lighting remain dimmed and noise kept to a minimum. The medical staff had had little experience of working this way and initially seemed reluctant to work without bright lighting and talk. The situation improved over time, with staff sharing a greater understanding of the role of anxiety in the birthing room and its effect on the overall impression of the birth with which the couple are left.

Skin to skin

The study required a period of 90 minutes of uninterrupted maternal-infant skin contact at birth, regardless of mode of birth or chosen feeding method. Babies were placed directly on their mothers' skin, dried and covered with warm towels.

They were left to organise themselves, controlling their warmth and breathing with remarkable results. The breastfed babies, due to their close proximity to the breast, invariably fed spontaneously with minimal direction from their mothers.

This time is precious and needs careful management within a busy consultant unit. It is not as effective just to place a baby on its mother's skin. In order to facilitate maternal-infant interaction, the room needs to be peaceful and warm with subdued lighting. This allows the new mother time to greet her baby, explore him and watch for his first feeding cues. This process can take at least 60 minutes and can be delayed if the woman has received pharmacological analgesia during labour. Levels of oxytocin rise dramatically following birth (Matthiesen et al 2001); therefore, women are biologically primed to fall in love with their babies and need a conducive environment to promote this interaction.

Tritten (2002) describes the first 60 minutes following birth as a 'critical time,' and refers to the birthing room

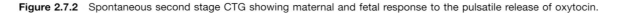

Figure 2.7.2 Spontaneous second stage CTG showing maternal and fetal response to the pulsatile release of oxytocin.

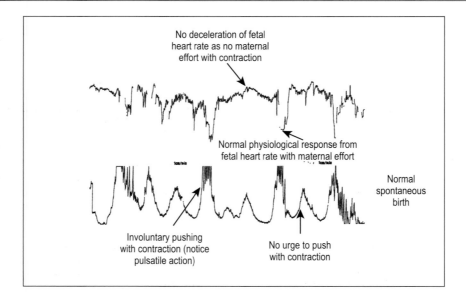

as 'sacred ground.' She birthed her baby at home and found the commotion and excitement of the midwives on their late arrival (although kindly meant) extremely disruptive – a lesson to us all, especially when creating this setting within a consultant unit.

Although it is well accepted that skin contact can support breastfeeding (Anderson 2003), we were careful to share its known benefits with all mother and baby partnerships.

Skin contact immediately following birth, for a period decided by the mother, is important as this early contact can help foster trust between mother and child and reduce stress (Christensson et al 1995). This unique contact following birth supports babies who have not been exposed to the usual positive stresses of labour. Babies born by elective caesarean section often take longer to organise themselves and initiate the first feed. Technology should not be seen as a barrier to this mother-infant interaction. Women experiencing more complex births should not be excluded as skin contact can offer equal benefits to themselves and to their babies.

Skin-to-skin contact following birth has been adopted as normal practice on our delivery suite and encouraged during the postnatal stay. It has impacted on the unit by the minimal use of cots and heaters, resulting in considerably fewer crying babies on the delivery suite! Christensson et al (1992) support this observation in their study looking at healthy full-term newborns and the increased crying reported when babies were left in cots as opposed to skin-to-skin care.

Implications for practice

The momentum of needing to prepare the unit to undertake the feasibilty study accelerated the change process and encouraged midwives to consider alternative ways of helping women cope with labour. The environmental changes were an important facet of the study and required team working and motivation from the midwives as well as support from management and the medical staff. The process of change took time and compromise, but the overall aim was to provide an improved childbirth experience for women and their families.

The midwives have established a 'promoting normal birth' group within the unit. The terms of reference for this group include:

- review and implementation of initiatives to improve normality within the unit
- disseminating information to colleagues
- sharing experiences of good practice
- the development of leaflets and posters to support and inform women.

GP surgeries are being approached and the promotional material displayed in all areas.

Another initiative that helps the free movement and promotion of normality for mothers with more complex pregnancies is the purchase of a mobile telemetry system.

In our experience, creating this conducive environment is as beneficial to mothers with low-risk pregnancies as it is for those needing more obstetric interventions – potentially reducing the need for those interventions in the first place. Integrating the environmental changes into a busy consultant unit has been a great achievement and team effort. Most mothers and babies are benefiting from skin to skin even if initial resuscitation is required.

Increased confidence and well-being has also been noted among the women and their partners, as well as increased satisfaction within the midwifery team.

REFERENCES

Aldrich C J, d'Antona D, Spencer J et al (1995). 'The effect of maternal pushing on fetal cerebral oxygenation and blood volume during the second stage of labour'. British Journal of Obstetrics and Gynaecology, 102: 448–453.

Anderson G (2003). 'A concept analysis of normal birth'. Evidence Based Midwifery, 1 (2): 48–54.

Berg M and Dahlberg K (1998). 'A phenomenological study of women's experiences of complicated childbirth'. Midwifery, 14 (1): 23–29.

Buckley S (2004). 'Unlocking the potential for normality'. The Practising Midwife, 7 (6): 15–16.

Christensson K, Cabrera T, Christensson E et al (1995). 'Separation distress call in human neonate in the absence of maternal body contact'. Acta Paediatr, 84: 468–473.

Christensson K, Siles C, Moreno L et al (1992). 'Temperature, metabolic adaptation and crying in healthy full term newborns cared for skin-to-skin or in a cot'. Acta Paediatr, 81: 488–493.

Edwards N (2003). 'Birth environments'. Midwifery Matters, 99: 17.

ENB (1999). Report on the Maternity Services (update), London: English National Board for Nursing Midwifery and Health Visiting.

Gaskin I M (2003). Ina May's Guide to Childbirth, New York: Bantam Dell.

Hansen S, Clark S and Foster J (2002). 'Active pushing versus passive fetal descent in the second stage of labor: a randomised controlled trial'. The American College of Obstetricians and Gynecologists, 99 (1): 29–34.

Howell C J (2000). 'Epidural versus non-epidural analgesia for pain relief in labour'. Cochrane Library (4) (update).

Klaus M, Kennell J, Robertson S et al (1986). 'Effects of social support during parturition on maternal and infant morbidity'. British Medical Journal, 293: 585–587.

McNabb M T (2003). 'Maternal and fetal responses to labour'. In: C Bates (ed), Midwifery Clinical Practice: the Fetus in Labour – the Baby at Birth, London: RCM Trust.

McNabb M T (2004). 'Biology of pregnancy and labour'. In: C Henderson and S McDonald (eds), Mayes' Midwifery, 13th edition, London: Elsevier Press, in press.

Matthiesen A et al (2001). 'Postpartum maternal oxytocin release by newborns: effects of infant hand massage and sucking'. Birth, 28 (1): 13–19.

Naakteborgen C (1989). 'The biology of childbirth' In: Effective Care in Pregnancy, vol 2, Oxford: OUP.

Norton D (1998). 'Holistic pregnancy and birth'. Positive Health, 28.

Odent M (1994). 'Labouring women are not marathon runners'. Midwifery Today, 31 (autumn): 23–24, 43, 51.

Odent M (2003). The Caesarean, London: Free Association Books.

Odent M (2004). The Caesarean, London: Free Association Books.

Page L (1995). 'Putting principles into practice'. In: L Page (ed), Effective Group Practice in Midwifery: Working with Women, Oxford: Blackwell Science.

Silverton L (1993). The Art and Science of Midwifery, London: Prentice Hall.

Thomson A M (1995). 'Maternal behaviour during spontaneous and directed pushing in the second stage of labour'. Journal of Advanced Nursing, 22 (6): 1027–1034.

Tritten J (2002). 'Sacred ground'. The Practising Midwife, 5 (6): 22.

The Practising Midwife 2005; 8(1): 18–20

The Practising Midwife 2005; 8(2): 25–27

Topics for further reflection

- The results of Tina Lavender and Jean Chapple's survey showed that the women involved in this study did not see midwives as being autonomous practitioners in the area of normal birth. How do you feel about this? Do you feel that this is an area which needs to be addressed and, if so, how could this be done?
- Do you feel that social attitudes to place of birth have changed over the time that you have been involved with birth (whether as a midwife, a parent or in some other capacity)? Do you feel they will change more during the next decade?
- Do you feel you offer a range of options to women about place of birth? Are there constraints on your ability to do this? How do women tend to respond to any information you offer them on this subject? Do you feel that there is any way in which your approach in this area could be altered to expand women's sense of their own choices, or do you feel that changes need to be made in other areas before more women realise that options like birth centres and home birth might be choices that are worth exploring?

Pregnancy

SECTION CONTENTS

Tell me a story

Lorna Davies

When my son was only two or three years of age, my husband created a fictional character who paid daily visits prior to bedtime. The character, called Jomu, was a boy from Hawaii who experienced exciting adventures with his friends and family. Jomu was an influential figure in my son's life, and he still makes the occasional visit even though Joe is now well into his ninth year.

The benefits of storytelling for children, such as those mentioned above, are well documented (Gussin Paley 1991, Shelley 1990). I believe that the Jomu stories have provided Joe with a multitude of life skills and attributes: they have helped him to develop listening skills, and taught him the rewards of concentration; they have given him a structure for his daydreams and fantasies, and have provided an opportunity for him to contribute his thoughts and ideas which may have helped him to establish self-worth and self-esteem. In short, Jomu has helped my little boy to make sense of his world, and I would even go as far as to say that the stories helped Joe to create values and beliefs that he may carry into adulthood.

Benefits for adults

The benefits for adults are also well recognised, and storytelling is being used by a wide range of professions from family therapists (Woodard 2003) to professors in business schools (Simmons 2002). The determined effort to reduce all knowledge to an analytic proposal, so prevalent in contemporary culture, is now seriously challenged (Denning 2000). The internet is awash with sites related to storytelling, and there is a plethora of courses available at all levels from basic technique to study at postgraduate level.

Stories can be used for many different purposes. They may be used to instil a sense of integration, understanding and pride in family and culture. The telling of stories can foster healing, offer new perspectives on one's own place in the world, and demonstrate a willingness to appreciate and celebrate the cultures of others. Stories put us in context and connect individual bits of information to the bigger picture, increasing our understanding of the details and the vision. By sharing and creating a common experience in storytelling, we are able to interpret events beyond our immediate experience (Baker and Green 1987). Storytelling even boasts worth epistemologically when valued as a way of knowing.

Words promote healing

Storytelling is currently gaining greater respect within the fields of medicine and allied health professions. We now know that words may have profound recuperative effects, promote healing, and create a more nurturing environment for people to deal with the trials of pain, suffering and grief. The Arts in Health Council website (2003) lists the projects where storytellers are invited into healthcare establishments to participate in therapeutic activities with patients.

In midwifery, authors such as Kirkham (in Kirkham and Perkins 1997) and McHugh (2001) have acknowledged the value of storytelling for women in the childbearing period of their lives. They emphasise the importance of recognising the value of stories in enabling women to make sense of the profound experience of birth and new parenthood for use in areas such as debriefing. England and Horowitz (1998) stress the significance of using storytelling in the antenatal period as part of the preparation for becoming a mother.

Traditionally, storytelling was the way in which women were prepared for the birth experience, and were able to make sense of the experience from the reflections of those who had been there already. Equally, midwifery was learnt by apprenticeship; the knowledge and skills required were passed down from generation to generation. The midwife's skills were largely acquired from the stories she was told (Sharp et al 2002). Perhaps we need to look back to the arts of our foremothers, and take heed.

The value of storytelling should certainly not be reserved for the women whom midwives serve. Midwives themselves benefit from the inclusion of storytelling, in its many guises, within midwifery education and practice. Kirkham and Perkins (1997) believes that our life experience is rendered meaningful and coherent only if it is created from stories. For example, reflective practice is the theoretical embodiment of storytelling, and its benefits for practice are manifold. As Judy Edmunds, an American midwife, eloquently states (1999):

Storytelling is right up there with love and support as far as seeming trivial but actually being hugely important. We are the torchbearers of truth, the weavers of courageous empowering visions to set before the women and families we serve. Our stories must be told often, until they become more compelling and convincing than the horrible 'you are weak and defective, prone to failure, need our technology, and might as well give up and give in now' myths people hear all around them.

Although we may be tentatively reaching out to reclaim the art and value of storytelling, in practice we all too sadly recognise that the reality of poor staffing levels and a ritualised approach to care frequently results in a story never told, or made meaningful.

Ticking time bombs

There are potential time bombs ticking away in midwifery practice. These days a midwife is expected to be self-aware (Hammett in Kirkham and Perkins 1997). Burnard (2002) believes that self-awareness is bound up with other relationships and therefore cannot be forced upon the individual but must be sought by her. If the midwife needs to understand the needs of women, she first has to understand her own needs and her own agenda. Midwives as women need to debrief, or defuse, as much as the women whom they support during this period.

Some years ago when I applied to the National Childbirth Trust (NCT) to become an antenatal teacher, I was invited to the home of the local tutor for what I imagined was going to be an interview. I was surprised when she asked me to talk about my own birth experiences. I was even more surprised how cathartic it was to talk about some aspects of the experiences that I realised I had locked away for some time.

Within the NCT philosophy, it is considered unreasonable to be expected to cope with other people's 'baggage' when you have not unpacked your own. However, in midwifery, at least in my own experience, we do not actively encourage this practice. Isn't this something we

should be introducing into our selection processes? Even if the applicant has not given birth herself, her values and beliefs surrounding birth have been formulated from a wide range of sources, and will irrefutably influence the sort of midwife she will come to be.

We recently introduced a 'hearts and minds' element to our induction programme at the university where I am employed. In one of the sessions, group members are asked to produce a life-steps chart on which they map their own life's journey, highlighting the events and incidents that link with their decision to become a midwife. It is a powerful exercise that leaves me ever more aware, as I listen to their stories, of the importance of the decision for many of the women and the sacrifices that they have made to achieve their goal. At the end of the session there is a much greater sense of unity and cohesion within the group – and I am convinced that this, albeit anecdotally, leads to greater tolerance and respect.

Gender issues

When I spoke to my husband about the exercise, he could not really grasp the relevance of such an event, which led me to reflect on whether there was a gender-related issue.

Feminists have long recognised that women's experience is different (Weiner 1994). Traditional epistemology has tended to exclude women by placing a boundary on knowledge, defining it through the means used to identify it – that is, objective, empirical and scientific.

As a midwife teacher, I observe women students draw upon a wide range of evidence, including anecdotal experience, homespun philosophy and intuition. Much of the subject matter discussed relates to the personal experiences from their own areas of practice as midwives.

Feminist educational theorists include personal experience as a basis for the production of knowledge, embracing the private sphere as a legitimate area of investigation (Kirby and McKenna 1989). Hooks (1989) states that feminist pedagogy includes a goal of justice for all humans, and allows students to be empowered through the recognition and validation of their own personal experience, and by encouraging them to draw on their personal experiences while learning about theory. Storytelling produces a vehicle for validating personal experience.

Pinkola Estes (1992), in her book *Women who run with the Wolves*, suggests that women have always used storytelling circles in order to create a space of their own and to develop a voice. Circles offer an opportunity to discuss freely and in detail the issues that are most important to them. Such gatherings may also offer warm encouragement to develop ideas and aspirations. Perhaps this is something that we need to take on board with regard to how we organise the learning environment. Our move into higher education has led, in my experience, to a more patriarchal approach to structure and practice. Large student group numbers militate against using group-structured interactive activities.

By adopting the ancient tradition of storytelling (Hughes 1995) and gathering in circles, we can create a safe and permissive environment that is women focused and serves as a positive role model for our students to take into practice to use in, for example, parent education.

Learning to learn

At my university, in spite of large group numbers, I believe that we still manage to achieve this to some degree, by employing Inquiry Based Learning (IBL). This is an adaptation of Problem Based Learning (PBL), a facilitative educational method that challenges students to 'learn to learn', working co-operatively in groups to seek solutions to real world problems.

It transfers control of the learning process from the teacher to the student. The students formulate and pursue their own learning objectives, and select those learning resources that are best suited to their current information needs. Teachers contribute to PBL by providing suggestions.

In problem-based learning, the traditional teacher and student roles change. The students assume increasing responsibility for their learning, giving them more motivation and more feelings of accomplishment, setting the pattern for them to become successful life-long learners. Teachers do not prescribe or dominate. The classical model consists of six to 10 students who need to resolve a phenomenon or a set of events that require explanation (Sadlo 1994). There is a strong emphasis on the use of group dynamics to facilitate motivation and the elaboration of an issue, which values the personal contribution of the student. IBL thereby promotes the sharing of stories, from the personal and professional lives of the participants.

Birth art

I also attempt to incorporate storytelling, in creative and resourceful ways, in other modules that I lead. For example, I have utilised the methods advocated by Pam England (1998) in *Birthing from Within*. Pam teaches antenatal educators the value of using birth art in parent education. Birth art encourages the group to explore their own ideas on what birth is about, and to begin to identify their own personal philosophies and to share birth stories.

I have used this approach with very experienced midwives, sometimes with profound effects.

Every picture tells a story, and the use of images of birth is a valuable tool in promoting discussion and the formulation of ideas. My own favourite way of achieving this is to use a slide presentation of birth accomplishment accompanied by appropriate music.

On occasions, I have asked each student to bring a birth story, either of their own birth (ie, as told by their mother), of the birth of one of their own children or of a birth from their practice experience that has a particular significance for them. They then tell their stories and share their feelings with the group. Clearly, this exercise requires a nurturing environment in which the students feel safe to share intimate parts of their life's experience, and will work only with small groups. The students start to link their own stories with their approach to practice.

This activity never ceases to amaze me inasmuch as many of the woman have never asked their mothers for their own birth story. Yet, when given 'permission', the mothers frequently come up with the most detailed accounts of their birthing experiences, 20, 30 or even 40 years before.

For me, this activity hammers home the message that the birthing experience has a profound impact on the life of women. Robinson (1998) says that, 'Letters about birth were different. They had an immediacy and clarity of expression which made them leap off the page. Even if the writer was poorly educated, descriptions of labour and birth were incredibly vivid. Women had intensity of recall for birth experiences which was different from other memories.'

The birth storytelling also gives participants a sense of who they are in the greater scheme of things, and this takes on particular significance for women if used in parent education sessions. We all need a sense of where we belong in the universe. The link with our past is said to take on greater significance in pregnancy (Hall 2000).

Creating trust and respect

In conclusion, by virtue of their role, midwives have the potential to share this incredibly important time in the lives of women and their families. By sharing some of the time on this journey into parenthood, the midwife may gain right of entry into the previously undisclosed world of the woman. As a result, she may share her hopes, fears, anxieties, dreams and expectations during the period of contact. The use of storytelling may provide a vehicle to facilitate the establishment of a trusting and mutually respectful relationship that allows both partners to gain and grow from the experience.

REFERENCES

Arts in Health (2003). http://www.nnah.org.uk/

Baker A and Green E (1987). Storytelling: Art and Technique (2nd Ed), New Jersey: R R Bowker.

Burnard P (2002). Learning Human Skills, London: Butterworth Heinemann.

Denning S (2000). The Springboard: How Storytelling Ignites Action in Knowledge, London: Butterworth Heinemann.

Edmunds J (1999). 'My top 10 favorite complementary modalities'. Midwifery Today, 52 (winter 1999): 9.

England P and Horowitz R (1998). Birthing from Within: an Extraordinary Guide to Childbirth Preparation, New Mexico: Partera Press.

Gussin Paley V (1991). The Boy Who Would Be a Helicopter: the Uses of Storytelling in the Classroom, Harvard University Press.

Hall J (2000). Midwifery: Mind, Body and Spirit, Hale, Cheshire: Books for Midwives.

Hooks B (1989). Talking Back: Thinking Feminist – Thinking Black, Boston, MA: South End Press.

Hughes, K (1995). 'Feminist pedagogy and feminist epistemology: an overview'. International Journal of Lifelong Learning, 14 (3): 214–230.

Kirby S and McKenna K (1989). Experience, Research, Social Change: Methods from the Margin, Toronto: Garamond.

Kirkham M and Perkins E (1997). Reflections on Midwifery Practice, London: Ballière Tindall.

McHugh N (2001). 'Story telling and its influence in passing birth culture through the generations'. Midwifery Matters, 89 (June): 15–17.

Pinkola Estes C (1992). Women Who Run With the Wolves, New York: Rider.

Sadlo G (1994). 'Problem-based learning in the development of an occupational therapy curriculum: the process of problem-based learning'. British Journal of Occupational Therapy, 57 (2): 49–53.

Sharp J, Cellier E, Trye M and Cody L (2002). Printed Writings 1641–1700: Part One: Writings on Medicine (Early Modern Englishwoman), Aldershot: Ashgate Publishing Limited.

Shelley M (1990). Telling Stories to Children, Oxford: Lion Publishing.

Simmons A (2002). The Story Factor: Inspiration, Influence and Persuasion Through the Art of Storytelling, Oxford: Perseus.

Weiner G (1994). Feminisms in Education: an Introduction, Buckingham: Open University Press.

Woodard J (2003). http://www.storyteller.net/tellers/storyjim

The Practising Midwife 2005; 7(7): 22–25

Getting parent education right

Kate Jackson

When the Royal Victoria Infirmary Maternity Unit in Newcastle-upon-Tyne appointed me as its Parent Education Coordinator it was to a brand-new post with a wonderfully open-ended remit.

I was aware that many of my midwifery colleagues felt ambivalent about parent education, so the first thing I did was to send a questionnaire to all of them to discover who would like to be part of the 'Teaching Team' and who wouldn't. We can't all be good at everything, and I think we would all agree that the outcome for anything is better if the person delivering the service has an interest – even a passion – for what they are doing. So 'hooray' for all the midwives who love the job they are doing – be it specialist or general – and let's agree that if we nurture that interest the end result will be happy for all concerned.

I identified a group of midwives with the skills and ability to impart information in group settings.

I also meet with every newly appointed midwife to introduce them to the Parent Education Department, discover their talents and recruit them if they are willing.

Midwives' fears, clients' needs

I listened to the criticisms my colleagues had about teaching. They disliked having to be taken from their clinical area to lead a session. This was detrimental both to clients and to fellow colleagues. They felt that if they came in on their own time they rarely got it back. They felt that there was little or no time available for preparation. They felt that there were limited resources to make teaching more varied. I looked at all of these concerns and devised a programme that would occupy a midwife for one 'late' shift a week for a four-week period, supernumerary to her usual place of work.

The next thing was to devise a questionnaire for our clients: we got 500 responses that helped to design the new courses. The results were interesting and confirmed

that what I thought would be the right things to include in course material were indeed what women wanted, too.

Developing courses

Over the next two years, we designed and offered the following courses to all our women and their families:

- **Tours of the unit** It is no surprise that 76 per cent of people want to have a look at the unit in which they have chosen to do the most intimate and amazing thing – give birth. So I looked at how we conducted the tours. Midwives in the various areas and wards were asked: 'What do you want people to know about your area?,' and I wrote a checklist for everyone who leads the twice-weekly tours of our unit. If we tell everyone not to bring the car seat up to the ward we save a needless trip for the birth partner – that sort of thing.
- **Courses for first-time parents** Included are new partnerships where one half has a child already, and people with a long gap who feel they would like to know how things have changed. This is a four-week course. The questionnaire revealed what these people wanted to know, and the content of these courses reflects this.
- **The all-day Sunday course** This is a one-stop condensed session from 11am–5pm on – naturally enough – a Sunday. It contains the same information as the four-week course, but condensed. The important stuff is there. While the four-week course meets an important social need as couples get to know one another, this course offers people with tricky time commitments a chance to receive information in a way that suits them.
- **The early pregnancy session** This course takes place between 12 and 18 weeks, and has been a real joy to

facilitate. A midwife and a physiotherapist are in the hot seat together. We are fortunate to have two marvellous Women's Service physiotherapists who are keen to be involved in a 'prevention is better than cure' way.

- **Breastfeeding Workshop** I inherited this course; it has been running successfully at the RVI for many years based on the Bloomsbury Breastfeeding Workshops. It has undergone several updates and offers a very comprehensive overview of breastfeeding and is an opportunity for staff training at the same time.
- **The back and pelvic pain group** This is run by the physios. They offer practical solutions to common problems at any stage of pregnancy in a 'one-off' session.
- **The toddler visit** I can't talk about this work for long without mentioning the toddler visit, such is the success of this session. And it wasn't even my idea! I read about a midwife in Sidcup who ran this at her unit. I wrote to her and she gave me all her best ideas. So, with thanks to midwife Anne Brunton, here is the gist of the toddler visit: children over two years old come with their mum, dad, gran or whoever to see the postnatal ward and play with a baby doll, bath and baby clothes. We might be lucky and see a baby in the distance, but stress that the visit is not about seeing babies – because that baby is someone else's new brother or sister, not theirs. We have appropriate books about new babies, we drink juice and eat fruit, do whatever they want to do – within reason – and each child goes home with a certificate saying they have been to the Big Sister or Big Brother Club at the RVI. Success assured. I could run this one every day. If you are thinking of doing this – remember that five is a good number to invite. More details about this one on request.
- **Elective section tour** This is exactly what it sounds like – a visit to theatre, recovery and the postnatal ward for women and partners booked for elective section. Our unit does 400 of these a year. Worth doing a special tour.
- **Active birth** Sixty-six per cent of the people who returned a questionnaire expressed interest in either staying or getting fit before and after birth. An active birth teacher, trained by Janet Balaskas, teaches a course for which a charge is made. This is currently £40 for six weeks – a bargain – and all of it is passed on to the teacher. We have a small room, so our top number is 10.
- **Postnatal yoga** The same wonderful woman offers this course for the same reasonable price. Support, stretching, baby massage and play, discussion and positive affirmation are all offered in this six-week course. One unexpected effect has been the emotional upheaval sometimes caused when women bring their six-week-old babies back to the unit in which they gave birth – when the memories of the event may not have been resolved. We found that the support of the teacher and the other women was of benefit here. This is also an appropriate moment to remind women of the Birth Reflections Service on offer to all women who give birth with us.
- **Diabetic women** This is a very small group, run as the need arises for these women and their partners. Women who have diabetes often have a very medical time during their pregnancy, and their general information and emotional needs may be poorly met. By chance, we had a midwife who was diabetic who designed and runs this group.
- **Using water for labour and birth** This is offered to women and partners who are curious to know more about water birth, or have made a decision and want to see the facilities.

Future possibilities

These following groups are in my mind only – and have been suggested by midwives and clients:

- **Pregnant again after pregnancy loss** Another specialist group that emerged as a need was expressed. This is in the planning stages.
- **Pregnant again after caesarean section** A VBAC group is planned for those women who want to try to achieve one. With reference to the NICE Guidelines, and designed with our consultants, this will offer the best advice possible to this group of women.
- **Bring your mother** We all know how much a mum can influence a daughter – not always positively! This is a suggested session to help the last generation realise how much has changed since they were new parents.
- **Interactive tours** This is going to be a great opportunity to help women and partners discover how to use what we have in delivery rooms to stay mobile and upright. This will be part of the large study into management of the second stage that is taking place in our unit at present.
- **Birth partners – what you can do** This session was requested by the women on the Active Birth course who felt that their partners were lacking in some basic support skills!

These may not all be implemented and they may not evolve as originally intended. That is the marvellous thing – to be able to respond to the needs of our clients and adapt courses and sessions in response to

Table 3.2.1

Session	Week one	Week two	Week three	Week four
1	Meet With me*	Big brother/Big sister club	Using water for labour and birth	Pregnant again after C/section
2	Early pregnancy	Big brother/Big sister club	Early pregnancy	Big brother/Big sister club
3	Primips 1	Primips 2	Primips 3	Primips 4

*This is the support, planning and preparation session midwives said they wanted

evaluations. We always evaluate with well-designed questionnaires, and take note of what they say!

We are enormously fortunate to have the unit and the people who work in it as the best 'teaching aid'. The way that we learn about anything will depend on how it is presented. Visual, aural and tactile is all part of it.

Maximising midwife time

So, back to the beginning. Table 3.2.1 shows how we offer all that and maximise midwife time. This happens every Thursday: if there are five Thursdays in a month, we have a week off.

Other courses are offered at different times through the week, facilitated by the physiotherapists, active birth teacher or me. So I spend some of my time teaching and some of it supporting other midwives to teach. Each interested midwife takes a whole month, and teaches once a year. The all-day course is facilitated by two midwives. Midwives teach this one about three or four times a year.

Every session we offer is taken up. We have a waiting list for many courses, especially the active birth and postnatal yoga. I am wondering how we can clone Lynn, our teacher!

We have a great team of community staff who offer courses in the local area for their own caseload. These are designed and run by the midwives, and are appropriate to our diverse client group. We met together to devise guidelines for teaching throughout the city – with adaptations built in to reflect local needs. Women and their partners can access a variety of sessions, from the more formal four-week course to a weekly 'drop in'. Breastfeeding workshops are held in the community, and our Sure Start midwives are involved in running many sessions to meet local needs.

Conclusion

I have learnt many things since taking up this specialist post. Here are some of my top tips:

1. Nurture your colleagues and share ideas about teaching – none of us know everything, and there are so many good ideas to build on.

2. When teaching, personal anecdotes have very limited value.
3. Asking 'Has anyone got any questions?' is the best way to ensure complete silence.
4. Use a variety of teaching styles to appeal to people who learn in different ways.
5. Encourage the social aspect of your courses – ask if people want to put their details on to 'contact lists' so that they can keep in touch outside the sessions. Social isolation can be difficult for many new parents.
6. Value your clients – they are giving up their time, so nice biscuits and proper cups show that you care for them. Super saver bargain Rich Tea and plastic cups of weak orange squash are more insulting than giving nothing!
7. Act on evaluations – if everyone says they hate playing the pain relief game, revise it or drop it.
8. Look at the written information you give to clients. Is it beautifully produced, evidence-based and relevant, or is it a fifth-generation photocopy with dodgy illustrations? Which would you rather have?
9. Enjoy teaching: if you don't, then switch to what you do enjoy. If that isn't possible and it's 'your turn', try to teach with someone else so you have someone to bounce ideas off.
10. Perfect planning prevents pathetic performance. The better prepared you are, the more relaxed you will be and the better the session will run. Leading Antenatal Classes (Schott and Priest 2002) has a good plan for organising classes.

If you have good ideas and know of something that works well, please let me know. Good luck!

REFERENCE

Schott J and Priest J (2002). Leading Antenatal Classes (2nd edition). Oxford: Books for Midwives.

The Practising Midwife 2005; 8(7): 32–34

Fears and feelings in second-time pregnancy

Mary Nolan

The psychology of second pregnancy is at least as complex and perhaps more so than the psychology of first. Women bring to their second pregnancies a whole range of lived experience, as well as the vicarious experiences that were so influential when they were expecting their first baby. The events of the first pregnancy, labour and birth, and of the early postnatal period, are now vividly revived in the memory and become the foundation from which the second experiences develop.

Anxiety levels may be lower for women having their second babies if their first pregnancy was enjoyable, unproblematic and led to the straightforward vaginal birth of a healthy term baby. For women whose first pregnancy was complicated by mental health or medical difficulties, the fears aroused by a positive pregnancy test may be very profound. Women with tocophobia, or who are simply very frightened of childbirth, may be anxious with due cause. A study (Saisto et al 1999) that compared 100 women who reported profound fear of childbirth with 100 who had no such fear found that there had been a high prevalence of emergency caesareans and assisted deliveries among the frightened women. Both first and second stages of labour had lasted longer than for those women in the control group. They had also, not surprisingly, received more epidural analgesia.

Adverse pregnancy events in the first pregnancy or at the first birth will often lead to a higher level of medical and midwifery input into the second pregnancy. Most women see this as very positive, and case studies (Clark 2004, Shenhav et al 2002) demonstrate that careful management of the second pregnancy generally results in a happy outcome. However, research (Elam-Evans et al 1997) suggests that women who delayed presenting for antenatal care until late in their first pregnancy often do the same second time round, even if the first pregnancy and birth were problematic.

Birth environment

Women who have been traumatised by their first experience of birth in hospital, with resultant loss of confidence in their bodies' ability to give birth and their own capacity as mothers, can be offered the chance to choose a different birth environment second time round. Provided there are no disqualifying medical complications, by booking into a birth centre or for a home birth these women's experiences of second pregnancy and birth can be transformed (Whiting 2003/04). Milan (2003: 145) explores the experience of three women who had had frightening first births:

All birthed their second babies at home. The quality of the care received was described as empowering, reassuring and emotionally supportive. The women framed their perception of the changes which had occurred in terms of reassessment of themselves and their capabilities in the light of the achievement of the (second) birth experience.

I recently took Laura to visit her local midwife-led birth centre. She had had a horrific first labour during which she had felt she had no control over what staff were doing to her, and was too frightened to ask any questions. She and her partner were astounded that such a comfortable, well-decorated, sensitively planned maternity unit could be available on the NHS! They were deeply impressed both by the professionalism and the loving concern of the midwives. Having booked into the unit, Laura was able to enjoy, if not a worry-free pregnancy, at least one where she did not spend every minute of every day worrying about the birth. In the event, her labour was short, mostly in water, straightforward and resulted in the arrival of a healthy 9.5lb baby girl.

Fears around birth weight

Women whose first baby was 'large', in their own view (and a 7lb baby may seem very 'large' to a woman who is

5' 0"!) or that of health professionals, often fear that their next baby will be even larger. This fear is reinforced by the popularly held view that each baby is heavier than the last. The evidence, in fact, is not so straightforward and can be cited to help reassure women for whom this issue is a major concern. A large study carried out in the East Midlands (Wilcox et al 1996) found that the mean crude birth weight difference between first and second pregnancies was 138g. However, nature tends to demonstrate regression towards the mean so that women whose first baby was more than 3,720g can expect to give birth to a lighter baby next time round. The authors concluded that clinical decisions should not be based on the assumption that a second baby will inevitably be heavier than a first.

Pre-eclampsia

Women who had pre-eclampsia with their first pregnancy may be fearful that it will occur again, while women who didn't may be unduly smug that they are not at risk this time! The evidence on recurrence rates for pre-eclampsia is complex. The risk of pre-eclampsia has generally been perceived as being lower in second pregnancies, unless the woman changes partner in between. The APEC website (Action on Pre-eclampsia) advises women that they are at higher risk if they have a new partner for their second baby. However, Skjaerven et al (2002: 38) have suggested that a more significant factor is the length of time between pregnancies:

The protective effect of previous pregnancy against pre-eclampsia is transient. After adjustment for the interval between births, a change in partner is not associated with an increased risk of pre-eclampsia.

Basso et al (2001: 624) concur:

Although partner change was associated with an increased risk of pre-eclampsia in women with no history of pre-eclampsia, this effect disappeared after adjustment for the interpregnancy interval.

A huge study of more than half a million women by Trogstad et al (2001) also found that it is the length of time between pregnancies that is the crucial factor in determining risk of pre-eclampsia. They concluded that women with no history of pre-eclampsia but who have a long gap between pregnancies are at increased risk of pre-eclampsia, while there is a tendency towards decreased risk with increasing time interval between pregnancies for women with a history of pre-eclampsia.

Premature birth and small for gestational age (SGA) babies

Women whose first baby was born prematurely and/or was small for dates are likely to be very concerned that they will have similar problems again. The research

Table 3.3.1 Adjusted odds ratios for low birthweight with subsequent baby

10.1	First baby premature and SGA
7.9	First baby premature but not SGA
6.3	First baby term but SGA

Figures from Bakewell et al 1997

certainly suggests that this is the case (Elam-Evans and Wilson 2000) although the chances of having a second low-birthweight (LBW) baby depend very largely on how early the first baby was born. The women most at risk are those whose first baby was born before 32 weeks (see Table 3.3.1 for odds ratios for low birthweight).

Women who are underweight before they start their second pregnancy are also at increased risk of having another LBW baby (Bakewell et al 1997).

These figures can be used to help the mother plan her second pregnancy realistically. Preparation for birth and for the possibility that her baby may need special care will need to take place early on so that the woman feels emotionally prepared and can put the necessary practical arrangements in place to minimise her anxiety if she does go into premature labour. She will appreciate midwives' straight talking about the possibility of a second premature birth, enabling her to feel more in control and better able to take responsibility for her own life.

Other common fears

Women who had a long first labour are very often fearful of a repeat experience. They may have been told that the first labour sets the pattern for subsequent labours. They may be struggling under a weight of family history which suggests to them that women in their family always have long labours. Research (Barton et al 1991) suggests that the duration of a second labour is likely to be less than the first, and that the need for oxytocin augmentation is much reduced.

Women who have turned 40 since having their first baby can be the victim of many insensitive comments from both friends and professionals about the difficulties (inevitable) that older women experience in giving birth. However, the study by Berryman et al (1991) of the experiences of women aged 40+ found that their experiences tended to contrast very markedly with the problem-centred approach that is the hallmark of much of the literature on later childbearing. It seems reasonable to anticipate that the vast majority of pregnancies and labours in older mothers will be straightforward, rather than insisting on a medical model of care where the prophecy that there will be problems so easily becomes a self-fulfilling one.

Conclusion

The recently issued NICE Guidelines (2003) on care in normal pregnancy suggest that a regime of seven antenatal visits is appropriate for women expecting their second baby, as opposed to the 10 recommended for primiparous women. While some women may be glad not to have to attend appointments so frequently, especially if they have a toddler in tow, others may feel that they are seen as 'less special' now that they are pregnant for the second time. It is important to remember that every woman, no matter what her previous obstetric history, does have such a history by the time she becomes pregnant again, and that history needs acknowledgement. Some women will require debriefing in order to be able to enjoy a happy and fearless second pregnancy and labour.

Sadly, antenatal classes for second-timers are rarely available although there is much valuable work that they could do. Midwives can help women in their care with the emotional work of second pregnancy by devoting time, whenever possible and certainly towards the end of pregnancy, to discussing their previous experiences. Women may also be able to attend 'refresher' classes with the National Childbirth Trust, with the Active Birth Centre, or with Yoga for Pregnancy teachers.

REFERENCES

Bakewell J M, Stockbauer J W and Schramm W F (1997). 'Factors associated with repetition of low birthweight: Missouri longitudinal study'. Paediatric and Perinatal Epidemiology, 11 (supplement 1): 119–129.

Barton D P J, Turner M J and Stronge J M (1991). 'Outcome of the second labour in patients whose first labour was prolonged'. European Journal of Obstetrics and Gynecology and Reproductive Biology, 42 (1): 15–18.

Basso O, Christensen K and Olsen J (2001). 'Higher risk of pre-eclampsia after change of partner. An effect of longer interpregnancy intervals?'. Epidemiology, 12 (6): 624–629.

Berryman JC and Windbridge K (1991). 'Having a baby after 40: a preliminary investigation of women's experience of motherhood'. Journal of Reproductive and Infant Psychology, 9 (1):19–33.

Clark K (2004). 'TTP and me'. The Practising Midwife, 7 (8): 13–17.

Elam-Evans L D, Adams M M and Delaney K M (1997). 'Patterns of prenatal care initiation in Georgia'. Obstetrics and Gynecology, 90 (1): 71–77.

Elam-Evans L D and Wilson H G (2000). 'Rates of and factors associated with recurrence of preterm delivery'. Journal of the American Medical Association, 283 (12): 1591–1596.

Milan M (2003). 'Childbirth as healing: three women's experience of independent midwife care'. Complementary Therapies in Nursing and Midwifery, 9 (3): 140–146.

NICE – National Institute for Clinical Excellence (2003). Routine Antenatal Care for Healthy Pregnant Women, London: NICE (www.nice.org.uk).

Saisto T, Ylikorkala O and Halmesmaki E (1999). 'Factors associated with fear of delivery in second pregnancies'. Obstetrics and Gynecology, 94 (5) part 1: 679–682.

Shenhav S, Gemer O and Schneider R (2002). 'Severe hyperlipidemia-associated pregnancy: prevention in subsequent pregnancy by diet'. Acta Obstetricia et Gynecologica Scandinavica, 81 (8): 788–790.

Skjaerven R, Wilcox A J and Lie R T (2002). 'The interval between pregnancies and the risk of preeclampsia'. New England Journal of Medicine, 346 (1): 33–38.

Trogstad L I S, Eskild A and Magnus P (2001). 'Changing paternity and time since last pregnancy; the impact on pre-eclampsia risk. A study of 547,238 women with and without previous pre-eclampsia'. International Journal of Epidemiology, 30 (6): 1317–1322.

Whiting R (2003/04). 'Through a glass darkly (into the light)'. AIMS Journal, 15 (4): 14–15.

Wilcox M A, Chang A M Z and Johnson I R (1996). 'The effects of parity on birthweight using successive pregnancies'. Acta Obstetricia et Gynecologica Scandinavica, 75 (5): 459–463.

Website Action on Pre-eclampsia: www.doorbar.co.uk/apec.html

The Practising Midwife 2005; 8(3): 26–28

Women's needs from antenatal care in three European countries

Ans G. Luyben, Valerie E.M. Fleming

Summary

Objective: to determine the important aspects of antenatal care from a woman's perspective in order to develop a woman-constructed conceptual model of antenatal care.

Design: grounded theory.

Setting: three European countries: Scotland, Switzerland and The Netherlands.

Participants: 23 women using routine antenatal care in the three countries were interviewed: seven women in Scotland, seven in Switzerland and nine in The Netherlands.

Measurements and findings: three main categories emerged: 'responsibility', 'establishing a sharing trust relationship' and 'support me to be responsible'. The category of 'responsibility', which incorporated the subcategories 'feeling confident' and 'feeling autonomous',

is reported. Despite the many aspects that the women had in common, a divergence of the categories in each of the countries was clearly observed. The main cross-cultural differences were within the subcategory of 'feeling autonomous'.

Key conclusions and implications for practice: responsibility is the main reason why women seek antenatal care. Feelings of confidence and autonomy are substantial attributes of this responsibility. The cultural background of the women seems to cause the differences within the categories. These findings have implications for both the provision and the evaluation of antenatal care.

Keywords

Women's views; Antenatal care; Europe; Grounded theory

Introduction

The concept of antenatal care in Western Europe has existed for just over 100 years, with the main aim being to reduce the high rate of infant mortality. The first programme was initiated in the UK in 1929, after a report was published by the Ministry of Health (Hall et al., 1985). According to Heringa (1998), other European countries were quick to follow this example, initiating similar programmes. With the exception of the introduction of more sophisticated diagnostic techniques, little has changed since this time (Oakley, 1982; Hall et al., 1985; Heringa, 1998).

Until the late 1970s, little systematic evaluation had been carried out to assess the effectiveness of the antenatal-care programmes (Hall et al., 1985; Heringa,

1998). According to Oakley (1982) and Hall et al. (1985), reduction in maternal and perinatal morbidity and mortality was seen by service providers and researchers as evidence of the value of these programmes, without taking into consideration other factors during this time, which may have affected these figures.

However, in the early 1980s, consumers and health-care providers began to call for an evaluation of the effectiveness of health-care services. As a result, antenatal-care programmes were the subject of considerable research in the 1980s and 1990s (Enkin and Chalmers, 1982; Hall et al., 1985; WHO, 1987; Garcia et al., 1989; Heringa, 1998; Haertsch et al., 1999; Langer et al., 1999; Villar et al., 2001; Villar et al., 2004). Some of these evaluations, particularly in the UK, included reports of women's experiences and satisfaction with antenatal care and childbirth. Women complained about organisational aspects, the information they were receiving, lack of continuity of care and the impersonal treatment at antenatal-care clinics (Hall et al., 1985; Reid and Garcia, 1989; Jacoby and Cartwright, 1990).

During the 1990s, research into antenatal care addressed the number of antenatal-care visits, the person best suited to provide the care, organisational aspects and screening procedures (Heringa, 1998; Villar et al., 2001; Gagnon, 2004; Hodnett, 2004; Villar et al., 2004). The findings of these studies showed that the effectiveness of each single screening procedure used in antenatal care still remained to be proven, and that a reduction of the antenatal visits was possible without a change in maternal and perinatal outcome. This, however, resulted in women being less satisfied with their care. Although continuity of care was shown to be beneficial, it remained to be proven whether this was due to the continuity or to the person providing the care. Researchers are, therefore, currently divided about the value of antenatal programmes in western Europe in reducing maternal and perinatal mortality and morbidity (Heringa, 1998; Langer et al., 1999; Haertsch et al., 1999; Villar et al., 2001).

The aim of this study was to evaluate the effectiveness of antenatal-care programmes in three European countries (Switzerland, Scotland and The Netherlands) from the perspective of the women who used the services. The objective was to develop a woman-constructed conceptual model of antenatal care.

Method

Approach

A grounded-theory approach, as proposed by Strauss and Corbin (1990), was chosen to address the objectives of this study. This is because it uses an inductive approach through developing a theory grounded in everyday reality. In this way, it takes into account the many factors that can influence antenatal care. Although grounded theory was introduced collaboratively by Glaser and Strauss (1967), the approach according to Strauss and Corbin (1990) emphasises the rigour of the method by developing categories through a systematic line-by-line reduction of the data.

Setting

Women were recruited to the study from three European countries: Scotland, Switzerland and The Netherlands. The regions involved were the west of Scotland, the German speaking part of Switzerland and the eastern and the western part of The Netherlands.

Sample

The participants were healthy women at different stages of uncomplicated pregnancies or women up to 6 months after giving birth. Routine antenatal care was defined as attending the normal number of visits as set by the health system of the country involved.

The first round of interviews was conducted using a convenience sample, and included five women from Scotland, five women from Switzerland and seven women from The Netherlands. Recruitment took place in Switzerland by AGL, in Scotland by both supervisors of the study and in The Netherlands by AGL and care providers.

After the first round of interviews, theoretical sampling was used to reflect the different kinds of care provider, and to demonstrate the evolving process throughout the subsequent pregnancies. This meant that, in The Netherlands, a woman in her third pregnancy was interviewed, and in Switzerland a woman during her first. The theoretical sample included three women from Scotland, three women from Switzerland and three women from The Netherlands. All women were recruited through care providers. In Scotland, two women were recruited through independent midwives; in The Netherlands, a woman was recruited who was cared for by medical practitioners; and in Switzerland, two women were recruited who were cared for by an obstetrician only. Also, in each of the countries, one of the women from the first sample was again interviewed to verify the results of the analysis.

Access and ethical considerations

The major ethical issues of this study were informed consent, anonymity and confidentiality. Ethical approval was obtained from the Ethics Committee of Glasgow Caledonian University and for the Scottish arm of the study from the Lanarkshire Ethics of Research Committee. Access to the participants did not require additional ethical approval in The Netherlands and Switzerland.

The women were provided with a document briefing them about the study, and were asked to contact the researcher if they were interested. No woman refused to participate, and none later withdrew consent.

All of the women gave written consent to the researcher before the interviews took place. Information and consent papers related to the study were translated by the researcher into the three languages used: English, German and Dutch. The translations were checked by individuals living in each of the countries involved.

Data collection

Data were collected through semi-structured interviews using an interview guideline as a reference. The leading interview question was 'If you could determine the content of care during pregnancy yourself, based on your needs and expectations, what would be important to you?' Following this question, the women were encouraged to tell their stories, during which some of the topics, such as expectations at the beginning of pregnancy, were introduced by the interviewer.

The data were collected in one-to-one audiotaped interviews by AGL at a convenient place for the women in either English, Dutch or German. No woman refused permission for the interview to be taped. Interviews lasted from 20–108 mins. Field notes were made after each interview, describing the interview situation and the main topics of the interview, in order to assist theoretical sampling and data collection.

Data analysis

The interviews were transcribed verbatim. Identifying data were removed. AGL undertook the analysis in each of the original languages. No qualitative computer database was used.

Open coding was performed by line-by-line analysis in order to create the smallest possible unit of analysis. The components which resulted from this analysis were examined and coded. These codes were grouped together in order to create categories. A number of different categories were identified and given a name in the original language, which fitted the meaning given by the women in the interviews (Strauss and Corbin, 1998). Only at this stage were the categories compared and integrated into the overall European sample (Boufoy-Bastick, 2002). The concepts within the categories were closely examined and compared for cross-cultural similarities and differences. In order to remain true to the meaning of the categories and concepts, dictionaries and individuals originating from the countries involved were consulted. The results of the total sample, as well as the questions that arose from the cross-cultural comparison, led the theoretical sampling. After open coding, axial coding took place with the results of the interviews of the theoretical sample, during which the existing concepts were rearranged, categories renamed and linked together. As saturation could not be achieved at this stage through cross-cultural differences within the categories, the study continued.

Findings

The total sample comprised 26 interviews with 23 women. Four women were interviewed during their first pregnancies. The interviews took place between 11 and 36 weeks of pregnancy. Three women were interviewed between 8 weeks and 5 months after the birth of their first child. One

of them had a previous miscarriage. Four women were interviewed between 8 weeks and 34 weeks of their second pregnancies. One of them had a previous miscarriage, and one of these women had a twin pregnancy. Seven women were interviewed between 2 weeks and 5 months after the birth of their second child. Three women were interviewed between 24 and 33 weeks of their third pregnancies. Two women were recruited between 4–5 months after having their third child. One of them had had two previous miscarriages. None of the women had a history of stillbirth.

The second interview took place with two women between 9 and 16 months after having their second baby, and one woman 16 months after having her third baby.

Most women were native inhabitants of the country in which they were interviewed, although in Scotland a woman originating from Germany and a woman originating from Canada were interviewed. In Switzerland, a woman of Dutch nationality was interviewed.

Four women in Scotland received 'shared care' from midwives and general practitioners, one of which had hospital-based care. Two women in the theoretical sample were cared for by an independent midwife. The nine women in the Dutch sample had care from independent midwives, although one of them received hospital-based medical care during childbirth and some part of the postnatal period. Eight Swiss women were cared for by private gynaecologists. Five of them were (informally) counselled by midwives. One woman in the Swiss sample received midwifery care only at a birth centre.

The term used for the participants of the study in this paper is 'women'. To ascertain anonymity, a list with culturally appropriate first names was made and one was assigned to each woman. These pseudonyms have been used in this paper. In accordance with the philosophy of the grounded theory used, the translation of Dutch and German are based on the meaning of texts (i.e. grounding them in their context [Strauss and Corbin, 1998]).

Three main categories emerged: 'responsibility'; 'establishing a sharing trust relationship'; and 'supporting me to feel responsible'. These initial categories and their relationships are presented in Figure 3.4.1. On further analysis, however, the category of 'responsibility' appeared to subsume the others, as 'establishing a sharing trust relationship' was the consequence of this feeling of 'responsibility', whereas 'supporting me to feel responsible' included the content the women needed from antenatal care in order to carry this responsibility.

The main category 'responsibility' incorporated two sub-categories: 'feeling confident' and 'feeling autonomous'. The women felt responsible for the experience of becoming mothers, for themselves and for their babies and family. As aspects of this experience were unknown to them, they felt they lacked confidence, and could there-

Figure 3.4.1   Women's needs from antenatal care in three European countries.

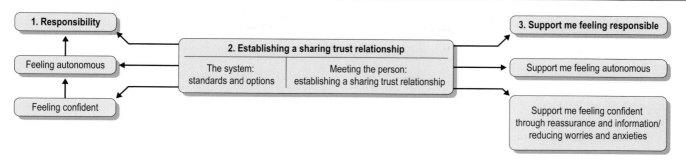

fore not act autonomously. During pregnancy, they aimed to regain a state of confidence in order to take over this responsibility.

The sub-categories of 'feeling confident' and 'feeling autonomous', consequently resulting in the main category of 'responsibility', are described.

Feeling confident

Most important concepts of 'feeling confident' were 'feelings' and 'knowledge'. Generally, most women regarded 'feelings' as a central concept during their pregnancies. They experienced a different feeling about their physical and mental health during pregnancy than normal:

I am less patient, and I will react much more emotionally concerning certain issues; that means that I think a lot more with my feelings, than I do with my head. (Ariane/The Netherlands)

That is, when I was pregnant, that was different. So now and then I did not recognise myself. (. . .) You know, when they played the hymn of the country, I cried. I mean, when ever do I during this hymn, when this hymn, no . . . really. You are different. You are just different. They are different emotions. (Paola/Switzerland)

Because women felt different, they were unsure of the things they were experiencing and lacked confidence. As they wanted to feel more confident, they tried to restore the balance by trying to find knowledge to counter what they felt. This feeling of uncertainty induced a reflective process ('thinking'), which meant trying to make sense of, and create a pattern from, all the knowledge that the women had available at that moment in their situation. A few women described this as 'becoming aware'. The process of thinking stopped, when the women felt confident again:

Interviewer: Are you comparing your feelings with your knowledge? (. . .) Or are you reflecting your feelings on your knowledge?

Woman: could be either way, I think, you know, sort of high blood pressure, I'm desperately going through all the possible reasons as to why I have a high blood pressure. (Jan/Scotland)

If the women remained remained unsure, the thinking process continued. This was called 'worrying' by the women. Reasons were the inability to share their worries about information they received and which had not been explained to their satisfaction. Some women tried to avoid this by consciously avoiding new information:

Why should we worry for 2 weeks, if you tell us the results, and we get a few days, then, this is enough time to worry, why should we worry if there is maybe no increased risk. (Megan/Scotland)

The types of knowledge upon which women reflected included cognitive knowledge, knowledge about their daily life and family, personal experiences about pregnancy and childbirth, and values, opinions, views and beliefs. Women also acquired knowledge through comparing their situations with stories from other women, family members and friends:

I liked it, that my mother had the same kind of story and my elder sister, that the first birth was more difficult and the second one was easier. I noticed that I could do something with that information. (Hannah/The Netherlands)

New information received by the women assisted them to feel confident because they had gained in understanding. In order to make this happen, information had to be explained so that it could be assimilated and linked to the knowledge they had about their situation and make it fit:

Well, I suppose knowledge is part of the process, isn't it? You have got to have knowledge. But to be able to do anything with knowledge you have got to have understanding. I suppose, that is the seam to your thinking. (Jan/Scotland)

Relationships also played a role in enabling women to feel confident. In the interaction between a woman and the people with whom she was involved in her world, the experience of pregnancy was 'shared'. This sharing included feelings and knowledge about being pregnant. All women shared their experiences with their partners or friends in order to be understood and not feel alone:

Also involving my husband a bit more in the pregnancy. And also sharing the knowledge that certain things are caused by pregnancy. . . . Something that one would not notice otherwise, or did not know, and blame it on a bad mood, or that it might cause tensions. That you can laugh about it together, and say, yes, we've gone through that, or so. (Sarah/Switzerland)

Knowledge about the health and condition of the baby formed part of this category. This knowledge derived through reading, hearing and seeing played a big role during the first part of the pregnancy. They emphasised the connection between themselves and their babies, and thus the influence of their physical and mental health on the health of the baby. The relationship to the baby, therefore, played an important role for the women.

As pregnancy continued, knowledge about the baby was gained through feeling it moving. The women wanted to use this knowledge to feel confident about the baby too. Therefore, they tried to ensure that the baby was healthy and tried to reduce all possible risks:

Because, when it is just about my own health I can take some medicine. Then it is only about me. But now it is also about someone else. (. . .) Or like eating, I think, when I eat something unhealthy, it is just about me, that is, well . . . But now there is someone else. Responsibility. (Rosemary/Switzerland)

The reflective process came full circle as the knowledge from the several sources was combined again with (personal) feelings. The reflective process stopped when women perceived that they felt confident, and thus relaxed:

I suppose, again your feelings reinforce, that yes, knowledge is there, this is what happens, because of this. So . . . Or this happening, because of this and that is fine. So relax about this. (Jan/Scotland)

On reaching this stage of feeling confident, some Dutch women talked about having a complete image (view), or a 'picture':

So that is what you take with you, in, in your total knowledge picture. (Laura/The Netherlands)

If the result of combining feelings and knowledge was not confidence but uncertainty, often the women experienced a need; they were lacking something. These were physical, emotional and social needs such as reassurance, confirmation, and information about certain issues, which were important to them; sharing their experience, especially the emotional side, including anxieties and worries; or finding encouragement and thus empowering them. With these needs, they went to antenatal care in order to feel confident afterwards:

I have always been looking forward to it. That, when I get home, I am a little bit further. I know exactly, what is till then, what is there, and . . . You go also with the expectation that everything is in order. You are also hoping for that, and, I have always been happy, and thought, well, everything is fine, and . . . (Verena/Switzerland)

If you are having worries all the time and you can share them. And maybe it is not strange, that you are having those worries. Or it appears that there is actually no reason to worry. And that can be made clear to you. Then it can, well, then it can put you at ease, yes. And it can give you a better feeling. Yes. (Hannah/The Netherlands)

As a strategy, when women did not feel confident after antenatal care, they tried to empower themselves through searching for information on their own:

I went to look for information from somebody else to get recognised. Or get an answer to what I felt. Or about what I thought I had to organise or . . . So I tried to solve it in a different way. But actually not with her. (Erin/The Netherlands)

Although women initially felt unsure at the beginning of their pregnancies, as it progressed they drew on various resources to regain a state of confidence, thus enabling them to feel autonomous.

Feeling autonomous

We chose 'autonomy' instead of 'control', because 'control' as a conscious act could be given away in confidence to someone the women trusted to preserve their feeling of autonomy. The Scottish women chose and confirmed the word 'control' as a central issue. The women from the other countries preferred 'autonomy'.

'Feeling autonomous' consisted mainly of 'making your own decisions', and 'feeling in control', which meant participants being able to do what they wanted or chose. This meant either women did things for themselves, or made sure that someone helped them to do what they wanted.

Important issues that resulted from the thinking process in 'feeling confident' were subjected to a decision-making process. Most often, the issues for these decisions in routine antenatal care were antenatal screening and the options for birth or postnatal care. However, in order to make such decisions, choices have to be available. The availability of choice was determined by the health-care system of the country and the information that was provided by the care provider. In The Netherlands, Hannah reflected on her need for advice on antenatal screening, and the ability to choose:

It is also caused by the media. As I get older, it is going to play a bigger role. And then I think it is also important, to get some specific advice on it.

And I want to choose for that, I'd like to have it in my hand, I think. Maybe it is also a bit a phenomenon of this time, but . . . I'd like to make a conscious choice about it. (Hannah/The Netherlands)

The decision-making process included 'thinking over' all the concepts already outlined in the 'feeling confident' category. Therefore, women had to consider all their knowledge on the issue and the options available. During 'thinking things over', risks are determined. These risks were then weighed against each other in order to set priorities and make a decision:

I thought, well, if there is no risk of dying, what is everyone worrying about, you know. Because all the same, I didn't want to be in a situation where I was going to put my own life at risk, cause that would be worse for Robin, than a bit of jealousy about this new baby. So, yeah, I think, you know, all sorts of different things, come in, come into play. (Vanessa/Scotland)

Expectations, wants and wishes resulting from the sub-category 'feeling confident', and issues on which decisions were made, were the topics of 'feeling in control'. Basically, the women expressed the wish that they would be supported in doing what they wanted to do, while they managed and organised their pregnancies themselves as much as possible:

So now I resolved, if it is, if it really stays in a breech position, I will not have a version. Then it just will be a caesarean section, likely with an epidural, then my husband can also be there. And then I can have my baby with me, that is what I want, that is what I think is important. (Ariane/The Netherlands)

Conversely, not all the women wanted to have all the control themselves. There were dimensions in the amount of control women sought. Although these dimensions were also visible across the three countries, there was an explicit cross-cultural difference:

I think emotionally, you know, you have to be in control of it as well. You have to be in control of your environment. And that is what is to be a pregnant mum, you just want to be in control. (Heather/Scotland)

Although, that was decided on by the midwife. (. . .) But that was actually all right. Cause, cause I had the confidence, that it would be okay. (Sarah/Scotland)

I don't want the responsibility of all this being in control. (Nora/Scotland)

Some of the Scottish and Dutch women described the necessary state of mind needed to be able to be in control:

I know what I feel, and until I see it reflected in print, I can't be totally confident enough. (. . .) Not just in print, but also with someone, other people's shared experience. You know, people who have seen it, done it. (Lynn/Scotland)

All women acknowledged that there would always be unexpected situations, during antenatal care and especially during birth. 'Feeling in control', and therefore remaining an autonomous person, required a 'strong attitude' ('feeling confident'). They suspected or knew that they would not have that attitude at birth, both physically and emotionally. Therefore, the women searched for someone they could trust and who shared their views, who helped them and spoke up for them. They needed a

person who could provide them with information, options and support. So then they felt in control throughout antenatal care, birth and postnatal care:

I think, if we had someone like that, a reference person, who, indeed a midwife, who maybe had spoken up, saying, maybe it is better that she goes home and walks around a bit, maybe we could try it this way. (. . .) Because she knows more about it. (Yvonne/Switzerland)

The presence of this person who would help them to gain confidence in themselves and in the care provider made it possible for participants to 'let go'. Some of the women explicitly said they 'surrendered' to the process, and not to the care provider as a person. The women mentioned the importance of being able to 'let go' in order to let the physical process of motherhood (pregnancy, birth) take place:

I can surrender to the process. Then I can let my control go, then it can happen. I think, it is very important during birth, to, to surrender to it. Literally. That is, you need the biggest surrender during birth, because it happens from your inside, and yes . . . I think I need all those conditions to really let go, that is so. (Kerstin/The Netherlands)

You still, well I certainly have a need of to sort of try to be in control. Though of course it is very difficult actually during labour itself. But . . . I think if you don't get the information sort of during labour, it certainly would make, makes me quite angry and uptight. Which of course in the end affects how labour actually progresses. I think, you probably have a lot easier labour, if you understand what is happening to you and, you know, you're sort of prepared with possible ways that it might go. (Jan/Scotland)

The experiences of being able to 'make one's own decision' and 'being able to do what you want' were combined with the feelings again in the subcategory of 'feeling autonomous':

And . . . There is the care again. They also give me there, the feeling that I, I can determine it myself. I like that very much. That just gives me a bit of peace. (Ariane/The Netherlands)

If women felt that their autonomy was not preserved during their own experience of becoming a mother, three strategies were described. These were 'balancing your wishes' or 'giving up' and 'empowering yourself through information':

Also I said to myself, give yourself time because, well, you don't have another choice. You also have to think about the work pressure, that they have. It just can't be different; you have to give it up. (Ariane/The Netherlands)

I'd rather be informed. I mean, I think it is like a patient, that is dying, you know, and do you tell them or not. And I, you know, most people would want to know, and, I think, better prepared and armed than not. (Jan/Scotland)

Finally, the third strategy involved women 'empowering yourself through another person'. In most instances, this was the partner or another care provider:

Which is one of my midwife's role as an advocate. To speak up for you. So that your wishes are known beforehand. And, she would discuss them with you. And you'd get it transferred over to the hospital, whatever that, and you'd still get as far as possible what you'd like. (Lynn/Scotland)

Responsibility

The category of 'responsibility' was generated as a result of collapsing both 'feeling confident' and 'feeling autonomous'. Some women talked about physical and emotional ownership of the experience.

And I think people need to make choices for themselves to have ownership of . . . of the problem, the grief whatever. (Lynn/Scotland)

The women talked about the responsibility they had for themselves, their babies and their environment during the pregnancy until childbirth and afterwards (biophysically as well as emotionally).

Ultimately, if I have made the decisions and things go wrong, the bus stops here. Yeah . . . If they have made the decision and things go wrong, how, how do you deal with that? (Lynn/Scotland)

So, just having to take the responsibility, when she would abort, because of the amniocentesis. (Lilian/Switzerland)

Immediately after childbirth, the women were happy that everything went physically well with the baby and themselves. After a while, they reflected on the physical, social and the emotional aspects of the experience. Again, they tried to relate the experience to their feelings. This process was part of antenatal care, as it included preparing for birth and the postpartum period. Thus, expectations of the experience (picture) were created:

The baby was fine, and, well, apart from jaundice, and the suturing done at the hospital. And . . . even that wasn't a problem. And I didn't realise that was an issue until afterwards. And it kind of worked out later; you're euphoric for the birth of a new baby. And that was fine for about 6 months. (Lynn/Scotland)

So I don't know if this is quite a common thing, you go in, and you think you are going to have an epidural and I was quite disappointed, not to receive an epidural. So that is one thing you know, if I would have a third child, I would maybe think about going private, because an epidural was very important to me. (Susan/Scotland)

Many women expressed the need to talk the experience over postpartum. The opportunity to do this would give them the missing information on the experience, but also the possibility of sharing the experience again:

Or also, it is not just about the burden, it is also about memories, about which, I had a feeling like, did this happen, or what did really happen there. Or, yes . . . (Sarah/Switzerland)

But I could still ask that kind of questions then. And that was very important to me, to get the picture complete. To, yes, let's say, to get the questions answered. So that I could leave it

behind. That it did not remain in (walk around) my mind, like I should have done that, or if I had done this. (Kerstin/The Netherlands)

Through this reflective process, the women aimed for 'the closure of their experience'. To close the experience and leave it behind in order to be able to move on, the women had to pull all their knowledge together and make it 'fit'. Their knowledge and experience were assigned to the category 'feeling confident' and in the sub-category 'knowledge' (experiences). For some women, it took longer than one pregnancy to reach their aim of making it all 'fit':

Yeah, I've come full circle. (. . .) I've got to the point, where I thought I would be embarking on motherhood. I suppose my expectations have now been met. (. . .) And it's been, it's happened the way I envisaged. But it's taken me quite a long time, a few years, to get to that point. (Lynn/Scotland)

A good experience empowered, whereas sometimes a bad experience created more anxieties. These feelings were part of their 'knowledge' in the next pregnancy. Some women called it 'emotional baggage'. A bad experience, however, could also empower. The experience most often made the women feel more confident:

If you go for the first time, for your first child actually you are just a lay person in that area, the further the pregnancy proceeds, the more you get to know actually, and now you are, I do not want to say an expert, but you just know an awful lot. (Marianne/The Netherlands)

And that is why I decided now, I am going to do this quite different. Now I am going to ask questions, now I will really, not think that I am a burden, now I am really going to demand time for me. (Ariane/The Netherlands)

Discussion

This exploratory study addressed antenatal care in three European countries from the woman's perspective using a grounded-theory approach. Two methodological limitations were encountered: organisational and linguistic. Organisationally, it was not possible to fly from one country to another to interview just one person. This problem was met by the assistance of the field notes for sampling and data collection. Thus, a balance could be made between organisational and financial aspects, and allowed an effective number of women to be interviewed in each sample.

The different languages did not limit organisation and data collection, but they did influence data analysis. Grounded theory demanded that data be being broken down into small parts, being closely examined and compared for similarities and differences during the stage of open coding (Strauss and Corbin, 1998; Dey, 1999). The analysis of small units of data is even more important when using different languages. The data collection and analysis was carried out by AGL in the original languages, which also increased theoretical sensitivity for each of the languages concerned.

In order to retain the meaning of what was being said for as long as possible, translation only took place at a later stage of analysis (Strauss and Corbin, 1998). Boufoy-Bastick (2002), in her study on academic attainments in English of different population groups on the Fiji Islands, described 'meta-concepts' to be compared in the anthropological use of grounded theory. These stages of analysis, in which labelling and coding took place in the original language and translation of the concepts at a category level, did not influence the construction of the categories, as these are 'meta-concepts'. Theoretical sampling was richer, as the theory about resulting categories, and also the comparison of the properties and dimensions of each category, created leads. Through the process of the grounded-theory approach, the meaning of these similarities and differences for the women in each of the countries could be verified and explored in depth in the next sample. The intensity of this process might, however, influence the number of women, and the duration of time needed to achieve the objectives, and thus saturation of the categories.

The emergence of similar categories from each country after the first interviews seemed to indicate that one overall model of antenatal care was developing in the three countries. Theoretical sampling, however, emphasised the similar and also the divergent data for each of the countries through which the saturation of the categories could not be obtained. Through the emphasis of these different categories, the most important cross-cultural differences were within the category of 'feeling autonomous'. A bias on behalf of the researcher could be excluded, as the new interviews from the theoretical sample were started with the leading interview question, which gave the women an opportunity to emphasise what they felt was important.

Women reflected on the knowledge they had of 'their worlds'; differences could be attributed to cultural backgrounds, which also include the medical and childbirth culture. The cross-cultural character of the study enriched and gave more depth to the research in different ways, such as the use of different terms for describing experiences and phenomena by the women in the different countries. This prompted a rethink about the meaning of each concept. The meaning of words were, therefore, subsequently checked in a dictionary and thesaurus in each of the languages used. Thus, it was discovered that, for instance, 'feel' had different meanings in the way these expressions were used by the women. In the Swiss data 'it is right/it fits' was used to indicate a balance between 'feelings' and 'knowledge', resulting in 'feelings' again; the Scottish expressions used did not make this clear.

After the first sample, both Swiss and Dutch women emphasised the relationship with the care provider ('to have someone who is always there for me' and 'listening'), whereas the Scottish women emphasised 'knowledge', 'information' and 'feeling in control'. A link between the countries in this respect was absent. Cross-cultural comparison indicated that the theoretical sample had to include women who were cared for by another kind of care provider, which was also mentioned in an interview by one of the Scottish women. This proved to be the right way to continue the constant comparative analysis.

During the interviews, the women seemed to fall back on the things they knew, even though they wanted something different. It proved to be hard to make them create a new solution, outside of the known, familiar system, in order to meet their wishes and expectations. Further research needs to address factors influencing this phenomenon.

Responsibility for themselves, their babies and the experiences of becoming mothers was the primary reason women sought antenatal care. Such responsibility included a feeling of confidence and autonomy. Garcia (1982 p. 89), in reviewing women's views, mentioned the woman's own responsibility and the obvious 'low regard' the antenatal-care system had for women's time and their own commitments; 'in order to act responsibly, pregnant women are expected to attend antenatal clinics and follow instructions' (p. 89). The women in the present study based their sense of responsibility on the results of their experience becoming an integral part of their worlds afterwards. The results indicated that the 'closure of the experience' by the women, through combining their new knowledge with their feelings, happened a long time after the formally defined postnatal period. These findings are important for the timing and the content of the evaluation of care.

The women in this study gained a feeling of confidence through knowledge and information, and through the relationship with the care provider. In this relationship, ideally the 'trust' the women gave is transferred into the 'confidence' that the women gained afterwards. Although information is an important aspect of this relationship, the reassurance included a degree of 'content', and also an 'attitude (behaviour)', which meant health professionals being interested, giving encouragement and reducing anxieties and worries through sharing them and simply 'being with' the women.

Van Manen (2002) highlighted that not much attention had been given to 'care-as-worry', and therefore 'being with', in the caring literature. This aspect of care was mentioned more by Dutch and Swiss women than by Scottish women. This finding is surprising, as 'being-with-women' is also part of the British midwifery philosophy (Wickham, 2004), which is supported by research addressing midwifery practice through interviews with Scottish midwives and clients (Fleming, 1998). In this study, a model of the midwife–client relationship, which also emphasised this interdependency between women and their midwives, was developed.

In her study about experiences of fears in pregnancy and childbirth in Finland, Melender (2002) described the importance of giving women the chance to express and discuss these feelings, with special attention to earlier negative experiences. The term used by women for talking about what and how they felt was 'trust'. In order to 'trust', the attitude or behaviour was more important than the continuity, although the latter was an important factor.

'Feeling autonomous' was another important attribute of 'responsibility'. 'Having choices', 'making decisions' and 'feeling in control' were important aspects of this category in Scotland and in The Netherlands, but hardly featured in Switzerland. It could be argued that the way each healthcare system was organised played a role here. The Swiss women described three levels of care; 'help', 'guidance' (or support) and care'. Although they could judge the content of 'help' and 'guidance', they could not make a judgement about the content of 'care'. An interpretation of the 'appropriate' knowledge level by the women themselves might be an explanation.

The women in The Netherlands referred to the standard care that the system provided them, and some of them wanted more options. Most of them, however, remained ambivalent about whether they should be allowed to have everything. All finally opted for just certain degrees of choice.

Other studies on women's views in Scotland described the importance of issues such as choice, decision-making and control (Hundley et al., 2001; Cheung, 2002). Although the cultural backgrounds could account for these phenomena, the findings of this study pointed in other directions. During antenatal care, a feeling of confidence was built up through knowledge, information and an encouraging attitude of the care providers. Antenatal classes were an important contributing factor greatly appreciated by the women, and, subsequently, expectations and wishes ('images') were created. Through fragmentation of the system, these 'images' were often not met. In order to gain 'control', the women were building up their own confidence ('a strong attitude') even more for possible future pregnancies.

Conclusion

The effectiveness of a programme has been defined as the 'achievement of the aims or objectives' of that programme (Long and Harrison, 1985). Several definitions of the aims of routine antenatal care currently exist. These aims all include the overall health of the mother and baby, but vary from 'reducing perinatal and maternal mortality and morbidity' to 'providing information, advice and reassurance' (Hall et al., 1985; Heringa, 1998; Villar et al., 2001). The aim Keirse (1989) defines for effective care in pregnancy and childbirth is 'what is of importance to mother and child'.

The aim of the women in this study was to be able to bear the responsibility of the experience of becoming a mother. Therefore, they needed to feel confident and to feel that their individual autonomy would be respected. Limitations in the methodological design of this study were of an organisational and linguistical nature, but they did not influence the findings. However, the cross-cultural aspect seems to overcome these limitations and gives even more depth to the study. Validity and reliability was increased through construction and comparison of the categories, and their properties and dimensions in each phase of the analysis, through which verification took place. Theoretical sensitivity was increased by the involvement of only one researcher for all three languages. Although many similarities in the study point towards one model of antenatal care, saturation could not be obtained, as diversities were also emphasised, particularly within the categories of 'autonomy' and 'confidence'. Further study is planned on the basis of the findings of this study, which will explore these differences.

REFERENCES

Boufoy-Bastick, B., 2002. A differential construct methodology for modelling predictive cultural values. The Qualitative Report 7, 1–11 Available from: http://www.nova.edu/sss/QR/QR7-3/boufoy.html.

Cheung, N.F., 2002. Choice and control as experienced by Chinese and Scottish childbearing women in Scotland. Midwifery 18, 200–213.

Dey, I., 1999. Grounding grounded theory. Guidelines for qualitative inquiry. Academic Press, San Diego.

Enkin, M., Chalmers, I., 1982. Effectiveness and satisfaction in antenatal care. Heinemann Medical Ltd, London.

Fleming, V.E.M., 1998. Women- with- women- with- women: a model of interdependence. Midwifery 14, 137–143.

Gagnon, A., 2004. Individual or group antenatal education for childbirth/parenthood. The Cochrane Library, Issue 2. Update Software Ltd, Oxford.

Garcia, J., 1982. Women's views on antenatal care. In: Enkin, M., Chalmers, I. (Eds.), Effectiveness and satisfaction in antenatal care. Heinemann Medical Ltd, London.

Garcia, J., Blondel, B., Saurel-Cubizolles, M.J., 1989. The needs of childbearing families: social policies and the organization of health care.

In: Chalmers, I., Enkin, M., Keirse, M.J.N.C. (Eds.), Effective care in pregnancy and childbirth. Oxford University Press, Oxford.

Glaser, B.G., Strauss, A.L., 1967. The discovery of grounded theory: strategies for qualitative research. Aldine Pub. Co, Chicago.

Hall, M., Macintyre, S., Porter, M., 1985. Antenatal care assessed: a case study of an innovation in Aberdeen. The University Press, Aberdeen.

Haertsch, M., Campbell, E., Sanson-Fisher, R., 1999. What is recommended for healthy pregnant women? A comparison of seven clinical practice guidelines documents. Birth 26, 24–30.

Heringa, M., 1998. Computer-ondersteunde screening in de prenatale zorg (computer-aided screening in anternatal care). Doctoral thesis, University of Groningen. Dijkhuizen Van Zanten bv, Groningen.

Hodnett, E.D., 2004. Continuity of caregivers for care during pregnancy and childbirth. The Cochrane Library, Issue 2. Update Software Ltd, Oxford.

Hundley, V., Ryan, M., Graham, W., 2001. Assessing women's preferences for intrapartum care. Birth 28, 254–263.

Jacoby, A., Cartwright, A., 1990. Finding out about the views and experiences of maternity-service users. In: Garcia, J., et al. (Eds.), The politics of maternity care services for childbearing women in 20th century Britain. Oxford University Press, Oxford.

Keirse, M.H.N.C., 1989. Augmentation of labour. In: Chalmers, I., Enkin, M., Keirse, M.J.N.C. (Eds.), Effective care in pregnancy and childbirth. Oxford University Press, Oxford.

Langer, B., Caneva, M.P., Schlaeder, G., 1999. Routine prenatal care in Europe: the comparative experience of nine departments of gynaecology and obstetrics in eight different countries. European Journal of Obstetrics, Gynecology and Reproductive Biology 85, 191–198.

Long, A.F., Harrison, S., 1985. Health services performance. Effectiveness and efficiency. Croom Helm, Beckenham.

Melender, H.L., 2002. Experiences of fears associated with pregnancy and childbirth: a study of 329 pregnant women. Birth 29, 101–111.

Oakley, A., 1982. The origins and development of antenatal care. In: Enkin, M., Chalmers, I. (Eds.), Effectiveness and satisfaction in antenatal care. Heinemann Medical Ltd, London.

Reid, M., Garcia, J., 1989. Women's views of care during pregnancy and childbirth. In: Chalmers, I., Enkin, M., Keirse, M.J.N.C. (Eds.), Effective care in pregnancy and childbirth. Oxford University Press, Oxford.

Strauss, A., Corbin, J., 1990. Basics of qualitative research. Techniques and procedures for developing grounded theory. Sage Publications, Thousand Oaks.

Strauss, A., Corbin, J., 1998. Basics of qualitative research. Techniques and procedures for developing grounded theory (2nd edn), Sage Publications, Thousand Oaks.

Van Manen, M., 2002. Care-as-worry, or 'Don't worry be happy'. Keynote address: Fifth International Qualitative Research Conference, Qualitative Health Research 12, 262–278.

Villar, J., Ba'aqeel, H., Piaggio, G., et al., 2001. WHO antenatal care randomised trial for the evaluation of a new model of routine antenatal care, Lancet 357, 1551–1564.

Villar, J., Carroli, G., Khan-Neelofur, D., et al., 2004. Patterns of routine antenatal care for low-risk pregnancy. The Cochrane Library, Issue 2. Update Software Ltd, Oxford.

WHO, 1987. Having a baby in Europe. Report on a study. Public Health in Europe 26. World Health Organization Regional Office for Europe, Copenhagen.

Wickham, S., 2004. Being with women. In: S. Wickham, Editor, Midwifery: Best Practice 2. Books for Midwives, London.

Midwifery 2005; 21(3): 212–223.

Women's experiences of unexpected ultrasound findings

Lisa M. Mitchell

Ultrasound imaging is an important screening and diagnostic tool in prenatal care, but for many couples in Canada and the United States, it is primarily a meaningful social ritual of seeing and meeting their baby. This article examines how women perceive ultrasound when they receive unexpected abnormal ultrasound findings. Drawing from qualitative analysis of semistructured interviews with 42 Canadian women, the article discusses women's reactions to receiving unexpected findings, and their perspectives on disclosure of results and on seeing the impaired fetus. Implications are discussed for practitioners regarding prescan counseling, informed choice, and disclosure of abnormal ultrasound findings.

Keywords: fetal ultrasonography, abnormalities, psychosocial aspects

Introduction

Ultrasound fetal imaging reassures most pregnant women. Yet this diagnostic tool includes the risk of detecting fetal demise or anomalies, of missing or falsely detecting anomalies, and of detecting variations in maternal or fetal physiology whose clinical significance is unclear (e.g., choroid plexus cysts or echogenic bowel). Relatively little research attention has dealt with women's responses to unexpected ultrasound findings, despite the widespread use of this technology. We do know that ultrasound is widely perceived by expectant women in North America more as a pleasant opportunity to see the baby than as a screening or diagnostic test.[1–3] Furthermore, there is evidence that women often undergo ultrasound without prescan counselling about its uses, limits, or risks.[1,2,4] In short, how ultrasound is provided to and understood by expectant women raises questions about how well prepared they are for something other than a picture of a normally developing fetus.

This article focuses on the role of the ultrasound in women's descriptions of receiving unexpected findings and seeing the impaired fetus. Women's narratives are drawn from a qualitative study of perinatal loss that examined women's experiences of unexpected ultrasound information. Findings are discussed in the context of current knowledge about the social meanings of ultrasound, parental responses to ultrasound-detected anomalies, and the limited use of informed consent for ultrasound. The ways in which women and their partners make sense of and make decisions following a diagnosis of impairment will be addressed in a subsequent article.

Literature review

Ultrasound imaging has been a key part of antenatal care in Canada, the United States, and Europe for decades.[5,6] One or two ultrasound scans per pregnancy are common. Several clinical trials, metanalyses, and reviews have failed to find either improved maternal or perinatal outcomes or reduced interventions with routine scanning (even when multiple fetuses and intrauterine growth retardation are detected).[7–10] The clinical efficacy and cost-effectiveness of ultrasound screening at 17 to 20 weeks for fetal structural and chromosomal abnormalities are also debated.[11–14] The ability of ultrasound to detect anomalies is affected by factors such as operator skill, equipment quality, timing of the scan, and type of anomaly.[4,7] Persistently high false-positive rates prompted the authors of one metanalysis to conclude, 'Though routine ultrasound scanning does not improve the outcome of pregnancy, it [does] expose pregnant women to the risk of false diagnosis of malformations.'[9]

Although other forms of prenatal testing, including amniocentesis and maternal serum screening, are used only after informed consent has been obtained, the same standard of practice is not routinely applied, apparently, to ultrasound. In a study of 49 women in Montreal undergoing their first routine ultrasound, none had prescan counseling, none reported being asked if they wanted an ultrasound, and none recalled being told what ultrasound could or could not detect.[2] Similar findings are reported elsewhere.[14] The inconsistent application of informed consent may be partially attributable to ultrasound's characterization as 'noninvasive,' without bioeffects or other risks. Some practitioners may resist implementing informed choice for ultrasound. In a study at two British hospitals, radiologist-sonographers were generally unsupportive of a leaflet discussing ultrasound's safety and efficacy and suggesting that ultrasound be offered not 'as routine but as one possible course of action.'[15] Sonographers questioned the quality of information and reasoned that discussing the leaflet with women might increase women's anxiety, cause bureaucratic problems, or be too time-consuming. Midwives in the same study did not share these concerns and supported providing the leaflet to implement informed consent.[15] Women who received the pamphlets were surprised by what they learned, but they expressed no increase in anxiety and were not deterred from having ultrasound.[15] Two separate studies confirm that providing reasons for and against having ultrasound does not necessarily decrease women's willingness to use this technology.[16,17]

Although there are numerous studies examining parental reactions and decision making following an elevated maternal serum screen result or abnormal amniocentesis result, comparable research about ultrasound is rare. Generally, studies of ultrasound-detected abnormalities do not address the specific role of ultrasound in parental experiences.[18–20] The manner of presenting abnormal findings to women, women's ability to see the impairment on screen, and the impact of dashed expectations for a happy 'baby's first picture' have not been systematically studied. There is indication that visualizing the anomaly may affect parental decision making and emotions. Two studies have identified a correlation between the decision to terminate a pregnancy and ultrasound visualization of the anomaly.[21,22] At least one study found more pronounced emotional trauma for women when a major anomaly is detected by routine ultrasound than when detected by amniocentesis.[23] A Belgian study of the psychological impact of ultrasound examinations found the 17 women with an ultrasound diagnosis of fetal anomaly were less satisfied with pregnancy and less reassured by ultrasound than the 26 women with normal findings.[24] A recent qualitative study of 24 women with false-positive results for ultrasound screening of chromosomal abnormalities found women were unprepared for the possibility of detecting a problem and two thirds continued to feel anxious even after a normal result was obtained.[25] Black's qualitative analysis, based on telephone interviews with women undergoing early ultrasound prior to chorionic villus sampling (CVS) or amniocentesis, sheds additional light on the role of ultrasound in women's experiences of pregnancy loss. Forty-four percent of the 105 women in her study felt 'viewing the fetus on ultrasound had made coping with the loss more difficult'; about 10% felt it made coping easier.[26] Studies among women with unproblematic pregnancies demonstrate that ultrasound evidence is widely assumed to be reliable and accurate, that sonographer's descriptions of the image influence women's perception of the state of the pregnancy and the fetus, and that even subtle changes in sonographers' behavior and language may be interpreted by women as meaningful indicators of fetal status.[2,3,27]

Methods

As part of a larger qualitative study of perinatal loss, 42 women were identified who had received unexpected ultrasound results indicating fetal demise or anomalies. Participants were interviewed between August 1998 and July 2001 in urban British Columbia, Canada. Ethics and human subjects' approval was obtained from the researcher's university and from the two research hospitals. Women identified from each hospital's fetal anomaly database were eligible to participate if a fetal demise or anomaly had been detected or suspected through ultrasound at least 1 year prior to recruitment and if they resided within a 1-hour drive from the contact hospitals. Of 201 potential participants identified in the databases, 186 women had current contact information and were notified of the larger study by telephone call or registered letter from hospital clinic staff and invited to contact the researcher if they wanted to participate. In this way, the recruitment procedure protected the identity of the potential participants until they decided to make contact with the researcher. Of the 86 women who contacted the researcher, 42 decided not to participate and 44 were interviewed. Another six women contacted the researcher after hearing about the study from their physician, magazine, or conference presentation. From the total group of 50 women interviewed about perinatal loss, the present article discusses only the 42 women who had unexpected abnormal ultrasound findings. Eight women are not discussed here because they did not have ultrasound or were referred for ultrasound because of elevated maternal serum screening or abnormal amniocentesis results.

The researcher obtained informed consent prior to conducting a 1- to 2-hour single interview with each woman, alone or with her male partner. Data from men's narratives are not included here. To allow the interviewee's story rather than the researcher's assumptions to dominate, an open-ended semistructured style of interviewing was used.[28,29] Interview tapes and field notes were transcribed, and identifying information was removed. To help ensure validity and reliability, the principle investigator and research assistants separately coded transcripts for keywords, emerging themes, and narrative patterns.[28,29] Analysis included descriptive statistics of demographic data and reproductive history and qualitative content analysis of the interviews.

Results

The women were mainly of Euro-Canadian background (93%), married (88%), had postsecondary education (93%), and were employed in professional (50%) or service occupations (40.5%). Mean age was 32.7 years; age range was 20 to 48 years. Nearly one quarter (24%) described themselves as not religious, whereas 43% said religion was important or very important to them.

Most of the initial ultrasounds were conducted at out-of-hospital clinics by a technician-sonographer. Nearly all women underwent at least one additional detailed scan conducted by a perinatologist or obstetrician. The average elapsed time from the ultrasound with unexpected results until interview was 22 months (range 0.5 to 46 months). The interviews focused on the most recent unexpected ultrasound findings (i.e., the results in the recruitment databases). For 14 (33.3%) of the 42 women, those most recent results occurred during a routine Level 1 second trimester scan in their first pregnancy. At the time of their most recent unexpected ultrasound findings, 12 (28.6%) women had one or more normal livebirths and no previous history of fetal loss, and 16 (38%) were multiparas with previous perinatal losses.

Based on the diagnostic information provided by the women, the most recent ultrasound results included a wide range of conditions – from choroid plexus cysts, cleft lip, and club feet to fetal demise, anencephaly, bilaterally absent kidneys, and severely malformed hearts. Slightly more than half of the women faced a lethal or potentially lethal fetal impairment (see Table 3.5.1), and termination was offered to most women. Table 3.5.2 summarizes the outcomes of the 42 women's pregnancies.

Table 3.5.1 Distribution of unexpected ultrasound findings in 42 women

Women's descriptions of ultrasound finding	N (%)
Lethal anomaly (e.g., anencephaly, renal agenesis)	23 (54.8)
Cognitive impairment (e.g., hydrocephaly)	5 (11.9)
Renal (non-lethal) anomaly (e.g., missing kidney, enlarged kidney)	5 (11.9)
Mobility impairment (e.g., spina bifida)	2 (4.8)
Other (e.g., club foot, cleft palate, choroid plexus cysts)	5 (11.9)
First trimester fetal demise	2 (4.8)

Table 3.5.2 Pregnancy outcomes in 42 women

Pregnancy outcome	Weeks N (%)*	Mean (range)
Pregnancy termination (includes 1 multifetus selective reduction)	17 (40.5)	19.2 (14–22.5)
Fetal demise (includes spontaneous loss of one fetus in each of two twin pregnancies)	6 (14.3)	25.4 (14–38)
Neonatal death	4 (9.5)	
Normal infant (includes 3 single fetuses from twin pregnancies)	8 (19)	
Infant with irreparable abnormality (e.g., only one functioning kidney, trisomy 21)	6 (14.3)	
Infants with repairable impairment (e.g., cleft palate)	4 (9.5)	

*Totals add up to more than 100% because of three cases involving both normal delivery of one fetus and loss or termination of other fetuses in the same pregnancy

Five major themes relating to unexpected ultrasound results emerged from the anthropological content analysis of interviews and are discussed in detail below. The themes are 'expecting ultrasound,' 'unexpected results,' 'interruption,' 'problems with disclosure,' and 'seeing the problem.'

Expecting ultrasound

None of the 42 women were asked if they wanted ultrasound. Most women (69%) recalled no prescan discussion with their practitioner about the reasons for having an ultrasound. This group included all 26 women with no previous history of fetal loss and 3 women with a previous loss. Women termed the purpose of the scan as 'making sure everything was alright with the baby' and 'seeing how it's growing.' Primarily, they anticipated ultrasound as a 'fun' or 'enjoyable' opportunity to see and 'meet' and get a picture of their baby. A husband or family member accompanied most women to the scan.

One of the most commonly voiced sentiments among the women was that they had not thought about ultrasound in terms of its potential to detect anomalies. This is reflected in comments from three different women:

We were so naive. We thought we were going to see the baby and get a nice photo.

I had the ultrasound. I did the tests. I couldn't believe it [fetal demise] had happened.

Grandma wanted to come . . . and the kids wanted to come, so they came with us. . . . So everybody's up, you know . . . like, 'Oh, let's go see the ultrasound. Let's go see the baby.'

Only four women said they felt apprehensive or worried beforehand; three of those women had undergone a previous loss. Only 7 of the 42 women (17%), including two preparing for amniocentesis because of maternal age, said that they had specifically discussed the possibility of detecting some problem with their partner before the ultrasound. Raising women's awareness that ultrasound 'isn't always fun' was one of the most frequently voiced responses to the question, 'What would you like to tell women about this experience?'

Unexpected results

Women were given the ultrasound findings in a variety of ways. Nearly two thirds of the women (25 of 42) received a diagnosis and statement of prognosis at ultrasound. Nearly one quarter (10 of 42) were told nothing more about the problem than 'we see something,' or 'there is a problem' or 'you need to see your doctor.' Another seven women (17%) first learned of the problem days later from their regular practitioner. Timing and method of disclosure were not related to either prognosis of abnormality or referral for a detailed fetal anomaly scan.

Even if they were not told that anything was out of the ordinary, women were particularly attuned to the way the scan was conducted and to the sonographer's behavior and comments. Several women felt the scan was taking 'too long' or that the sonographer spent a 'long time' looking at one part of the fetus. The women also reported a range of the sonographer's behavior that alerted them to a problem: 'a look,' 'she was quiet,' 'she turned the screen away,' or 'she looked really frustrated.' Four women who were not told of any problem at the ultrasound recounted that the sonographer had made unsettling comments. For example, one woman recalled that the sonographer kept shaking her head and saying, 'Oh my God.' Another woman recounted:

I said to her [the sonographer], something to the effect of, you know, 'This must be so fun and exciting and everything else.' . . . She made some kind of comment that, you know, like it's not always fun to do. Not everybody gets a healthy baby.

Interruption

As they recounted the abnormal ultrasound, nearly all individuals made reference to a rupture in the taken-for-granted nature of the world, saying, for example, that 'the world stopped,' or 'after I heard that, it was all a blur.' One woman described her ultrasound:

. . . it started out okay . . . [and then the technician's] just like 'Oh, I'll be right back. I've just got to go and talk to the doctor about something.' So we're all sitting there like not breathing, making little jokes: 'Oh she probably can't figure it out. Stupid girl,' you know. And he [the physician] came back and looked

at it for like 30 seconds and looked at me and he just stood back and he said, 'Your baby has what we call anencephaly, which means that it has part of a brainstem, but no brain.' And that was all he said.

Another woman said:

I felt quite in shock. I could hardly breathe. My chest felt tight and I just felt like I wasn't really there. It even felt unreal. . . . You know, it was like it was happening to somebody else. I remember looking at his [the physician's] lips and seeing his lips move and thinking, I can't believe this. It was really hard to breathe.

Although this sense of interruption was undeniably more pronounced for women faced with a lethal or potentially lethal fetal anomaly, it was also experienced when a correctable problem was detected. One participant recounted hearing the diagnosis of cleft palate and lip:

And then, as soon as he started to talk, I could just feel the sense of dread, like 'Oh my God!' I was just, sorta like, my heart was sorta pounding, and it's that scenario where they're talking but you're, you're kind of absorbing it, but not really. You think, 'I can't believe this is happening to me.'

Problems with disclosure

The dissatisfaction voiced about how the scan results were disclosed was particularly marked among women who left the ultrasound assuming everything was fine or knowing only that a problem had been seen. One woman describes what she calls 'my death at 20 weeks':

We went for the 20-week scan. It was all laugh, laugh, smile, smile, and then nothing. The technician said, 'There's a problem; you need to get hold of your doctor as soon as possible.' Well, that was Friday afternoon. So we waited all weekend in a complete panic. First thing Monday morning, I called the doctor. She tells me, over the phone for god's sake, 'Your baby won't survive.'

Similarly, three women described themselves as dismayed and confused when they learned of the problem 'accidentally.' In one case, the replacement for a woman's regular physician began discussing the lethal fetal condition, which had not yet been disclosed to her. Another woman, told by her doctor only that a repeat ultrasound was needed, later saw the first ultrasound report of 'severe oligohydramnios.' And, after admitting that the obstetrician did not want to tell her, one ultrasound technician told a woman she would be called about genetic counseling because choroid plexus cysts had been detected.

Seeing the problem

Ultrasound images of the fetus were incorporated into women's narratives about the disclosure of unexpected results in a variety of ways. Many women remarked that they didn't get to 'see the baby,' that is, the fetal image was not described to them in the expected and often sentimentalized terms used by sonographers to describe 'the baby's' anatomy and activity. Rather, the image was used by sonographers primarily to explain and show the impairment or to explain why further investigation was needed. For some women, ultrasound enabled them to make unfamiliar diagnostic terms meaningful with both an image of and a reference to something concrete and known. Women recounted seeing 'the pear-shaped head' (hydrocephalus), 'a lot of gray area' (teratoma), 'her whole body was swollen' (cystic hygroma), a bowel appearing like 'sausages linked' (duodenal atresia), and a kidney that 'looked like Swiss cheese' (multicystic kidney). In some cases, ultrasound offered a literal picture of the impaired fetus to take home, place in a keepsake box, and show during the interview.

In addition to the ultrasound image as evidence of the impairment, women made sense of the image in a variety of ways, including kinship ties, a vulnerable fetus, a 'good decision,' being a mother, and an image preferable to what might be seen of the physical fetus. A diversity of meanings is evident in the following excerpts from the interviews with four women.

When I saw it, I thought, 'This isn't messed up chromosomes or an elevated triple screen level. This is a real, live baby.'

You could see the head, the legs, and arms moving around. I was really happy. You know it's come up that people ask if I would have done an abortion. You know, 'cause of all them problems. But I didn't even think about it. It was my baby in there.

I remember one thing that upset me. . . . I remember he was trying to get the baby to move, and the baby, like he knows that the baby, like there was decreased fluid and that was part of the problems with the baby. And, um, so he kept . . . he kept jiggling my abdomen with it [the transducer], like trying to get the baby to move. . . . I just didn't like that he was trying to make that baby move.

[Did you want to see the fetus after delivery?] No, I knew. I'd seen the ultrasound, seen her waving. That's my image.

Few women questioned the accuracy of ultrasound findings. Initial ambiguity or uncertainty by sonographers about the nature or extent of the abnormality tended to be explained by women as a problem of the ultrasound equipment. Women whose unexpected findings turned out to be false positives and those whose final diagnoses were different from the initial one blamed the sonographer. A few women, including two who were concerned about diagnostic error, said they 'never really saw' the anomaly. Not all women wanted to see the impairment on screen:

I didn't want to see it. I was like, 'No, I don't want to' . . . at that point [the doctor] said, 'Look at the monitor.' He made me look so he could show me what was wrong with the baby.

Discussion

The women in this study experienced considerable disjuncture between their expectations for a pleasurable picture of the baby and the anxiety, grief, and anger of unexpected ultrasound results. The sense of disruption, and the associated emotional turmoil, is common to other stories of loss and suffering such as the death of a family member, the diagnosis of life-threatening illness, and an abnormal amniocentesis result.[27,30] Unexpected results are particularly unsettling and distressing. However, this study indicates that current practices of ultrasound scanning may contribute to that distress.

Detecting fetal abnormality by ultrasound is 'unexpected,' not only because of the unpredictable nature of genetic and developmental changes and the low likelihood of a problem resulting but also because of the social meanings in which ultrasound is provided to and experienced by women. Ultrasound's location in women's lives as both a device for, and a social ritual of, communication and pleasure makes it a distinctive form of prenatal testing. The social meanings of this technology dominate its medical uses. Ultrasound is strongly associated with 'seeing the baby,' 'getting a picture,' and parental 'bonding' with the baby. Women are not unaware of ultrasound's diagnostic potential, but when they talk about ultrasound as a prenatal test, it is regarded as a source of reassurance rather than a potential source of bad news, as amniocentesis would be.

Ultrasound's association with pleasure and reassurance is perpetuated when there is no discussion between a woman and her practitioner about the pros and cons of this examination. Not only did women in this study and elsewhere say they felt 'unprepared' for the possibility of fetal abnormality,[14,25] but the absence of informed consent and prescan discussion about ultrasound precludes that preparation. Women are not alerted to the potential ramifications of having ultrasound when they are asked if they have booked a scan or when providers say, 'It will show how the baby is doing.' Arguably, many women undergo ultrasound, not because they have made an informed choice to do so but because ultrasound is so much a part of prenatal care and parental expectations that it has become a test that does not require a decision.[14] Stapleton et al.[31] use the term 'informed compliance' to describe a similar situation with maternal serum screening.

Precisely because it is a technology of visualization, ultrasound provides women with an image of the impaired, threatened, or lost fetus. To what extent 'seeing' the fetus and/or the diagnosed condition influenced the decisions of the women/couples interviewed by this author is difficult to assess given the small sample size, the variability of detected conditions, and the lack of a control group. Literature on the impact of seeing is limited, but this study's finding indicates that having a visual image of the problem may be used in diverse ways. Seeing the condition on screen can make its existence 'real,' and as Drugan et al.[21] observe 'can have a considerable impact on helping the parents absorb and comprehend the situation.' Yet, just what 'the situation' is and what is being made 'real' are neither inherent in nor obvious from the ultrasound image. In this study, being told about the presence of a lethal anomaly meant different things to different women: 'not a keeper,' 'a mistake,' 'a baby in need of protection,' 'a fighter,' 'a test sent by God,' and 'something you don't want to see.' This sort of diversity of meanings should not be regarded as evidence of women's failure to grasp 'the reality' of the ultrasound image. Rather, the meaning of the ultrasound image is deeply shaped by a variety of factors including, among others, the sonographer's word choices and behavior, the way in which the clinician describes an impairment's severity, prognosis, and treatment, and the particular beliefs, experiences, and social circumstances of the woman.

The diverse ways in which unexpected findings were revealed to women in this study cannot be explained by either severity of abnormality or diagnostic uncertainty. Different policies at different clinics are probably a key factor, but reports of delays, partial or accidental disclosure, and bluntly worded presentation by sonographers raise questions about those policies.

Conclusion

Eliminating the anxiety and anguish following a diagnosis of fetal abnormality is impossible. However, on the basis of the findings of this study, the following measures might mitigate women's distress.

First, several suggestions arise for practitioners conducting ultrasounds and disclosing results. This study indicates that women want to know during ultrasound if a problem has been detected. Women should not leave the ultrasound thinking all is well, if it is not. Clinic policies should ensure that, if possible, women be given a name and description of the problem and some statement of prognosis before they leave. In addition, sonographers need to be mindful that women continually evaluate their actions and comments. When a problem is seen, it may be helpful for a sonographer to say, 'I'm going to be quiet while I do the examination and then I'll bring in a physician to talk to you about it.' Seeing the scanned impairment may be helpful, but women should be given the chance to decline.

Second, several implications emerge for postscan counseling. To minimize the distress created by waiting for answers, women should be able to talk at length with a provider as soon as possible after a problem has been detected. Ensuring that women have accurate information about the detected problem is essential, but postscan counseling should also provide women with an opportunity to voice their priorities, perspectives, and concerns. Providers might begin with 'Tell me about your ultrasound' or 'Tell me what happened at the ultrasound.' Encouraging women to talk about their sense of 'shock' or 'unreality' may enable them to voice their concern over how the findings were disclosed, their distress about the loss of a hoped-for child, their sense of isolation or stigma, and anxiety about parenting a child with a disability. As well, they may express what Landsman has referred to as 'the fundamental unfairness of bearing infants with disabilities despite . . . prenatal testing . . .and the mother's compliance with the best scientific prescriptions for producing positive pregnancy outcomes.'[32] Some women may benefit from thinking about this sense of interruption as an opportunity to focus on what is happening and make the necessary decisions.

Third, the current findings support and reinforce Baillie et al.[25] in calling for informed choice for ultrasound. Midwifery's woman-centered and non-directive approach to informed choice merits attention as a model for all health care practitioners who refer women for ultrasound[33,34] (Luba Lyons Richardson, unpublished manuscript, 2003). Informed choice should provide women and couples an opportunity to ask questions, to learn about its limitations, and to confront the small but real possibility of detecting a problem and needing to make difficult decisions. Ideally, a practitioner-initiated discussion would occur before the first ultrasound is scheduled. The discussion and written information might include not only reasons for having ultrasound but also the possibility of unwanted findings that may need follow-up testing, the potential and limitations of ultrasound to detect specific types of anomalies, and the risk of false positives and false negatives. Increased awareness of the screening and diagnostic aspect of ultrasound might encourage women and their partners to discuss the ramifications of parenting a child with health problems or disabilities. These discussions are important for fostering more positive images of people with disabilities, better-informed health care consumers, and alternatives to litigation, particularly around 'wrongful birth.' As supporters of women-centered health care have been saying for years, encouraging informed choice leads to reflection, engaged thinking, empowerment, and active participation in life's decisions. Those truly are 'improved outcomes' for pregnancy care.

Acknowledgments

A version of this manuscript was originally presented by the author as Invited Speaker to the 2000 Annual General Meeting of the College of Midwives of British Columbia. The research on which the article draws was funded by the British Columbia Medical Services Foundation and the National Institutes of Health. The author thanks the research participants and three anonymous reviewers.

REFERENCES

1. Green J. Women's experiences of prenatal screening and diagnosis. In: Abramsky L, Chapple J, editors. Prenatal diagnosis: The human side. New York: Chapman and Halls, 1994:36–53.
2. Mitchell LM. Baby's first picture: Ultrasound and the politics of fetal subjects. Toronto: University of Toronto Press, 2001.
3. Sandelowski M. Channel of desire: Fetal ultrasonography in two use-contexts. Qual Health Res 1994;4:262–280.
4. Chitty L. Ultrasound screening for fetal abnormalities. Prenat Diagn 1995;15:1241–1257.
5. Anderson G. An analysis of temporal and regional trends in the use of prenatal ultrasonography. Ottawa: Royal Commission on New Reproductive Technologies, 1992.
6. Levi S. Routine ultrasound screening of congenital anomalies. Ann N Y Acad Sci 1998;847:86–98.
7. Green C, Hadorn D, Bassett K, Kazanjian A. Routine ultrasound imaging in pregnancy: How evidence-based are the guidelines? Victoria: BC Office of Health Technology Assessment 96 2D, 1996.
8. RADIUS Study Group, Ewigman BG, Crane JP, Frigoletto FD, LeFevre ML, Bain RP, McNellis D. Effect of prenatal ultrasound screening on perinatal outcome. N Engl J Med 1993;329:821–827.
9. Bucher H, Schmidt J. Does routine ultrasound improve outcome in pregnancy? Meta-analysis of various outcome measures. BMJ 1993;307:13–17.
10. Bricker L, Garcia J, Henderson J, Mugford M, Neilson J, et al. Ultrasound screening in pregnancy: A systematic review of the clinical effectiveness, cost-effectiveness and women's views. Health Technol Assess 2000;4(16).
11. Levi S, Chervenak F, editors. Ultrasound screening for fetal anomalies: Is it worth it? Ann N Y Acad Sci 1998;847.
12. Getz L, Kirkengen AL. Ultrasound screening in pregnancy: Advancing technology, soft markers for fetal chromosomal aberrations, and unacknowledged ethical dilemmas. Soc Sci Med 2003;56:2045–2057.
13. Smith-Bindman R, Hosmer W, Feldstein V, Deeks J, Goldberg J. Second-trimester ultrasound to detect fetuses with Down syndrome. JAMA 2001;285:1044–1055.
14. Smith DK, Marteau TM. Detecting fetal abnormality: Serum screening and fetal anomaly scans. Br J Midwifery 1995;3:133–136.
15. Oliver S, Rajan L, Turner H, Oakley A, Entwhistle V, Watt I, et al. Informed choice for users of health services: Views on ultrasonography leaflets of women in early pregnancy, midwives, and ultrasonographers. BMJ 1996;313:1215–1255.
16. McFayden A, Gledhill J, Whitlow B, Economides D. First trimester ultrasound screening carries ethical and psychological implications [editorial]. BMJ 1998;317:694–695.
17. Crang S, Valenius E, Dykes AK, Jorgensen C. Women's informed choice of prenatal diagnosis: Early ultrasound examination routine ultrasound examination age-independent amniocentesis. Fetal Diagn 1996;11:20–25.
18. Hunfeld JA, Wladimiroff JW, Passchiere J, Uniken Venema-Van Uden M, Frets PG, Verhage F. Emotional reactions in women in late pregnancy (24 weeks or longer) following the ultrasound diagnosis of a severe or lethal fetal malformation. Prenat Diagn 1993;13:603–612.
19. Jorgensen C, Uddenberg N, Ursing I. Ultrasound diagnosis of fetal malformation in the second trimester. The psychological reactions of the women. J Psychosom Obstet Gynaecol 1985;4:31–40.
20. Salvesen KA, Øyen L, Schmidt N, Malt UF, Eik-Nes SH. Comparison of long-term psychological response of women after pregnancy termination due to fetal anomalies and after perinatal loss. Ultrasound Obstet Gynecol 1997;9:80–85.
21. Drugan A, Greb A, Johnson MP. Determinants of parental decision to abort for chromosome abnormalities. Prenat Diagn 1990;10:483–490.
22. Holmes-Siedle M, Ryynanen M, Lindenbaum R. Parental decisions regarding termination of pregnancy following prenatal detection of sex chromosome abnormality. Prenat Diagn 1987;7:239–244.
23. Dallaire L, Lortie G. Parental reactions and adaptability to the prenatal diagnosis of genetic disease leading to pregnancy termination. Prenatal Diagnosis: Background and impact on individuals. Royal Commission on New Reproductive Technologies. Research Studies 1993;12:495–529.
24. Detraux J, Gillot-DeVries FR, Vanden Eynde S, Courtois A, Desmet A. Psychological impact of the announcement of a fetal abnormality on pregnant women and on professionals. Ann N Y Acad Sci 1998;847:210–219.
25. Baillie C, Smith J, Hewison J, Mason G. Ultrasound screening for chromosomal abnormality: Women's reactions to false positive results. Br J Health Psychol 2000;5:377–394.
26. Black RB. Seeing the baby: The impact of ultrasound technology. J Genet Couns 1992;1:45–54.
27. Rapp R. Testing women, testing the fetus: The social impact of amniocentesis in America. New York: Routledge, 1999.
28. Denizen N, Lincoln Y, editors. Collecting and interpreting qualitative materials. Thousand Oaks (CA): Sage, 1998.
29. LeCompte M, Schensul J. Analyzing and interpreting ethnographic data. Walnut Creek (CA): Altamira Press, 1999.
30. Becker G. Disrupted lives: How people create meaning in a chaotic world. Berkeley (CA): University of California Press, 1997.
31. Stapleton H, Kirkha M, Thomas G. Qualitative study of evidence based leaflets in maternity care. [Internet] BMJ 2002;324:639–644. [cited March 16, 2002] Available from: http://www.bmj.com.
32. Landsmen G. Reconstructing motherhood in the age of 'perfect babies': Mothers of infants and toddlers with disabilities. Signs 1998;24:69–99.
33. College of Midwives of British Columbia. Informed choice policy. Vancouver (BC): CMBC, 1997.
34. International Confederation of Midwives. International code of ethics for midwives: Do they fit your practice? [Internet] Midwifery Today 1996;40(winter). Available from: http://www.midwiferytoday.com.

Journal of Midwifery & Women's Health 2004; 49(3): 228–234

(Reprinted with permission from Journal of Midwifery & Women's Health)

TTP and me

Kirstin Clark

Thrombotic thrombocytopenic purpura (TTP) is an extremely rare blood condition characterised by: fever, microangiopathic haemolytic anaemia, thrombocytopenia, and neurological and renal abnormalities.

The thrombi are composed primarily of platelets with relatively large amounts of von Willebrand factor (vWF). vWF is an integral component of the process resulting in platelet adhesion and aggregation which is vital for normal clotting of the blood. Ultra-large molecules of the factor are especially sticky but are not usually found circulating in the blood. They are normally broken down to smaller sizes by vWF cleaving protease, so vWF retains its adhesive properties without binding inappropriately to platelets and causing undesired clots.

In TTP, vWF is synthesised normally, but its subsequent breakdown is defective due to a lack of vWF cleaving protease. This deficiency may be inherited or due to an acquired inhibitor.

The adult form affects 1–3 per million per year. The cause is unknown but it often follows infection or, in women, oral contraception or pregnancy. Young adults from 20 to 50 years are predominantly affected, with women twice as likely to develop TTP as men. There are cases of so-called congenital TTP, which classically presents in infancy or early childhood. In these patients there is no circulating inhibitor, but vWF cleaving activity appears to be absent per se.

Plasma exchange: a lifeline

Before the introduction of plasma exchange, mortality rates approached 100 per cent. However, survival rates are now in the region of 80–90 per cent. Plasma exchange involves the removal of a patient's plasma and its replacement by donor plasma. This removes circulating antibody against vWF cleaving protease, and provides plasma with normal vWF cleaving protease activity. The procedure usually needs to be performed daily for at least five days to be effective.

I'd never heard of this condition until I was 25 weeks pregnant and found out that my extreme tiredness wasn't due to being severely anaemic but because I was seriously ill with TTP. We didn't know whether I would survive or not.

The only problem I had at the beginning of my pregnancy was severe exhaustion. I was slightly anaemic, and by taking Spatone (natural spa water with a high iron content) and a couple of weeks off work the tiredness subsided to coping levels.

By 25 weeks the tiredness had got worse. I had my blood checked at work, thinking I was just anaemic. The haematologist appeared out of nowhere. My haemoglobin (Hb) was only 8, and my platelets were on the low side, so she wanted to re-check everything and I would get the results after lunch. I was offered a wheelchair to go down to the canteen, but my colleagues would never have let me off the ward if they had known what the real problem was!

My platelets were only 10. I had TTP, but it was curable. That was a relief, as I thought I had something incurable, which frightened me. I was admitted immediately. My baby wasn't that active, but he never was during the day – only at night – so I wasn't too worried. I knew I was having a boy from my 20-week scan. The fetal heart (FH) was okay. My consultant explained briefly what would happen. I would be transferred to the intensive therapy unit (ITU) to have the plasma exchange, but he didn't intend to deliver the baby yet. I was given steroids. Rhodri, my husband, had rushed in, after being told he needed to come immediately. Following a chat with the renal specialist who was in charge of my plasma treatment, I was transferred to ITU.

I didn't feel that ill, just tired. I would have walked to ITU, but the nurses didn't think that was a good idea! I thought I was being transferred because that was where the treatment was done. I had no idea what was really going on, let alone what was about to happen. I thought the treatment would get me to 28 weeks and then the baby would be born. A femoral line was inserted that evening, and my treatment started. The process took three hours to exchange three litres, and the only problem I had was that I fainted because my blood pressure (BP) plummeted.

'The worst moment of my life'

That night I didn't sleep. My baby didn't move, and I was too frightened to ask for one of the midwives to visit. I didn't want what I knew to be confirmed. One of my colleagues did visit at the end of the night. As predicted, no FH. She went to get another sonicaid, the scanner and the registrar. Having the death of my baby confirmed by ultrasound scan was the worst moment of my life. Then all hell let loose. My consultant was called, and Rhodri came rushing in. My mother had rung, and my consultant had spoken to her; he told me that my parents were on their way.

My blood picture was worsening. I was given six units of blood, but I couldn't have platelets as they would clot together. My baby was lying in the transverse, but I was told that the induction would turn him, and I would have Cervogem every two hours until I gave birth. The induction started once my family had arrived from Hampshire. They had been told that they needed to get to the hospital immediately.

There was a high risk of me having a massive postpartum haemorrhage (PPH), so I would need a Syntocinon drip for 24 hours, and I had to give my consent for an immediate hysterectomy if I started to bleed. The underlying implication was that I might not survive, and I did realise that. I gave my consent, but I knew that although God had taken away my baby He wasn't going to take me as well. Apparently I had also said that if anything was to happen I held a donor card. I have absolutely no recollection of saying this, but when my mother told my consultant I carried a donor card he said that I had already told him.

Thirteen hours after the start of the induction I gave birth to my perfect son, Ifan Morgan Clark, at 01.58 on 13 December 2000. It was very emotional. My mother and sister stayed for the birth. Rhodri had waited right up until I had to push, then he went outside. These were the longest few minutes of his life. He said there was a horror film on TV while he was waiting for me to give birth, and it didn't help his anxiety. He was relieved when my sister told him to come back in. And I did not bleed!

I had all the usual photos taken, and I am very grateful that I have got them all. The medical photographer took a lot for me, as the ward camera packed up.

The plasma exchange continued and, now that I had given birth, my blood picture improved rapidly. I left ITU the day after the birth, and went into a side room on the gynae day unit so that Rhodri could stay over until I was discharged. The only problem I had with the plasma exchange was that during my final treatment I had a blood reaction. The doctor was amazed that I didn't know what my symptoms were but, as I said to him, I'd never seen anyone react to blood before. Now I know what it's like!

As I improved, I was told more about what was going on. I knew my consultant hadn't left the hospital for more than 24 hours, until he knew I was out of danger. What I didn't know was that a theatre and staff were on standby once I was in labour until it was certain I wasn't going to have a massive PPH. The next risk was a potential massive stroke, which could have killed me, as I was still forming clots. As my blood picture improved, that danger lessened.

I recovered from the TTP very quickly after I had given birth. I only had six treatments of plasma exchange, with three litres of plasma exchanged each time. All the investigations to find a cause didn't show anything, so the conclusion was that the TTP occurred because of the pregnancy.

It was decided that I shouldn't go back on the combined oral contraceptive pill, and the risk of TTP happening again in another pregnancy was unknown. But I was given the support of all the doctors involved in my case if we decided to try again. We had absolutely no doubts that we would. I finally left hospital two days before Christmas, much quicker than anyone had expected. I was still having regular checks of my full blood count (FBC). Next, I had to come to terms with was the loss of Ifan, and cope with Christmas and New Year.

Future risks in pregnancy

I was reviewed by the haematologists six weeks later. We needed to find out more about future risks in pregnancy, so they decided to check my vWF multimer levels. I was told I had large vWF multimers, which required further investigation, so I needed to see a TTP specialist in London. In the meantime I was not to get pregnant. I was devastated at this news, but it made us both think of what we would do if I was told I should never risk getting pregnant again.

We saw the specialist a month later, and he thoroughly explained the condition to us – including all the risks. We were also told that it was definitely the pregnancy that had caused the condition. He saw 200–300 cases of TTP a year, two or three of them pregnancy or estrogen related. As mine was in this category, it meant I would never be able to take the combined OCP, or hormone replacement therapy later on, as these might lead to another bout of TTP.

The main concern was that TTP could cause a massive stroke, which would probably be fatal. The specialist wanted to find out whether I was at risk of TTP recurring by checking the enzyme that breaks down the vWF. If the enzyme was present, then I had a one in five chance of TTP reccurring in another pregnancy. They would then monitor my blood picture carefully and treat if necessary. If the enzyme was missing, then it would be a completely different picture. I would be at very high risk of the TTP reccurring (I wasn't given a risk factor), but with careful treatment he was hopeful that it could be prevented and I could have a successful pregnancy. It would mean daily aspirin and heparin injections and, from 12 weeks, fortnightly plasma exchange. I would also have to give birth by 37 weeks. In addition, there would be a risk of the TTP occurring following birth.

We asked if he had ever done this treatment in pregnancy before. He had, once, and the woman concerned had already been showing signs of TTP. But her pregnancy had been successful and had gone to term. He was confident that we could also be successful, but there were no guarantees.

We came away a lot more hopeful than we had been when we went in. The blood results showed that I was missing the enzyme, so I would need all the treatment that had been talked about. I discussed everything with my obstetrician and haematologist. I could remain at my local hospital rather than going to Liverpool, which I was highly relieved about. I didn't want to have to travel and be looked after by people I didn't know. I had the support of all concerned, and now all I needed to do was to get pregnant again.

The next pregnancy

I realised I was pregnant again when I was on nights at the end of June 2002. Waves of nausea kept coming over me throughout the shift! I was really excited again, but there was also the trepidation of what was about to happen. Rhodri was pleased, but also very worried. I saw my consultant at six weeks. I was scanned, and a heartbeat was seen. The haematologist was contacted, and I was prescribed enoxaparin 20mg daily. The dose was increased to 40mg at 22 weeks of pregnancy, in accordance with guidelines on high-risk pregnancies with clotting problems. My consultant also informed the renal specialist that I was pregnant, so that he could arrange for the dialysis line to be inserted and the plasma exchange to start.

Although I knew I was going to be seen regularly by my consultant, I also saw my community midwife. She knew me well from my last pregnancy, and we felt it was important to keep midwifery support throughout this pregnancy.

Pregnancy-wise, everything went okay – no severe exhaustion. I was tired, but nothing like last time. I saw my midwife as normal, but was also checked by the consultant every fortnight. He scanned me each time to check on the growth of the baby. It was great for me, as I got to see how my baby was doing, and I had lots of pictures. I am aware of the debate about whether too many scans are harmful to the fetus, but to me it was extremely reassuring. The only thing the scan picked up was a low-lying placenta. At 31 weeks a blood vessel was seen touching the cervix. I really didn't want a caesarean section, but it looked as though I would have to prepare myself for one. However, three weeks later the radiographer said that all was clear – c-section avoided, so I thought.

Preparing for plasma exchange

At 12 weeks I had my dialysis line inserted. It is usually done under sedation and under X-ray control, but the renal doctor didn't want to risk sedating me so I just had plenty of local anaesthetic and minimal X-ray exposure. The line goes in through the right internal jugular vein, into the right atrium. The exit site is buried under the skin, so all you see are the venous and arterial ports, which are used to connect up to the dialysis machine. Everything went well. For a couple of days afterwards it was extremely painful – I felt as though my neck had been hit with a sledgehammer! Two days later the plasma exchange started.

I was given three litres of Octaplas over three hours. Octaplas is made by pooling plasma from donors and treating it with solvent to reduce the increased risk of viruses caused by pooling, and has been shown to reduce the risk of transfusion-related acute lung injury. The renal nurses were great. They don't often do plasma exchange, so they had to come to terms with a different machine, but at least they would all be 'experts' by the end of my pregnancy. I was weighed at each visit, and blood was taken for FBC, clotting, LFTs (liver function tests), U&Es (urea and electrolyte) and LDH (lactate dehydrogenase) levels. I had half-hourly blood observations carried out during the exchange.

The only problem I had with the first treatments was that my BP plummeted and I almost passed out. I also experienced a lot of tingling in my face and hands. This was down to a lack of calcium, so I needed calcium infusions during the exchange. It was also decided that three litres of Octaplas was too much of an exchange at the beginning of my pregnancy, so it was reduced to two litres initially, then increased to two-and-a-half and eventually to three.

The fortnightly plasma exchange proceeded well. My blood was checked weekly, and the platelets remained within normal limits throughout my pregnancy. After each treatment I went up to the antenatal ward to check the FH. Although I could feel movements from 13–14 weeks, it was very reassuring to hear the heartbeat. We knew that the plasma exchange didn't pass through the fetal blood system, but nobody actually knew whether this regular treatment would affect the baby in any way. Also, with my BP plummeting during the first few treatments, it seemed safer to get checked over afterwards.

I stopped working at 16 weeks as it was all getting too much – much to the relief of my colleagues! My consultant was also pleased, as from 12 weeks he had been asking me at each visit when I would be giving up work. I had no problems until I reached 22 weeks, when the line became infected and I needed two weeks of antibiotics. From then on I started having weekly plasma exchange.

The dialysis line needed changing twice due to infection. The first time was at 24 weeks, when the Staphylococcus infection didn't clear up. I had 48 hours of IV antibiotics, going home on oral ones, and the tunnelled line was removed and replaced with a left subclavian line.

Midwife support

I was now beginning to get very edgy, as it was coming up to the time when everything had gone wrong with Ifan. Once I was out of hospital I couldn't feel the baby move, and I panicked. My community midwife was excellent. She visited daily to listen in until I was over my crisis point, which only lasted a week, then I relaxed again as the movement went back to normal. She would have continued visiting every day until I gave birth if I wanted her to, and it was really reassuring to know that she was there for me as and when I needed her.

The next infection occurred at 30 weeks, over New Year. Initially I had 48 hours of IV antibiotics, and went home on oral ones. But a week later I was readmitted with a temperature of 40 degrees and rigors. The line was immediately removed, and I had more IV antibiotics. I was given steroids, but it was felt that it was best not to give birth yet.

Once my temperature was back to normal, I had another tunnelled line inserted on my right side. This time it was felt safe to sedate me, but the line insertion turned out not to be a simple procedure. There were three attempts to get it in, and as it went into the right atrium I felt as though I was going to die – I suddenly couldn't breathe, and my heart was racing away. Luckily I didn't have a pneumothorax, just muscular spasms which weren't helped by me panicking. But it did have everyone very worried. So much so that when this line stopped working three weeks later the renal doctor didn't want to put a new line in unless it was absolutely necessary. That experience finally put me off ever risking another

pregnancy again, no matter what the result of this one would be.

I saw my haematologist at 33 weeks. She was pleased that everything was going well, and said that I was very lucky. I had my enzyme levels checked to see whether I would need to continue with plasma exchange after birth.

My third line stopped working after three weeks, and as I was now 35 weeks pregnant it was decided that I should come in to be induced that day. I was highly relieved as I was now getting scared of things going wrong at the last minute, and had been planning to ask to be induced at 36 weeks.

The induction failed – I had no tightening at all – so after 24 hours we decided to have a caesarean section.

After a couple of attempts at getting the spinal in, and my waters breaking in the anaesthetic room, my son, Gwion Morgan, was born on 1 February 2003 at 21.16, weighing 6lb. He came out crying, which was extremely reassuring, but it brought back a lot of memories of Ifan – why couldn't he have been born crying? It was all very emotional. I think my colleagues were looking through the theatre doors to make sure everything was okay – at least, I was told I had an audience at the doors and that I should charge a fee! Rhodri cut the cord, and then ran round taking lots of photos.

Everything had gone well. Gwion ended up in SCBU overnight because he was grunting, but he was back with me in the morning. He was tube-fed for the first few days, but once he pulled his tube out he breastfed well until I stopped feeding him at three months.

A lucky escape

I recovered from the surgery well. I had very little pain. In fact, I used more analgesia after having my lines put in than I did after the section. I discovered that it was a good thing that Gwion had been born instead of waiting another week or two as the placenta had started to separate at the edges. The histology report showed that 20 to 25 per cent of blood volume had been lost – yet I had had no pain or any PV (per vaginam) bleeding. A lucky escape.

The enzyme results came back from London, showing that the levels were still well below normal. They did not return to normal when mixed with plasma, which meant that I didn't have an inhibitor to the enzyme. This meant that the plasma exchanges had been working to stop me developing TTP; without them, the TTP would almost certainly have returned. The advice was for me to continue having plasma exchange for another six weeks, as there was still a risk of occurrence in the postnatal period. However, my doctors decided against this because of the difficulties putting the line in, which would mean that I would have to have a femoral line inserted – not ideal. Also, my blood was absolutely normal, there was no sign of the TTP occurring, and in my previous pregnancy I had recovered from the TTP very quickly after the birth so it was felt that there wasn't a great risk of TTP occurring in the postnatal period.

I stayed in for 10 days. My blood was checked daily and it remained normal. It continued to be closely monitored for the postnatal period because of the risk of TTP reccurring, but thankfully it never did. I remained on Clexane for three months. I worked out that throughout my pregnancy I had 50 litres of Octaplas.

A thriving baby

Eighteen months on and all is well.

Gwion is thriving. The whole experience was much more stressful than I had ever anticipated, but I'm very glad I did take a risk and that the outcome was very good. I was lucky this time, but I'm not going to risk getting pregnant again; the outcome might be very different.

Initially I was monitored every three months by the haematologists, and now it's yearly. I naturally have low levels of the enzyme, rather than having developed an inhibitor to it, which I think means I have a congenital form of TTP. I had haemolytic anaemia as a baby, and the haematologists now think that this was almost certainly TTP, as the blood results were very similar to those in TTP. Hopefully TTP will never recur, but I don't worry about that. Whether Gwion will develop TTP we don't know, but we have been told that it is very unlikely that he will.

Losing Ifan was very hard, and there are still difficult days. But his death saved my life, and in turn it is the reason we have Gwion. Looking upon it that way was the only way for us to come to terms with Ifan's death.

I am a member of a very good internet support group for TTP. They have all been very interested in my pregnancy, and it has given hope to a few of them. One American asked me how I could afford all this treatment throughout my pregnancy. I answered, 'because of a wonderful system called the NHS'.

I would like to thank everyone involved in my care. But I would especially like to thank all those anonymous blood donors, because without them neither my son nor I would be here today.

End note

It is now seven years since we lost Ifan. Gwion is now 5, and two years ago we adopted a baby girl from China, Ceinwen, who is now 3. We now have a wonderful family.

I have since become a Stillbirth and Neonatal Death Society (SANDS) befriender and I try to help other families that have lost babies.

I still have annual check ups for TTP, and thankfully it has never reoccurred. Because we don't know what will trigger it, when I had surgery recently, I was given a plasma transfusion prior to going into theatre, as a precaution.

Ifan is still very much in our hearts and thoughts. Both children know that they had an older brother. They often ask to go and visit him at the Marble Church, where he is buried, and whenever we drive past, they always shout out 'Hello Ifan, goodbye Ifan', which always makes me smile. Ifan will never be forgotten.

REFERENCE

Information about TTP is taken from a factsheet written by Dr Sarah Allford, research registrar, and Professor Samuel Machin, professor of haematology, at UCH: http://www.netdoctor.co.uk/diseases/facts/ttp.htm

OTHER USEFUL WEBSITES

http://www.TTPNetwork.org.uk
http://moon.ouhsc.edu/jgeorge

The Practising Midwife 2004; 7(8): 13–17

A guide to less common antenatal blood tests

Kath McKay

There is evidence to suggest that, for women with a pre-existing medical disorder or a pregnancy-induced complication, pregnancy outcome is more likely to be adversely affected (RCOG 2001). As part of her role, the midwife has a duty to refer a woman for medical opinion if she has detected an abnormality in the progress of the pregnancy (UKCC 1998). In addition, she requires knowledge of such complications and the care that may be involved in order to provide appropriate information to the women and her family (NMC 2002).

In contemporary midwifery practice, there are so many blood tests available to inform antenatal care that it is easy to feel overwhelmed. The aim of this article is to discuss some of the less common, specialised tests that may be used, and for which women and their families will require an explanation. Earlier articles in this series relate specifically to pre-eclampsia and iron deficiency anaemia (McKay 1999, 2000).

The tests to be discussed here are related to familiar medical complications encountered by the midwife: diabetes, hypertension and thrombosis.

Glycated haemoglobin (HbA1c): monitoring glycaemic control in diabetes mellitus

As part of the care given to pregnant women with Type 1 diabetes, frequent estimations are done of the blood levels of HbA1c.

Type 1 diabetes is defined as an autoimmune disorder that causes destruction of the beta cells in the pancreas and results in a failure to produce insulin by the individual (Atkinson and Eisenbarth 2001). As insulin has a role in transporting glucose from the blood into the body's cells, a lack of it will result in an abnormally high blood glucose level. One of the aims, therefore, in managing Type 1 diabetes is to 'normalise' the blood glucose levels by using an exogenous source of insulin provided via a Novopen or syringe.

In any non-diabetic individual, as a natural occurrence, a particular percentage of the haemoglobin in the blood is modified and becomes attached to carbohydrate molecules circulating in the blood. This type of haemoglobin is then termed glycated or glycosylated. There are subdivisions to adult haemoglobin (HbA), and it is HbA1c that binds to glucose.

Thus, measuring the level of HbA1c in an individual is considered to be helpful in monitoring glycaemic control. For example, a high HbA1c indicates a higher percentage of glycated Hb, which suggests that there has been a high blood glucose level present.

As red blood cells have a lifespan of approximately 120 days with a constant turnover, the HbA1c measurement reflects blood glucose levels over the six to eight weeks prior to the test (Kilpatrick et al 1994). If glycaemic control is good, then HbA1c levels will approach non-diabetic levels.

In clinical practice, normal reference ranges may vary between areas. In an audit of 22 maternity units, the 'norm' for HbA1c estimation ranged from 4.6–8.2 per cent (Penney and Pearson 2000). It is recommended that the HbA1c estimation is best carried out at four- to six-week intervals, which will indicate long-term control. In pregnancy, however, HbA1c is often carried out more frequently as the aim is to keep strict glycaemic control within a very narrow range (blood glucose 5–6mmol/L), and insulin demands change as gestation progresses (Mitchell 2001). Therefore, monitoring of glycaemic control in pregnancy is more intense than in the non-pregnant diabetic population.

It has been suggested, however, that there are limitations in using glycated Hb as a monitoring test. According to Kilpatrick (2000), two individuals may have the same HbA1c levels over a six-week period, but self-monitoring of blood glucose may indicate large fluctuations in blood glucose levels in one individual and tight control with little variation in another. Also, some individuals are noted to be faster 'glycators' than others, so it may be more useful to monitor an individual's own serial measurements over time, rather than a 'one level fits all' approach. Other lifestyle factors, such as smoking and age, have also been found to influence variations between individuals (Kilpatrick 2000).

The values of HbA1c during pregnancy in healthy women have been shown in some studies to be lower in the first and second trimesters. In other studies, values were found to be similar to those of non-pregnant women (Ramsay et al 1996).

Hypertension of unknown origin: the detection of phaeochromocytoma

In clinical practice, pregnant women with a history of hypertension at any time in pregnancy warrant further investigation as it is an abnormal deviation from the adaptive changes normally observed. Raised blood pressure (BP) is a sign of potential pathology, and the cause needs to be established in order to provide appropriate management.

The most common cause of hypertension in pregnancy detected by midwives is pre-eclampsia. However, other causes of hypertension that are not pregnancy-induced need to be excluded. In order to do this, a vanillymandelic acid (VMA) test may be requested to explore the differential diagnoses in women with raised BP and to exclude the presence of phaeochromocytoma, a tumour of the adrenal medulla. This is a rare disease, with the incidence estimated to be 1/50,000 term pregnancies (Smith and Wigent 1998).

A phaeochromocytoma secretes additional adrenaline and noradrenaline in excess of the normal production of the adrenal medulla. The tumour can be malignant or benign. As adrenaline and noradrenaline have an effect on the cardiovascular system, resulting in changes in heart rate, an over-production of these substances can manifest itself with persistent hypertension (Thabrew and Ayling 2001). VMA is a breakdown product of the catecholamines adrenaline and noradrenaline, and is excreted in urine.

As the symptom may also be caused by pre-eclampsia, a measurement of VMA may be carried out to exclude the presence of a phaeochromocytoma. The test involves a 24-hour urine collection, with increased levels suggesting the presence of a tumour. Foods including walnuts, bananas and vanilla may cause a false positive, and should be avoided around the time of testing. Due to the nature of the test and the risk of malignancy, great sensitivity needs to be used to explain the significance of the test to a woman.

Drug therapy to control the hypertension and surgical removal of the tumour are the available treatments. The timing of these treatments is individualised for the woman

and depends on gestation of the pregnancy, location of the tumour and stabilisation of the disease. Antenatal diagnosis and treatment have been associated with improved outcomes for the woman and the fetus (Smith and Wigent 1998).

Investigations into the nature of hypertension in pregnancy are important as raised blood pressure is an important sign of potential maternal and perinatal complications; identifying the cause is vital in order to guide the appropriate management. Together, hypertensive and thromboembolic disorders account for 50 of the 106 total direct maternal deaths documented in the most recent Confidential Enquiries into Maternal Deaths (RCOG 2001).

Blood tests relating to the diagnosis of deep venous thrombosis

Thrombosis and pulmonary embolism continue to be the most common cause of direct maternal deaths. Thirty-five direct deaths were recorded in the most recent report on maternal death (RCOG 2001).

The reasons why women are at increased risk of such disorders are well established, and recommendations have been made in this report to reduce the risk further (RCOG 2001). However, an area of continued concern is the difficulty in prompt diagnosis.

For example, the clinical features of deep venous thrombosis (DVT), including redness/discoloration, swelling, pain/positive Homans' sign and warmth or coolness depending on the vein obstructed are not always evident. Even when these symptoms are present, they have a low detection rate (Gorman et al 2000).

As a prompt diagnosis is crucial, other non-invasive tests may be used. One of the dominant tools for diagnosis of DVT is Doppler ultrasound (Girling 2001). However, a combination of non-invasive diagnostic approaches is often used, involving ultrasound with blood tests – for example, D-dimer and physical clinical examination (Gorman et al 2000).

D-dimer measurement

D-dimer is a product of fibrinolysis, and levels can be measured from a venous blood sample. Raised levels are suggestive of increased fibrinolytic activity, which may arise from increased fibrin (clot) formation and be suggestive of a thrombosis.

However, levels of D-dimer can also be raised in many conditions, including infection, inflammation and trauma (Egermayer et al 1998). Therefore, on their own, raised D-dimer levels cannot be used to diagnose venous thromboembolism but may be useful in informing clinical scenario, together with clinical signs and results of ultrasound findings. Different laboratories use different assay techniques to measure D-dimer – there is no single standard numerical reference range. Results are usually described as D-dimer positive or D-dimer negative, the former suggesting raised levels.

However, in pregnancy, D-dimer may be elevated as a result of the prothrombotic changes that occur (Girling 2001). It could therefore be argued that raised levels should not be considered relevant in pregnancy as all pregnant women would have elevated levels. If, however, a modified 'normal' measurement for pregnancy is available, D-dimer measurement could aid diagnosis. Therefore, if D-dimer levels are to be used in any way to inform clinical decisions, they ought to be viewed in the context of the pregnant state and not on non-pregnant ranges.

Antiphospholipid antibodies: anticardiolipin and lupus anticoagulant

When a pregnant woman is admitted to hospital with a suspected DVT, a blood test for antiphospholipid antibodies may be requested. Obstetric problems such as thrombosis, pre-eclampsia and recurrent pregnancy losses are an indication for testing for the presence of such antibodies (Hewell and Hammer 1997). The presence of these antibodies is not diagnostic of thromboembolism, but provides insights into the possible origins of the problem.

In certain individuals, the presence of one or both of these antibodies in their blood may be suggestive of an increased risk of arterial and venous thrombosis. The antibodies in question are called anticardiolipin and lupus anticoagulant (the term lupus anticoagulant is a misnomer, as it does not prolong bleeding but causes thrombosis). These autoantibodies are produced by the individual and are active against coagulation proteins. The presence of one or both is indicative of a much broader phenomenon called Antiphospholipid Syndrome (APS), an autoimmune disease associated with thrombophilia (Atterbury et al 1997). Women who have this syndrome have an increased risk of arterial or venous thromboembolism, recurrent pregnancy loss or thrombocytopaenia. The results of such tests will be considered in the context of the total clinical scenario.

Conclusion

This article has provided an explanation of specific, less common blood tests that relate to potential complications in pregnancy. With more understanding of the rationale for these particular tests, the midwife can feel more confident in providing information and support to women who may require them as part of their care in pregnancy. Although the tests described form a very small part of the overall care pregnant women with diabetes, hypertension or a suspected DVT may require, clearer understanding will enhance midwifery care.

REFERENCES

Atkinson M A and Eisenbarth G B (2001). 'Type 1 diabetes: new perspectives on disease pathogenesis and treatment'. The Lancet, 358: 221–229.

Atterbury J L, Munn M B, Groome L J and Yarnell J A (1997). 'The antiphospholipid antibody syndrome: an overview'. Journal of Obstetric, Gynecologic & Neonatal Nursing, 26 (5): 522–530.

Egermayer P, Town G I, Turner J G et al (1998). 'Usefulness of D-dimer, blood gas and respiratory rate measurements for excluding pulmonary embolism'. Thorax, 53: 830–834.

Girling J (2001). 'Thromboembolism and thrombophilia'. Online: http://www.sciencedirect.com/science/journal. [17.2.04]

Gorman W P, Davis K R and Donnelly R (2000). 'Swollen lower limb – 1: general assessment and deep vein thrombosis'. British Medical Journal, 320: 1453–1456.

Hewell S W and Hammer R H (1997). 'Antiphospholipid antibodies: a threat throughout pregnancy'. Journal of Obstetric, Gynecologic & Neonatal Nursing, 26 (2): 162–168.

Kilpatrick E S (2000). 'Glycated haemoglobin in the year 2000'. Journal of Clinical Pathology, 53: 335–339.

Kilpatrick E S, Rumley A G, Dominiczak M H and Small M (1994). 'Glycated haemoglobin values: problems in assessing blood glucose control in diabetes mellitus'. British Medical Journal, 309: 983–986.

McKay K (1999). 'Biochemical and blood tests in midwifery practice (1) – pre-eclampsia'. The Practising Midwife, 2 (8): 28–31.

McKay K (2000). 'Blood tests in pregnancy (2) – iron deficiency anaemia'. The Practising Midwife, 3 (4): 25–27.

Mitchell M (2001). 'Improving maternity care for pregnant diabetics'. British Journal of Midwifery, 8 (9): 560–564.

Nursing and Midwifery Council (2002). Code of professional conduct, London: Nursing and Midwifery Council.

Penney G C and Pearson D (2000). 'A national audit to monitor and promote the uptake of clinical guidelines on the management of diabetes in pregnancy'. http://proquest.umi.com/pqdweb [9.9.03].

Ramsay M M, James D K, Steer P J et al (1996). Normal values in pregnancy, London: WB Saunders.

Royal College of Obstetricians and Gynaecologists (2001). Why mothers die: 1997–1999, the fifth report of the Confidential Enquiries, London: Royal College of Obstetricians and Gynaecologists Press.

Smith C M and Wigent P J (1998). 'Phaeochromocytoma in pregnancy: considerations for the advanced practice nurse'. Journal of Perinatal & Neonatal Nursing, 12 (2): 11–25.

Thabrew I and Ayling R M (2001). Biochemistry for clinical medicine, London: Greenwich Medical Media Ltd.

United Kingdom Central Council for Nursing, Midwifery and Health Visiting (1998). Midwives' rules and code of practice, London: United Kingdom Central Council for Nursing, Midwifery and Health Visiting.

The assisted conception pregnancy

Jo Morgan

Many previously infertile couples have been enabled to achieve a pregnancy following the scientific and clinical advances in reproductive technologies. The development of in vitro fertilisation (IVF) and allied assisted conception techniques over the past three decades have attracted considerable media interest and drawn public attention to infertility. Since the birth in 1978 of Louise Brown, the first 'test tube baby' conceived by IVF (Denton 1996), public awareness of what can be achieved has led to an increase in demand for infertility treatment.

As infertility affects approximately one in six of all couples attempting to start a family, 25 per cent of whom will be helped by IVF and its allied assisted techniques (Joels and Wardle 1994), the impact on midwives is becoming significant. Pregnancies resulting from this technology present a number of unique problems. This article will explore the psychological, physiological and emotional needs that the midwife may encounter while caring antenatally for a woman and her family who have finally achieved a pregnancy following one of these treatments.

It will be assumed that the pregnancy is that of a single fetus, and that donor gametes have not been used, as the many issues that arise from multiple pregnancy or the use of either ovum or sperm from a donor justify a separate article. There are many different techniques of assisted conception based on IVF and using the same principles – differing merely by the site at which the gametes are placed and at what stage of development they are returned to the body. The main methods are shown in Box 3.8.1, and the care discussed in this article could apply to any one of these techniques.

Pregnancy confirmed

The infertility centre at which the woman has received treatment usually makes a pregnancy diagnosis much earlier than following a normal conception as the woman's

Box 3.8.1	IVF and allied assisted conception
GIFT	Gamete intrafallopian transfer
ZIFT	Zygote intrafallopian transfer
DIPI	Direct intraperitoneal insemination
DOT	Direct oocyte transfer
POST	Peritoneal oocyte and sperm transfer
ICSI	Intracytoplasmic sperm injection

cycle is monitored so carefully. Once a positive test has been achieved, an early ultrasound scan will be carried out, usually between six and eight weeks' gestation (Sidebotham 1997). This is carried out, first, to ensure that it is not an ectopic pregnancy; and, second, it is a legal obligation of the Human Fertilisation and Embryology Authority (HFEA) to maintain a register of the outcome of all treatment cycles resulting in a pregnancy. Its definition of a clinical pregnancy is the presence of a fetal heart on an ultrasound scan (HFEA 1995).

Once a diagnosis has been made and the ultrasound scan done, the woman's care is usually passed to the maternity services in the area in which she lives. This change can often lead to a sense of abandonment as the healthcare professionals with whom she now has contact may not have her full history and therefore have no concept of the years of investigations and treatment that she and her partner have endured or the stress with which they have had to cope.

The couple will be acutely aware of the possibility of pregnancy failure after, often, a long history of unsuccessful attempts at conception and the subsequent feelings of loss and bereavement (Bryan 2000). Dunnington and Glazer (1991) suggest that the pregnancy may even be denied in its early stages as emotional protection against failure. When the couple are slotted into the 'routine' antenatal care system they may be unable to express their doubts and fears with carers who see only the success of a pregnancy. In addition, the woman may struggle to lose her infertile identity, particularly as this infertility has not been corrected, merely bypassed by the IVF treatment, and once the baby is born she will return to being the infertile woman that she has seen herself as being for so long. This can have a detrimental effect on maternal-fetal bonding (Dunnington and Glazer 1991).

If the midwife is sufficiently knowledgeable about the psychological effects of infertility, and can competently and compassionately impart information to the woman and her partner while allowing them to discuss their fears and worries, she can help the couple to accept and enjoy this pregnancy. Reassuring them that most people experience some of the same fears, regardless of conceptual origin, can often help them to see themselves as 'normal'.

Confidentiality and continuity

Some people may choose not to reveal the method of conception. The HFEA (1993) demands that confidentiality be maintained and that the licensed infertility centre cannot pass on information without the parents' consent. The couple may be happy to inform the named midwife of the type of conception but request that this is not recorded on the antenatal notes; the midwife must comply with this request carefully in order to meet both the Nursing and Midwifery Council Code of Professional Conduct (2002) demand that she protects confidential information and the couple's own request. However, if the couple are open about the method of conception, care can be thoroughly planned in conjunction with the infertility centre.

Sidebotham (1997) advocates that continuity of care is essential to build up a trusting relationship. The woman's care should be carefully planned at the booking interview: the named midwife or lead professional may wish to liaise with the councillors at the infertility centre who may, together with the couple, suggest how the woman can make the transition from seeing herself as an infertile woman to a healthy woman expecting a baby.

Screening

Screening for fetal abnormality can pose further problems for the couple. They will need careful counselling before any screening procedures, relying on medical staff to give accurate information on all screening techniques and the implications of their results. A trusting relationship with a midwife who can offer fully informed choice in a caring and sensitive manner will assist them with their painful dilemmas (Sidebotham 1997).

When there has been a delay in conceiving, women are more likely to be in the higher age bracket and thus considered at risk of certain fetal abnormalities. They will be offered the same routine screening as all pregnant women (Joels and Wardle 1994). This may be the triple test or a nuchal fold scan: these are non-invasive screening tests that will give the couple a clearer knowledge of the individual risk of carrying a child with Down's syndrome or spina bifida (Sidebotham 1997).

Should the projected risk of the baby being affected be above accepted limits, they will then have to make the difficult decision whether to go ahead with invasive tests such as amniocentesis, which increases the risk of miscarriage, or to have no further tests. Whatever the couple decide they will need a great deal of support and understanding. An older mother who has been subjected to years of fertility treatment and finally achieves a pregnancy may wish to decline all tests and go ahead with the pregnancy regardless of outcome; she should be able to discuss all the implications with the midwife in a non-judgemental atmosphere (Denton 1996). The midwife must also be able to refer her to the appropriate support agencies should the outcome of these testing procedures indicate any abnormalities.

A relatively new issue these pregnant women and their families face is that of medical research studies making newspaper and television headlines – sometimes regardless of their size or validity. A recent study by Kurinczuk (2002) looked at the rate of major defects in babies born after IVF and ICSI, and found that children conceived through these two methods were twice as likely to have a birth defect. Several possible explanations were put forward, including the underlying cause of the original infertility, drugs taken to encourage or maintain ovulation, and some aspects of the actual techniques used. However, fertility experts have cautioned that these findings contradict other studies that failed to find any increased risk of birth defects, and that further studies are needed to confirm the findings (Gottlieb 2002).

Such studies add to parents' anxieties and fears; the midwife caring for them will be in the frontline to supply them with information, and will need to be aware of what has been published and its validity. The National Electronic Library for Health website (www.nelh.nhs.uk) has a useful 'Hitting the headlines' link that analyses the research that has led to newspaper articles. Access to this may enable the midwife to gain valuable information to help support parents.

Antenatal care

Antenatal care for the woman with an IVF or allied assisted conception of a single fetus is, in principle, the same as that for a naturally conceived pregnancy – following the normal pattern of antenatal clinic visits, ultrasound scans, blood tests and home visits. However, Joels and Wardle (1994) argue that the midwife must be aware that these woman and their partners do have increased psychological and emotional needs, and may be much more anxious than usual. The midwife therefore has the important role of assisting them to control their fears and anxieties, and helping them to form a bond with the fetus.

As mentioned earlier, many couples use denial of the pregnancy as emotional protection against failure. This must be resolved during pregnancy and, with the midwife's help, the couple can prepare realistically for life with a new baby and reduce the possibility of postnatal depression. Denton (1996) suggests that they may have spent many years avoiding being with parents of young babies because of the pain it caused them. They should be encouraged to join antenatal classes and mix with other pregnant women. Friendships often form at this point that can provide an invaluable support network after the baby is born, and classes also enable the parents to discuss their child development with other parents and realise that their child is really no different from the rest, despite its more unusual conception (Sidebotham 1997).

Increased risks

Joels and Wardle (1994) report that pregnancies resulting from IVF and allied assisted conceptions carry increased risks for both mother and baby during the antenatal period. These are often associated with the underlying cause of the couple's infertility. Polycystic ovarian syndrome (PCOS) can cause an increased secretion of luteinising hormone (LH), which increases the risk of miscarriage in IVF pregnancies by 28 per cent. Women with PCOS also have increased insulin resistance, and are therefore more likely to develop gestational diabetes and hypertensive disorders of pregnancy.

Treatment with gonadotrophin-releasing hormone analogues and gonadotrophins to stimulate multiple follicular development for assisted conception can cause ovarian hyperstimulation syndrome in which the ovaries swell dramatically and exude fluid into the peritoneal cavity. This leads to major changes in the woman's electrolyte balance and coagulation. The woman will experience nausea, vomiting, abdominal distension and breathlessness; this may persist for several weeks into the pregnancy, and in some cases require treatment in hospital. As already noted, women with an IVF pregnancy are often older, and there is an increased risk of early miscarriage in those over 40 (Joels and Wardle 1994). Recent research by Wang et al (2002) indicates that gestational hypertension and pre-eclampsia are more common in women implanted with an oocyte fertilised with surgically obtained sperm rather than with their partners' ejaculated sperm.

The midwife should quickly be able to recognise any potential deviation from the norm that may indicate these problems, and sensitively refer the woman to the appropriate professional. However, as Sidebotham (1997) points out, because of the woman's often increased anxiety levels any extra medical attention could prove worrying rather than reassuring. Care should therefore be taken to discuss any symptoms thoroughly in an attempt to achieve a happy medium of care. The midwife should also ensure that the woman and her partner are kept fully informed and involved in all decision-making throughout.

Women who have entered their pregnancies with high levels of anxiety often misinterpret the normal physiological signs of pregnancy, such as backache or associated aches and pains, as an indication of something more serious caused by the way in which they achieved this conception (Bryan 2000). While recognising that there are some increased risks, the midwife must sensitively reassure the woman when her symptoms are normal.

A search of the literature reveals that few pieces of research have been undertaken examining the symptomology of pregnancy, and that the work that has been done would appear to be somewhat contradictory. A 1982 study by Becker et al (cited in Bryan 2000) that examined clinic records and symptom questionnaires of 655 women noted that previously infertile women had 90 per cent more pregnancy-related complaints than the control group of fertile pregnant women. The conclusion was that they had raised anxiety levels.

While it should be recognised that this is an old study, and that more recent research (Holdtich-Davis et al 1995, Klock and Greenfield 2000, Stanton and Golombok 1993) indicates that women who conceived after IVF did not have higher anxiety levels than those who conceived spontaneously, these more recent studies are based on very small numbers, and their validity must therefore be questioned.

Quantitative research undertaken by McMahon et al (1999) based on questionnaires and interviews concluded that IVF mothers were more likely to deny the significance of any problems in pregnancy and less likely to seek information about the pregnancy. They interpreted this as the mothers not allowing the discomforts of pregnancy to affect the relief and joy at expecting a baby. The authors point out that health professionals need to be aware that these women may have adopted different coping strategies as they tried and failed to conceive: these may present as keeping a tight control of their emotions and happiness to protect themselves from further disappointment.

While this study had some limitations, it does give the midwife further insight into the complex issues that these women face. The midwife should therefore be prepared to support the woman and her family through these symptoms, whether imagined or real.

Sidebotham (1997) advocates that the midwife can increase the woman's sense of wellbeing by helping her to maintain optimum health during her pregnancy, offering advice on diet, exercise and lifestyle. This helps her to gain self-confidence, enabling her to accept her body's ability to nurture the pregnancy. Taking a holistic approach and looking at the whole woman can enable the midwife to help her to improve her perception of herself and her body's abilities, despite the years of what she may see as its failures.

Conclusion

Sidebotham (1997) believes that the challenge for the midwife in caring antenatally for a woman and her family who have achieved a pregnancy following assisted conception is to allow them to be partners in their own care. They may have experienced years of feeling passive or powerless during treatments and interventions: the midwife's role is to undo some of these negative experiences, restoring their sense of dignity, building their confidence and enabling them to form a meaningful relationship with their fetus which will in turn help the bonding process following birth.

The majority of midwives will have encountered few women who have conceived in this way, but as demand increases so, too, will the number of women seeking antenatal care. Although the literature appears to be inconclusive as to whether these women do have greater anxieties, they present unique biological, psychological and psychosocial problems. A sophisticated level of care is therefore required to meet their demands.

Today's midwife must be able to meet these demands, recognising that there are complex psychological factors surrounding the assisted conception pregnancy. A high standard of professional care, support and additional sensitivity for the potential difficulties that these women and their families face are required. While, fundamentally, such a pregnancy is the same as any other, emotionally it may be very different. As such, it may require a more challenging level of care.

REFERENCES

Becker R, Stauber M and Stadler C (1982). 'Psychosomatic aspects in pregnancy and delivery of former sterility patients'. Advances in Psychosomatic Obstetrics and Gynaecology, 222–223.
Bryan A (2000). 'The psychosocial effects of infertility and the implications for midwifery practice'. MIDIRS Midwifery Digest, 10 (1): 8–12.
Denton J (1996). 'Pregnancy after treatment for infertility'. In: J Alexander, J Levy and S Roch (eds). Midwifery practice; Core Topics 1, Basingstoke, Macmillan, 95–115.
Dunnington R and Glazer G (1991). 'Maternal identity and early mothering behaviour in previously infertile women'. Journal of Obstetric, Gynaecological and Neonatal Nursing, 20 (4): 309–316.
Gottlieb S (2002). 'Assisted reproduction increases risk of birth defects, study says'. British Medical Journal, 324: 633.
HFEA (1993). Code of Practice, London, HFEA.
HFEA (1995). The Role of the HFEA, London, HFEA.
Holdtich-Davis D, Black B P and Sandelowski M (1995). 'Fertility status and symptoms in childbearing couples'. Research in Nursing and Health, 18 (5): 417–426.
Joels L A and Wardle P G (1994). 'Assisted conception and the midwife'. British Journal of Midwifery, 12 (9): 429–435.

Klock S C and Greenfield B A (2000). 'Psychological status of in vitro fertilisation patients during pregnancy: a longitudinal study'. Fertility and Sterility, 73 (6): 1159–1164.
Kurinczuk J (2002). 'Birth defects after assisted reproduction'. New England Journal of Medicine, 341: 725–730.
McMahon C, Tennant C and Ungerer J (1999). '"Don't count your chickens": a comparative study of the experience of pregnancy after IVF conception'. Journal of Reproductive and Infant Psychology, 17 (4): 345–356.
NMC (2002). Code of Professional Conduct, London, NMC.
Sidebotham M (1997). 'Pregnancy following assisted conception'. In: I Karger and S Hunt (eds). Challenges in Midwifery Care, Basingstoke, Macmillan, 115–131.
Stanton F and Golombok S (1993). 'Maternal-fetal attachment during pregnancy following in vitro fertilisation'. Journal of Psychosomatic Obstetrics and Gynaecology, 14: 153–158.
Wang J X, Knottnerus A, Schuit G et al (2002). 'Surgically obtained sperm and the risk of gestational hypertension and pre-eclampsia'. The Lancet, 359: 673–674.

The Practising Midwife 2004; 7(8): 18–21

Asking the question: antenatal domestic violence

Sally Price, Kathleen Baird, Debra Salmon

Background

The need for midwives to address domestic violence in pregnancy has been clearly identified (Department of Health 2000, 1999). It is well documented that living with violence has the potential to seriously impact on maternal and fetal health (Hillard 1985, McWilliams and McKiernan 1993, Mezey and Bewley 1997, Mooney 1993, Salzman 1990). Domestic violence is also relevant to the midwife's role in child protection, as it is associated with a significant number of child deaths in the UK (Hester and Pearson 1998, Hester et al 1998).

Current policy and professional guidelines recommend that women should be given the opportunity to disclose their experiences of domestic violence (Department of Health 2004, NICE 2001, 2003, RCM 1997). However, it has been thought that women are unlikely to tell health professionals unless they are asked. Some evidence suggests that women want to be asked about their experiences of abuse (Davidson et al 2000). Bacchus et al (2002) found that routine antenatal enquiry for domestic violence is acceptable to women if conducted in a safe confidential environment by a trained health professional who is empathetic and non-judgemental.

Despite this evidence, midwives are concerned. Some feel they lack knowledge or skills to be able to make either a routine enquiry or a specific one if they suspect a woman of being abused (Price and Baird 2001).

The Bristol Pregnancy and Domestic Violence Programme

The Bristol Pregnancy and Domestic Violence Programme (BPDVP) was introduced at North Bristol NHS Trust in April 2003. It aimed to equip midwives with the knowledge and confidence to effectively enquire about domestic violence in the antenatal period. The programme consisted of attending a seven-and-a-half-hour training day with ongoing support for professional practice. This support was provided through a specifically designed website, statutory midwifery supervision, and evidence-based practice guidelines that promote a multi-agency approach to dealing with domestic violence and describe the availability of local organisations and agencies.

The training was provided by two experienced trainers and underpinned by national and international evidence (Bacchus et al 2001, Bacchus et al 2002, Helton et al 1987, Hester et al 1998, Humphreys et al 2000, Richardson et al 2002). As well as providing an opportunity to develop awareness and understanding of domestic violence, the programme provided relevant information and practical advice around inter-agency working. However, the main focus of the day was on the development of skills to ask women directly about domestic violence. 'Asking' appears to be the most contentious issue for practitioners and, according to UK studies, the most difficult role for midwives to take on (Mezey et al 2003, Price and Baird 2003, Scobie and McGuire 1999). Skills were developed by rehearsal of questioning through role-play, examining case studies and in-depth discussion in a safe environment, allowing for constructive feedback from colleagues and trainers.

Evaluation methods

The evaluation of the BPDVP was multi-faceted and has been reported elsewhere in full (Salmon et al 2004). A key aspect of the evaluation was to describe and analyse the experiences of the 79 community-based midwives taking part in the programme.

Individual and focus group interviews were used to explore the process of programme introduction. Thirty-four midwives who were interviewed had attended the programme, had had the opportunity to access support and were implementing routine antenatal enquiry for domestic violence. Fourteen midwives were interviewed at three months post introduction of the programme and 20 at six months. Two midwives were also interviewed in relation to the specific issues around antenatal enquiry with women from black and ethnic minority communities. Data was collected on the following areas: the degree to which the programme met educational goals and support; the midwives' experiences associated with asking about domestic violence in pregnancy; implications for service and educational development; and potential barriers to successful implementation.

Findings

The programme was viewed very positively. The training day clearly identified that leadership, support and advice had facilitated the successful implementation of routine enquiry:

It gave you enough confidence to go out there and ask women, whereas before I didn't have the confidence in myself to do that.

The midwives found that the programme raised awareness, presented good information from credible sources and supported the development of practical skills and confidence in relation to asking women about their experiences of violence. Midwives identified that it was the opportunity to practise questioning skills which built up their confidence and made them feel more comfortable in their interactions with women:

It was difficult initially . . . to know how to word it. And I changed my wording, how I approached it after a while.

I know it was difficult the first few times . . . the first few times you're not really quite fluent. I think really for me it was just getting the words right rather than feeling awkward about bringing it up as an issue.

Attendance on the programme combined with routine integration of enquiry into the booking visit helped practitioners to develop their practice. Initially asking the question caused some anxiety among most of the midwives interviewed, despite their considerable midwifery experience (mean 14.8 years). Explaining to women that certain questions were being put to all women as a matter of policy helped midwives to feel more at ease:

It certainly helps because the questioning is standard throughout the Trust. You're not picking up on just one family . . . because it's a global thing, it's much easier. A number of people have actually seen it on TV.

The most significant difficulty associated with asking the question was the attendance of male partners at consultations.

Midwives felt particularly anxious about trying to see women alone if there was a known history of domestic violence. However, they were unwilling to engineer opportunities to see the woman without her partner:

I can see that if someone really was having problems and if the partner was always coming to a point where your sixth sense did start to trigger . . . then you might have to . . . be slightly devious. But really up until that point I think I wouldn't want to be pulling someone aside and saying 'by the way . . .' and sort of whispering behind people's backs. You just wouldn't do that. It just wouldn't be suitable.

Midwives also identified the need to improve guidance within the programme in relation to recording responses to the question about domestic violence. Other perceived barriers included shortages of staff, in particular those associated with the recruitment and retention of midwifery staff, lone working, and the potential threat of violence. Three midwives described how windows had been smashed and rubbish thrown at the antenatal clinic since the introduction of the routine enquiry.

Further anxieties about receiving a positive response were expressed:

That was the one thing when I thought about it, I wouldn't know what to do if someone said 'Yes'. I wouldn't know how to deal with that or where to go first.

Participants questioned how far midwives should go in their interventions. The majority said that they felt happy to help women by giving information about support services, but few felt confident about supporting women in long-term violent relationships. Midwives also lacked confidence in the capacity of other agencies to effectively support these women. They were concerned about the degree to which others would be able to respond quickly and effectively to those needing help. Despite these reservations, midwives were clear that they did have a role in dealing with domestic violence, believing that the midwifery role should include more social and public health aspects of care to women:

I think it has to be part of our role, yes . . . The reasons why there is a high maternal morbidity and mortality rates isn't so much now from medical problems; it's the social problems. I think we have to be addressing these sorts of issues and mental health problems.

At six months post training, practitioners were becoming more forceful in their view that their role should be limited to enquiry and information giving and not extended to in-depth support. Concerns were raised about the level of emotional energy and practical skill required to manage complex social problems:

It's easy to do the clinical stuff; it's the support for social problems that you require support for.

All those interviewed were very clear about the range and quality of support on offer to them, and how to access this:

You've always got your line manager, you've got your peers and your supervisor. So depending on whether it's a Saturday night, you've got a supervisor on call haven't you if you have an issue. So I couldn't tell you exactly what that flow chart says but then I know who I would go to.

While two midwives commented that the information provided by the website had been excellent, many more said that they did not have computer access within their work base and so could not access this information.

Midwives identified the specific need for developments in relation to minority ethnic women. There was a feeling that the needs of women with limited English remained largely unmet. The use of family members as interpreters was identified as problematic, with difficulties experienced in obtaining professional interpreter services:

I think we feel the concern of missing something . . . I would really kick myself because I would think: 'Well, why didn't I pick up on that?' It's a worry because there is only so much you can do when you haven't got the language there.

The midwives felt that the programme should place an increased emphasis on cultural sensitivity, and that more resources were required to effectively support ethnic minority women in relation to domestic violence. The greatest resource requirement for all women was felt to be for more midwifery time. Disclosures of experiences of violence were found to require considerable time, with most midwives reporting more than an hour spent with the woman, and in two cases more than three hours. However, eight midwives reported that dealing with disclosure took less than 30 minutes. Reasons for these differences are unclear, although it could be suggested that individualisation of care means that there can be no standardisation of the midwifery time required to effectively deal with women's disclosures.

Discussion

The midwives in this study felt that not only was domestic violence a priority for health services but one in which they should take a lead role. The overall findings suggest the training has a strong impact on practice. This confirms the work of Taket et al (2003) that routine enquiry cannot be effectively implemented without in-depth training. Midwives around the UK are receiving training with many examples of good practice (Breslin et al 2003, Mezey et al 2003, Ward and Spence 2002). However, a key aspect of this programme was the emphasis on skills development practised through role play, case presentations and in-depth discussion. Without innovative and diverse teaching methods to develop skills, midwives may not have confidence in their ability to question women about domestic violence. Consideration must be given to the financial costs of providing such in-depth

training. These could be reduced by linking domestic violence with mandatory child protection training that already has a high priority in the health service.

It is also important to acknowledge how supporting women who experience domestic violence may be professionally challenging and demanding. Midwives need to have clear support mechanisms in place for both the women and themselves, combined with adequate resources particularly in terms of midwifery time. Without this, routine enquiry may not be effective or sustainable. Other studies also show a failure to maintain routine enquiry is linked to organisation failure in adequately supporting staff (Davidson et al 2000, Mezey et al 2003, Taket et al 2003).

The need for training to be integrated with the planning and service development within maternity services is apparent. Midwives identified that clear leadership was essential for successful implementation. It may be essential to create specialist posts in this area to support practice and develop inter-agency links. A lack of regular interagency contact meant that the midwives in this study were unclear about the resources available to support women, and lacked confidence in the referrals they made. A specialist midwifery post could enhance this with readily available advice, support and guidance in complex situations, although this study also confirms the role of statutory midwifery supervision in supporting professional practice.

Conclusion

With domestic violence an issue for maternity services, it is important to recognise that midwives and service managers are faced with professional challenges to ensure practice is effective. Preparation and training should focus on skill development, in particular asking the routine question about domestic violence, policy and procedures and the evidence to support practice. The need to adopt a multi-agency approach tailored to meet individual women's needs and have clear support mechanisms in place for both the women and midwives is essential if the introduction of routine enquiry is to be effective. Midwives must be aware of the support and safety mechanisms that can sustain them in their work and be clear about the parameters of their role in supporting women who live with violence.

Acknowledgement

The authors would like to thank the community-based midwives from North Bristol NHS Trust who participated in this study, and their managers who gave their full support.

REFERENCES

Bacchus L, Bewley S and Mezey G (2001). 'Domestic violence and pregnancy'. The Obstetrician and Gynaecologist, 3 (2): 56–59.

Bacchus L, Mezey G and Bewley S (2002). 'Women's perceptions and experiences of routine enquiry for domestic violence in a maternity service'. International Journal of Obstetrics and Gynaecology, 109: 9–16.

Breslin R, Kelly L and Regan L (2003). First Interim Report of the Portsmouth Domestic Violence Early Intervention Project Evaluation, Child and Woman Abuse Studies Unit, London Metropolitan University.

Davidson L, King V, Garcia J et al (2000). Reducing Domestic Violence . . . What Works?, Health services Policing and Reducing Crime. Briefing Note, London: Home Office.

Department of Health (1999). Making a Difference, London: Department of Health.

Department of Health (2000). Domestic Violence: a Resource Manual for Healthcare Professionals, London: Department of Health.

Department of Health (2004). National Service Framework for Children, Young People and Maternity Services – Maternity Module, London: Department of Health and Department for Education and Skills.

Helton A, McFarlane J and Anderson E (1987). 'Battered and pregnant: a prevalence study'. American Journal Public Health, 77 (10): 1337–1339.

Hester M and Pearson C (1998). Preventing Child Abuse. Monitoring Domestic Violence, Bristol: The Policy Press.

Hester M, Pearson C and Harwin N (1998). Making An Impact: Children and Domestic Violence, London: Department of Health, School for Policy Studies, University of Bristol, NSPCC, Barnardos.

Hillard P (1985). 'Physical abuse in pregnancy'. Obstetrician and Gynaecologist, 66: 185–190.

Humphreys C, Hague G, Hester M et al (2000). Domestic Violence Good Practice Indicators, University of Warwick: The Centre for the Study of Well-Being.

McWilliams M and McKiernan J (1993). Bringing It Out Into The Open, Belfast: HMSO.

Mezey G and Bewley S (1997). 'Domestic violence and pregnancy'. British Journal of Obstetrics and Gynaecology, 104: 528–531.

Mezey G, Bacchus L, Haworth A et al (2003). 'Midwives' perceptions and experiences of routine enquiry for domestic violence'. British Journal of Obstetrics and Gynaecology, 110: 744–752.

Mooney J (1993). The Hidden Figures: The North London Domestic Violence Survey, Middlesex: Middlesex University Centre for Criminology.

National Institute for Clinical Excellence, The Scottish Executive Health Department and The Department of Health Social Services and Public Safety: Northern Ireland (2001). The Confidential Enquiries into Maternal Deaths in the United Kingdom. Why Mothers Die 1997–1999, London: RCOG Press.

National Institute for Clinical Excellence (2003). CG6 Antenatal Care – Routine Care of the Healthy Pregnant Woman, NICE Guideline: www.nice.org.uk

Price S and Baird K (2001). 'Domestic violence in pregnancy. What midwives need to know'. The Practising Midwife, 4 (7): 12–14.

Price S and Baird K (2003). 'Domestic violence in pregnancy. An audit of professional practice'. The Practising Midwife, 6 (3): 15–18.

Richardson J, Coid J, Petruckevitch A et al (2002). 'Identifying domestic violence: cross sectional study in primary care'. British Medical Journal, 324: 274.

Royal College of Midwives (1997). 'Domestic abuse in pregnancy'. Position Paper 19, London: RCM.

Salmon D, Baird K, Price S et al (2004). An Evaluation of the Bristol Pregnancy and Domestic Violence Programme to Promote the Introduction of Routine Antenatal Enquiry for Domestic Violence at North Bristol NHS Trust, Bristol: Faculty of Health and Social Care, University of the West of England.

Salzman L (1990). 'Battering during pregnancy: a role for physicians'. Atlanta Medicine, 65: 45–48. In: Hunt S and Martin A (2001). Pregnant Women, Violent Men: What Midwives Need to Know, Oxford: Books for Midwives Press.

Scobie J and McGuire M (1999). 'The silent enemy: domestic violence in pregnancy'. British Journal of Midwifery, 7 (4): 259–262.

Taket A, Nurse J, Smith K et al (2003). 'Routinely asking women about domestic violence in health settings'. British Medical Journal, 327: 673–676.

Ward S and Spence A (2002). 'Training midwives to screen for domestic violence'. Midirs Midwifery Digest, 12 (supplement): 17–18.

The Practising Midwife 2005; 8(3): 21–25

Preventing infant allergies

Belinda Blake

The subject of food allergy is often in the news. More people are discovering that certain foods may be contributing to their health problems. Conditions such as irritable bowel syndrome (IBS) and migraines can commonly be traced back to dietary triggers. Food allergy should also be an important consideration when it comes to planning for a baby, pregnancy and breastfeeding, as the symptoms and consequences of food allergy in both the mother and unborn child are complex and can be far-reaching.

Allergies or food sensitivities?

An allergy is a disorder that occurs when the body becomes hypersensitive to a particular stimulant or allergen. Contact with the allergen triggers the production of antibodies into the blood stream. In classic allergy this involves the immunoglobulin type E (IgE), which then attaches to mast cells and triggers the release of pro-inflammatory chemicals, including histamine. Classic, or 'Type I', allergy is caused by a genetic fault in fatty acid metabolism (affecting the delta-6-desaturase enzyme), resulting in an impaired ability to calm inflammation in the body through the production of anti-inflammatory prostaglandins. It is referred to as atopy.

Evidence shows that this genetic tendency towards increased sensitivity to allergens is likely to be inherited by the baby (one parent with atopy carries a 50 per cent risk; two parents with atopy carries a 75 per cent risk), although, interestingly, the baby may not necessarily react to the same allergens or with the same symptoms as its mother. Most people who have IgE-type allergies are aware of their triggers (eg, strawberries, peanuts or shellfish), as the reaction is immediate and often severe. As a result, they are more likely to avoid these foods.

However, other types of allergy – sometimes described as 'food sensitivity' – are less obvious to the sufferer. This 'Type II' allergy involves other immune mechanisms, notably the IgG antibody which, rather than attaching to mast cells, forms circulating immune complexes with any over-sized food molecules. It is the accumulation of these large molecules in the blood and body tissues that eventually triggers the release of proinflammatory chemicals. As a consequence, symptoms of food sensitivity may not manifest immediately after eating, but can take hours or even days and thus can be more difficult to identify.

Why do food sensitivities develop?

It is still unclear why certain individuals develop food sensitivities, but the incidence is rising. According to Shepperson Mills and Vernon (2002), 'Food sensitivity or intolerance is more common now than true food allergies: around 24 million American adults are affected by the foods they consume.'

The allergy specialist Dr James Braly explains that 'delayed food allergy appears to be simply the inability of your digestive tract to prevent large quantities of partially digested food from entering the blood stream' (Braly 1992). Inefficient digestion and a damaged gut wall, alongside an inability to detoxify and eliminate waste efficiently from the body, are key considerations. Foresight, the association for promotion of preconceptual care, also cites Candidiasis, an overgrowth of the yeast *Candida albicans*, as a key factor in the cause of food sensitivity and, subsequently, fertility problems through its ability to damage gut integrity (Barnes and Bradley 1990).

Overexposure to a limited number of foods may also contribute to an increased risk of sensitivity. Wheat, dairy and soya are now ubiquitous in the British diet (Hourihane 1998); and these, alongside peanuts (Rance 1999), are high on the list of key food allergens in the UK.

Early exposure to a number of potentially highly allergenic foods, either through breast milk, formula or baby foods, may also precipitate allergy development.

According to allergist-immunologist Dr John James, 'studies suggest that mothers from families with a history of allergies should refrain from eating peanuts through the duration of breastfeeding to avoid introducing peanut proteins to their offspring . . . A nursing mother should also avoid eating other foods that a baby is allergic to, which most commonly are eggs and cows' milk' (Sampson 2002).

Impact of food allergies on conception and pregnancy

The constant activity of an immune system attacking regular deliveries of food allergens is exhausting for the body, keeping it in a constant state of stress. The ability of circulating immune complexes to penetrate all tissues of the body means that symptoms can be far-reaching (delayed-onset food allergy has been linked to more than 100 medical conditions and to some 100 different allergic symptoms (York Nutritional Laboratories 2004)). These cause the individual a great deal of distress and may involve taking regular medication, such as NSAIDs, to help ease symptoms. These, in turn, may exacerbate damage to the mucous membrane lining to the gut wall.

Disturbances in the gut environment (through the presence of food allergies, an overgrowth of Candida, or through persistent over-use of NSAIDs or antibiotics, for example) may also deplete levels of the protective bifidobacteria that inhabit the bowel. These beneficial bacteria are known to play an important role in supporting good immune health, both for the mother and for her baby. An important study published in The Lancet (Kalliomäki et al 2001) demonstrated a direct link between the reduction in the development of allergies in 'susceptible' children and the administration of probiotics given to the expectant mothers during the last few weeks of their pregnancies.

Another Norwegian study also demonstrated an increase in the risk of developing allergies in predisposed children (ie, those born to mothers with allergies) born by caesarean section (Eggesbø et al 2003), suggesting that factors that interfere with the natural colonisation process of a baby's sterile gut may well play a role in the development of food allergy. With the rise in popularity of caesarean births in this country, the role of these friendly bacteria in helping to prevent food allergy and establishing a strong immune system in the baby should not be underestimated.

Perhaps the most important implication of food allergies or sensitivities is that they are likely to lead to nutrient deficiencies. Braly (1992) found zinc deficiency to be extremely common among allergy sufferers, and much research now links low levels of zinc to decreased fertility, increased risk of miscarriage, low birth-weight babies

(Hurley 1991) and a higher risk of postnatal depression (Bryce-Smith and Hodgkinson 1987). In addition, it has been demonstrated that 'morning sickness' during pregnancy can be eased in many women by increasing levels of both zinc and vitamin B6 (Pheiffer 1975), suggesting again that it may be a deficiency symptom.

Undiagnosed coeliac disease (CD) is now considered a major threat to fertility and pregnancy. Erosion of the gut villi caused by gluten sensitivity is known to cause malabsorption of many nutrients essential for pregnancy (including iron, which can lead to severe and persistent anaemia during pregnancy), and has been linked to an increased risk of miscarriage, fetal growth restriction and unfavourable pregnancy outcomes. Both gluten and yeast sensitivity have been linked to infertility caused by blocked fallopian tubes. With an estimated 1 in 300 people in the UK, US and Europe suffering from coeliac disease (British Nutrition Foundation 2000), this is a growing problem. Italian obstetricians have recently found undetected coeliac disease to be so common among women with problem pregnancies that they are recommending that all pregnant women should be routinely scanned for gluten allergy (Ciacci et al 1996).

Sensitivity to dairy products has been shown to exacerbate problems associated with atopic conditions such as asthma (James 2003). Since asthma may naturally worsen for many women during pregnancy, ingestion of dairy products may make this condition more unstable, threatening the oxygen supply to the growing fetus.

Effects of food allergy on the baby

There is some evidence to suggest that food sensitivities carried through into pregnancy and throughout breastfeeding may also directly affect the baby. Research now suggests that the fetus begins producing antibodies to allergenic substances from as early as 11 weeks into pregnancy (Braly 1992). Whilst it is known that 'breast milk provides the ideal nutritional, immunologic, and physiologic nourishment for all newborns' and 'components of breast milk enhance natural defenses and promote immunoregulation' (Zeiger 2003), Zeiger goes on to explain that 'debate still exists today regarding the degree to which breastfeeding prevents, reduces, delays, or increases the development of allergic disease'. A meta-analysis of studies exploring the benefits of maternal avoidance of food allergens throughout lactation concluded that the elimination diets 'may substantially reduce the development of eczema in their child in early childhood' (Kramer 2000). In cases of colic the possibility of maternal dairy sensitivity should be of primary consideration (Jacobsson and Lindberg 1987).

Babies born to coeliac mothers have a 10 per cent chance of inheriting this disease. Physically, they may develop a swollen tummy, with wasted arms and legs, and are likely to experience symptoms such as persistent vomiting and diarrhoea. Much evidence now also strongly suggests a link between food allergy and autism (especially gluten in wheat and casein in milk products), and it has been found that 'parents or siblings of autistic children are far more likely to suffer from milk or gluten allergy' (Holford 2003). Cow's milk allergy has also been linked to increased risk of developing juvenile diabetes (Virtanen et al 1999) and ADHD (Holford 2003).

It is important to differentiate here between dairy sensitivity and lactose intolerance. Lactose intolerance is not related to an immune response, but rather to a genetic inability to produce the enzyme lactase, required for the digestion of lactose (milk sugar). This is a very common condition, particularly in people of African, Indian and Asian descent, and can lead to symptoms such as diarrhoea, abdominal cramps (colic) and vomiting in the new baby. Unlike dairy sensitivity, respiratory symptoms are not provoked by lactose intolerance.

Identification and treatment

There are a number of ways of identifying a food allergy or sensitivity and, ideally, this should always be explored prior to pregnancy.

As a nutritionist, one of my first ports of call is clinical history. Often, symptoms may have been present for years and, in many cases, may date back to childhood – for example, a strong childhood dislike of milk or a history of days off school with unexplained 'tummy upsets' or recurrent ear infections. Commonly, these people also have a family history of atopy.

Food cravings may also be indicative of food sensitivity, as the body responds to the bombardment of circulating immune complexes by producing a range of chemical mediators, including the opioids, in order to mask symptoms. Fragments of proteins, or peptides, can also mimic our own endorphins in the brain, triggering addictive tendencies – the 'opioid effect' from these 'exorphins' may also account for symptoms associated with autism (Reichelt et al 1981, Shattock and Savery 1997).

Keeping a simple food diary (a record of food eaten and subsequent symptoms) may well help an individual identify food triggers. An elimination diet, removing one or more suspect foods, can provide good results but must be carefully monitored if implemented to ensure that no major nutrients become deficient as a result. In those women considered to be a likely candidate for food sensitivity or allergy, a gradual reduction of suspect foods may well be a more cautious approach during pregnancy, since an individual may often experience an initial deterioration in symptoms as the body is able to detoxify allergenic debris.

Laboratory testing offers an alternative. While the NHS can arrange for an IgE allergy test and can identify markers for coeliac disease (anti-endomysial antibodies), IgG sensitivities are generally not tested for. Private laboratories do offer blood tests for both IgE and IgG allergies (see resources) and, although expensive, these can be a valuable and less time-consuming option.

In the case of babies, allergy testing is not recommended for children under the age of 18 months. As well as being an invasive test, the immune system is still forming and so would not provide worthwhile information (IgG antibodies pass readily across the placenta and give the fetus and newborn baby protection against infection; the baby usually starts producing his own IgG at around three months). So, for a baby suffering from symptoms such as colic, unexplained vomiting, eczema or hyperactivity, the careful elimination of key potential allergens (first, cow's milk) both from the mother's diet (if breastfeeding) and from the baby's (if taking formula or whole milk) would be the best line of investigation, ideally under the guidance of a nutritionist or other health professional.

The good news is that food sensitivity can be a short-term problem. Unlike the lifelong IgE marker that triggers classic allergy, the IgG marker has a relatively short-term 'memory'. Therefore, a period of approximately three to six months' strict avoidance of the offending food should allow it once again to be consumed, in moderation, without re-triggering symptoms – as long as the gut has had a chance to heal fully.

For mothers and older children supplements including the amino acid L-glutamine, essential fatty acids, vitamin A and zinc, and a diet rich in these nutrients (including fresh fruit and vegetables, eggs, nuts, seeds and some oily fish), have been shown to be effective in helping to heal the gut wall and so prevent further sensitivity. For babies and young children a probiotic supplement specially formulated for babies and children may be beneficial in helping to relieve symptoms such as colic.

The way forward

Currently, 39 per cent of children and 30 per cent of adults have been diagnosed with one or more atopic conditions. Treatments for asthma and other allergenic disorders currently account for 10 per cent of primary care prescribing costs, while direct NHS costs for managing allergenic problems are estimated at more than £1 billion per annum (Gupta et al 2004).

Although not fully conclusive there is plenty of evidence to suggest that food allergies and sensitivities should be a primary consideration prior to conception, alongside other key factors such as smoking and alcohol consumption, not only for the health and wellbeing of the mother, but also for the healthy development of the baby.

Increasing awareness, I feel, is essential. All future mothers need to be encouraged to enjoy a varied diet which includes a good range of different freshly prepared foods (where possible and practicable), rather than relying on common food allergens at every meal. Emphasis on the importance of good preconceptual care may help increase awareness of potentially allergenic foods prior to conception. There needs to be awareness of symptoms, in both the mother and child (especially those considered to be high risk), which may be linked to food allergy/sensitivity. Finally, the encouragement of breastfeeding, which although potentially linked to sensitizing the baby, offers the best support and protection for a newly developing immune system.

REFERENCES

Barnes B and Bradley S G (1990). Planning For A Healthy Baby, Vermillion, pp. 155–156.

Braly J (1992). Dr Braly's Food Allergy & Nutrition Revolution, Connecticut: Keates Publishing Inc.

British Nutrition Foundation (2000). Information supplied.

Bryce-Smith D and Hodgkinson L (1987). The Zinc Solution, Century Arrow.

Ciacci C et al (1996). 'Celiac disease and pregnancy outcome'. Am J Gastroenterol, 91 (4): 718–72.

Eggesbø M et al (2003). 'Is delivery by caesarean section a risk factor for food allergy?'. Journal of Allergy and Clinical Immunology, 12 (2): 420–426.

Gupta R et al (2004). 'Burden of allergenic disease in the UK: secondary analyses of national databases'. Clinical Experimental Allergy, 34 (4): 520–526.

Holford P (2003). Optimum Nutrition for the Mind, London: Piatkus.

Hourihane J O (1998). 'Prevalence and severity of food allergy – need for control'. Allergy, 53 (46 supp): 84–88.

Hurley L S (1991). 'Teratogenic aspects of manganese, zinc and copper nutrition'. Physiological Reviews, 61: 249–295.

Jacobsson I and Lindberg T (1987). 'Cow's milk proteins cause infantile colic in breast-fed infants: a double-blind crossover study'. Pediatric, 71: 286.

James J (2003). 'Respiratory manifestations of food allergy'. Pediatric, 111 (6): 1625–1630.

Kalliomäki M et al (2001). 'Probiotics in primary prevention of atopic disease'. Lancet, 357: 1076–1079.

Kramer M S (2000). 'Maternal antigen avoidance during lactation for preventing atopic disease in infants of women at high risk'. Cochrane Database Syst Rev (2): CD000132.

Pheiffer C C (1975). Mental and Elemental Nutrients, USA, Keates, p. 227.

Rance F (1999). 'Food hypersensitivity in children: clinical aspects and distribution of allergens'. Pediatric Allergy and Immunology, 10 (1): 33–38.

Reichlet K-L, Hole K, Hamberger A et al (1981). 'Biologically active peptide containing fractions in schizophrenia and childhood autism'. Advances in Biochemical Psychopharmacology, 28: 627–643.

Sampson H A (2002). 'Peanut allergy'. New England Journal of Medicine, 346: 1294–1299.

Shattock P and Savery D (1997). Autism as a metabolic disorder. Autism Research Unit, University of Sunderland, Sunderland, UK.

Shepperson Mills D and Vernon M (2002). Endometriosis – A Key to Healing Through Nutrition, London: Thorsons, p. 205.

Virtanen S M et al (1999). 'Infant feeding, early weight gain, and risk of type I diabetes'. Diabetes Care, 22: 1961–1965.

York Nutritional Laboratories (2004). Information supplied.

Zeiger R S (2003). 'Food allergen avoidance in the prevention of food allergy in infants and children'. Pediatric, 111 (6): 1662–1671.

RESOURCES

YorkTest Laboratories provides a home-test kit that tests for both food and chemical IgG mediated allergies, requiring a simple pin-prick blood sample. Tel: 01904 410410; www.yorktest.com

Individual Wellbeing can test for allergies and food sensitivities (including IgE and IgG markers) but requires a blood sample taken professionally. Tel: 020 7730 7010; www.individual-wellbeing.co.uk

Common food allergens and alternatives

Allergen: wheat

Found in: bread, biscuits, pastries, many confectionery bars, pasta, pizza bases, many cereals, pancakes, ice-cream cones, couscous, bulgur wheat, semolina, stock cubes, soya sauce, mustard, sausages, spelt, kamut, plus many ready meals and baby foods – check labels for cereal starch, cereal binders, cereal fillers.

Alternatives: rye (bread or crackers), gluten-free breads, oats (oat cakes, porridge), rice (rice flour, brown or white rice, rice cakes, rice pasta or noodles), corn (corn or polenta flour, corn crackers, polenta, corn pasta, corn tacos, popcorn), quinoa (quinoa flour, puffed quinoa cereals), millet, buckwheat (flour, noodles), legumes (legume pasta), amaranth (flour, puffed cereals), Tamari soya sauce, Marigold Swiss Bouillon stock, plus a large range of gluten-free breads, biscuits, cakes and cereals available in most supermarkets.

Those with gluten allergy/coeliac disease need to avoid all foods containing wheat, spelt, kamut, rye, oats and barley.

Allergen: dairy

Found in: cow's milk products (milk, formula milk, cheese, yogurt, cream, butter, ice cream) plus products containing these foods, including some breads, cakes, biscuits, instant mashed potato, soups, ready meals, processed meats and sausages, custard, puddings, sauces, chocolate and confectionery – check labels for lactose, milk solids, casein, caseinate, hydrolysed casein, lactose, lactalbumin.

Alternatives*: goat's milk (milk, cream, butter, cheese (eg, chevre), yogurt, Nanny Goat infant formula and follow-on milk (often better tolerated than cow's milk, but may still trigger problems in some individuals), sheep's milk (yogurt, cheese – eg, feta), soya milk (milk, yogurt, cream, ice cream, cheese), rice milk (milk, cheese), oat milk, nut milk (eg, almond), quinoa milk, coconut milk (milk, cream).

*Milk alternatives are only advocated for use by older children and mothers suspected of dairy sensitivity. They are not suitable for babies and are no replacement for breastfeeding.

Common symptoms of food sensitivity

- Arthritis/joint pain
- Autism
- Chest infections
- Colic
- Constipation
- Dark circles around eyes
- Depression
- Diarrhoea/nappy rash
- Earache/middle ear infections
- Headaches/migraine
- Hyperactivity
- Insomnia
- Learning difficulties
- Panic attacks/anxiety
- Fatigue
- Flatulence
- Nausea
- Sinusitis/excess mucus
- Skin rashes
- More than 100 different symptoms have been associated with food sensitivity

Common symptoms of atopic allergy

- Allergic rhinitis (hay fever)
- Anaphylaxis
- Asthma
- Eczema/dermatitis
- Food allergy
- Urticaria/angio-oedema

The Practising Midwife 2005; 8(10): 20–23

Topics for further reflection

As Ans Luyben and Valerie Fleming discuss, the concept of antenatal care is relatively new, and little has changed since its inception, except for the realisation that there as a need to evaluate the effectiveness of antenatal care, which was the aim of their study. Among other things, their findings highlight the emphasis that women put on their feelings and confirm the importance of the midwife's role in helping women to feel confident. Several of the other articles in this section relate to this area, and show how this is a key goal for many midwives as well.

- Do you agree with Lorna Davies' suggestion that storytelling can enhance midwifery practice and education? In what ways do you currently use stories in your practice? Do you have 'favourite' stories that you share with women in different situations, and have you seen other midwives use storytelling as a tool? Do you feel that this is beneficial to women and, if so, how?
- Kate Jackson lists a number of current and possible future topics for parent education sessions. How many of these topics are covered within your locality? Which of the ones that aren't (if any) do you feel would be the most useful? If you were planning a programme of parent education and had an abundance of resources, would you add other topics to the list?
- As Sally Price and her colleagues raise in the article about domestic violence, asking women questions about their experiences in this area is one of the most contentious issues for practitioners. Is this an area of practice that you have previously considered? How do your own feelings and experiences relate to the issues raised in this article?
- The authors of several of the articles in this section make suggestions for practice (either directly or indirectly). Which, if any, of these articles do you feel has made you think about your own practice the most, and why is this? Have any of the articles caused you to think that you might adapt your practice in a particular area?
- Looking at the overall content of the articles in this section, which could be said to be a cross-section of current thinking in this area, can you identify any other recurrent themes which reflect the way that our thinking is moving in the current decade? What would you see as the recent key issues in this area?

Focus on . . .
Women, Midwives and Risk

Blood transfusion: the hidden dangers

Tricia Anderson

Most of us are aware of the potential hazards of blood transfusions for our own health, particularly with the rise in awareness of a wide variety of blood-borne diseases such as HIV, hepatitis and the new variants of CJD. We confidently reassure women that all donated blood is now thoroughly screened for all known viruses, and that their health is not at risk.

But how many of us pause to think of the potential dangers of a blood transfusion for the health not of the mother but of her future children? As every midwife knows, there are particular concerns about antibodies for women in their reproductive years, as they have the potential to cross the placental barrier and invade in utero a baby who may have a different blood type. And as any midwife who has seen a baby with severe hydrops fetalis knows, the consequences can be fatal.

We all ask women about blood transfusions when taking a medical history, but do we really understand why? All *Mayes' Midwifery* has to offer is that 'details of any blood transfusion are important, including the reason and any adverse reaction' (Sweet 1997), but it doesn't say why it is important, and I'm not sure that as a student I really understood. I do now, because of Julie.

A true story

Julie's first baby had been born by forceps two years previously. She suffered a modest haemorrhage from a large episiotomy which left her feeling drained and with a postnatal haemoglobin of 7.8g/dl. She was offered a blood transfusion on the postnatal ward which both the midwife and the senior house officer said would give her a quick 'pick-me-up. Exhausted and pale, Julie agreed, and had a straightforward two-unit blood transfusion. She did indeed feel better, and was happy with the decision she had made.

Two years later, Julie is pregnant with her second baby. A routine blood test in early pregnancy has confirmed her blood group to be O Rh neg. But there are some unexpected and unwelcome little newcomers in Julie's blood that had not been detected during her last pregnancy. Julie now has anti-Kell antibodies at a titre of 1 : 8.

The midwife has to explain that, quite possibly, the rogue antibodies were caused by the blood transfusion that Julie had two years ago. The midwife then has the even more difficult task of explaining that if the father of Julie's baby is Kell-positive (a reasonably high chance of 1 in 10) and Julie's baby is Kell-positive (a likelihood of 1 in 20), the health of her newborn could be seriously, even fatally, compromised.

A blood sample is taken from Julie's partner, and an anxious two-week wait for the results begins.

What is Kell?

The Kell blood group system was first found in 1946 by Coombs, when he isolated a new antibody in the blood of a Mrs Kelleher who had just given birth to a baby with severe haemolytic disease (Goh et al 1993). The Kell blood group is comprised of more than 20 antigens, of which Kell (written as K1 or KEL) is the strongest (Redman and Lee 1995).

As with the Rhesus factor, the Kell antigen is a protein on the red blood cells and is very potent in terms of eliciting a maternal antibody response. Anti-Kell antibodies have been known to cause Haemolytic Disease of the Newborn and Fetus (HDNF) for more than 20 years (McKenna et al 1999). With the decline in Rhesus iso-immunisation as a result of rhesus immunoglobulin pro-phylaxis, anti-Kell is now the most important cause of non-Rhesus HDNF (Goh et al 1993).

Revisiting the physiology of isoimmunisation

If a woman receives even a small amount of foreign blood into her blood circulation, either through blood transfusion or more commonly through a transfer of fetal red cells through the placenta and into the maternal circulation, she may produce antibodies that cause agglutination and destruction of the foreign red cells. Unfortunately, during a subsequent pregnancy these antibodies do not remain confined to the maternal system. They can, in turn, pass through the placenta to the fetus where, if the fetus is of a different blood group to the mother, they will continue their haemolytic activity. This haemolysis breaks down the fetal red cells and causes a state of fetal anaemia and hyperbilirubinaemia.

In the case of anti-Kell antibodies, it seems that the antibodies cause suppression of the creation of red blood cells (erythropoiesis) rather than red cell destruction (Vaughan et al 1998), although McKenna et al (1999) consider that both modes (suppression and destruction) are present. Whatever the mode, severe fetal anaemia is the result. This may lead to a condition called hydrops fetalis, where there is severe ascites, pericardial and pleural effusion and oedema, with enlargement of the liver and spleen which eventually results in death. Polyhydramnios is also commonly present (Babinszki et al 1998).

The constant haemolysis in Rh disease may also cause bilirubin staining of the amniotic fluid as well as severe jaundice in the newborn. The bone marrow responds to this state of anaemia by releasing immature red blood cells into the circulation (Sweet 1997).

The impact of anti-Kell isoimmunisation on fetal well-being

The incidence of anti-Kell immunisation in the overall population is low – between 0.1 and 0.2 per cent – and is largely reported to be as a result of maternal blood transfusion (Grant et al 2000). Ninety-one per cent of the population are Kell-negative; of those, only 5 per cent will go on to produce anti-Kell antibodies in response to a transfusion of Kell-positive blood (Redman and Lee 1995). Julie was unlucky: she was in that 5 per cent.

The Kell antigen is present on the fetal red blood cells of a Kell-positive baby from 12 weeks' gestation, and antibody screening should therefore take place before this. If the father is Kell-positive, there is a 50 per cent chance that the fetus will be affected (McKenna et al 1999). The father will be heterozygous (Kk) or homozygous (KK) for the KEL gene: 98 per cent of men will be heterozygous, and 2 per cent will be homozygous (Bowman et al 1992).

The perinatal mortality rate of babies in anti-Kell pregnancies has been reported as being between 1.5 and 3.9 per cent (Grant et al 2000).

Once it has been established that a woman has anti-Kell antibodies and that the father is Kell-positive, the central question is, 'How affected is the fetus?'. Some fetuses will be unaffected, whereas others will be severely compromised. One of the challenges with anti-Kell is that there appears to be no clear link between the severity of fetal anaemia and the commonly used tests such as maternal antibody level or amniotic fluid optical density estimation (Grant et al 2000). The only direct method of monitoring fetal well-being is by intrauterine cordocentesis, when fetal haemoglobin and presence of maternal antibodies can be directly assessed.

Amniocentesis allows for the identification of the fetal genotype – and, in the case of Kell-negative fetuses, allows the pregnancy to proceed without concern. However, the amniotic fluid optical density test which assesses the presence of bilirubin may be misleading or of little value (Babinszki et al 1998), as the anaemia may be caused by suppression of red blood cell production, not their destruction.

The number of affected pregnancies is very small. A midwife may come across this situation only once or twice in her career. Grant et al (2000) analysed the outcome of pregnancies in Kell alloimmunisation in the West Midlands over a 13-year period between 1984 and 1996 by retrospectively analysing case notes. Sixty-five pregnancies were identified in 52 Kell-sensitised women with Kell-positive partners. The alloimmunisation was related to a previous blood transfusion in 45 per cent of cases (29 pregnancies), and had been induced by a previous pregnancy in 33 cases. Of the 65 pregnancies, 22 fetuses were proven to be Kell-positive, and 18 of these were affected. Five of the 18 were affected as a result of a previous maternal blood transfusion.

Very severe disease occurred in 50 per cent of the affected fetuses (nine of the 18). Of the nine severely affected fetuses, one died at 21 weeks despite two intrauterine blood transfusions, having had a haemoglobin of 1.2g/dl at the initial cordocentesis. The others survived, but were born prematurely and needed blood transfusions both during pregnancy and postnatally.

Grant et al (2000) stress the importance of using Kell-negative blood for transfusions in all women of childbearing age, which would reduce the incidence of this rare but severe disease by 45 per cent.

Another study, by McKenna et al (1999), analysed 156 pregnancies complicated with anti-Kell isoimmunisation at Ohio State University between 1956 and 1995. Twenty-one fetuses (24 per cent) were affected, eight severely, and two died. Leggat et al (1991) found 194 pregnancies affected by anti-Kell in Newcastle upon Tyne over a 25-year period between 1965 and 1989. Bowman et al (1992) found 459 affected pregnancies in Manitoba, Canada, between 1944 and 1990. Babinszki et al (1998) analysed the cases referred to the Maternal-Fetal Medicine Center at the Mount Sinai Medical Center in New York over a 13-year period from 1985–1998. Five fetuses from four mothers were severely compromised by anti-Kell isoim-munisation. All underwent intensive medical treatment, and all survived.

What are also to be found in the literature are a few very sad case studies, such as that reported by Goh et al (1993). They present the case of a fetal death as a result of hydrops fetalis in a Kell-affected pregnancy. A gravida 4 para 3, the mother said she had never had a blood transfusion, and all her pregnancies were by the same partner, who was Kell-positive. Her first pregnancy had been uneventful. Anti-Kell antibodies were detected in her second pregnancy, but no action was taken and she went on to have a normal birth at term with a healthy baby. In her third pregnancy she suffered a placental abruption and fetal death in utero, but on post-mortem no cord blood studies were performed as there were no visual signs of hydrops fetalis.

In her fourth pregnancy a closer eye was kept on her anti-Kell antibodies, which remained between 1:1,024 and 1:2,048. Fortnightly ultrasound scans watched for signs of hydrops, but at 27 weeks she was admitted with reduced fetal movements. A cardiotocograph showed signs of fetal compromise, and a hydropic male infant in poor condition was delivered by caesarean section. The baby died after a 40-minute attempt at resuscitation. Autopsy findings showed signs of severe haemolytic anaemia, and the cord haemoglobin value was 2.5g/dl.

A medical success: two case studies

Recent advances in fetal medicine mean that not all these stories now have sad outcomes. Blakley Huntley gives a detailed personal account of her experience of being an anti-Kell antibody carrier in the United States (Huntley 2001). She had a happy first pregnancy and birth, but was found to have anti-Kell antibodies early in her second pregnancy. Her husband was wrongly tested for Kell antibodies – not for the presence of the Kell antigen. By the time the mistake was discovered, her baby had died in utero, for her husband did turn out to be Kell-positive.

For her third pregnancy she was cared for from a very early stage by an expert in blood incompatibility at the University of North Carolina. The medical regimen she underwent was intense. First, she had three treatments of plasmapheresis (plasma exchange transfusion) between weeks 10 and 16 to help keep her antibody titre low. She received a weekly transfusion of a blood product called Intravenous Immune Globulin (IVIG) between weeks 10 and 20. The procedure took from three to seven hours, and often made her feel ill for days afterwards.

At 16 weeks, an amniocentesis confirmed that the baby had inherited the Kell antigen from its father. Regular ultrasound Doppler flows showed that the baby was not

thriving. Blakley underwent yet more plasmapheresis, and the baby had a total of six intrauterine blood transfusions – at 22, 23, 24, 27, 30 and 34 weeks' gestation. During each of these fetal blood transfusions, Blakley was given terbutaline to stop contractions and a sedative to keep her and the baby calm, as a large team of doctors and nurses administered the transfusion through the uterus and into the umbilical vein.

Regular scans and fetal heart monitorings were done until she reached 38 weeks, when she was induced and gave birth to an 8lb 3oz baby girl. The baby had two further blood transfusions in the neonatal intensive care unit, and is now fit and well. As Blakley says, 'My pregnancy was hard, but I would do it again. I am inexpressively thankful to be living in a time when such a feat was possible' (Huntley 2001).

A similarly inspiring case study is related by Babinszki et al (1998) from the Maternal-Fetal Medicine Center at Mount Sinai Hospital, New York. A woman in her second pregnancy was referred to them with an anti-Kell titre of 1:256. The father was Kell-positive and homozygous for the Kell antigen: therefore, the fetus had to be Kell-positive, too. The woman's titre level was monitored and rose steadily to 1:4,096 at 20 weeks. At 21 weeks it fell to 1:1,024 where it remained for the rest of the pregnancy.

She had twice-weekly ultrasound scans, and a cord blood sample at 20 weeks was satisfactory. However, at 28 weeks she was admitted with a fever and uterine contractions, and the CTG showed a sinusoidal fetal heart rate pattern. An urgent fetal blood sample was obtained and showed a very low haematocrit of 12.4 per cent. An immediate intrauterine transfusion of packed red blood cells was started and the sinusoidal rhythm disappeared.

Two further intrauterine blood transfusions took place, at 29 and at 32 weeks, and the woman remained on tocolytic therapy until 33 weeks. At 35.5 weeks, following spontaneous rupture of membranes, a healthy male infant weighing 2,030g was delivered by caesarean section. He had one further blood transfusion, and was allowed home eight days later.

Recommended care

All midwives are aware of the importance of maternal antibody screening. They should ensure that maternal blood is taken for antibody screening before 12 weeks' gestation, as this is when the antigens are detectable on the fetal red blood cells – this is especially important in a woman who has had a blood transfusion.

1. If a woman presents with anti-Kell antibodies, check the Kell antigen status of the father of the baby as

quickly as possible. Ninety-one per cent will be Kell-negative, and therefore the maternal antibodies can be ignored.

2. If the father of the baby is Kell-positive, either heterozygous (Kk) or homozygous (KK), or if paternity is unknown or uncertain, there should be immediate referral to a tertiary centre or fetal medicine unit. There should be no delay.

3. The care they will offer may vary, as advances in fetal medicine are occurring rapidly. It is likely to include some of the following:
   a. amniocentesis to assess fetal genotype. If the fetal blood group is Kell-negative, the pregnancy can continue without concern. If Kell-positive, proceed to:
   b. amniotic fluid optical density measurement to assess hyperbilirubinaemia (although there is disagreement as to how predictive this measurement is)
   c. regular antibody tests to monitor maternal antibody titre (although there is disagreement as to how predictive this level is)
   d. cordocentesis to assess fetal haemoglobin and the presence of maternal antibodies
   e. maternal plasmapheresis
   f. intrauterine blood transfusions into the umbilical vein
   g. serial ultrasound scans and cardiotocography to monitor fetal well-being and assess for development of hydrops fetalis
   h. early delivery if evidence of fetal compromise.

4. A high degree of alertness needs to be maintained. As the process is not a purely haemolytic one as with anti-D isoimmunisation, the suppressive nature of the anti-Kell antibody on red cell production – and hence the severity of the fetal anaemia – may not be detected in the usual tests (b) and (c) above.

5. The woman will need supportive midwifery care as she negotiates the roller-coaster of suddenly becoming a very 'high-risk' pregnancy.

6. Issues that arise when paternity is in doubt need to be handled extremely sensitively. The midwife needs to explain to the woman, in private, that if there is any doubt whatsoever over the paternity of the baby she needs to say so, as it could have profound implications for the well-being of her unborn baby.

7. If the woman did generate her anti-Kell antibodies as a result of a Kell-positive blood transfusion, she will need a great deal of supportive care, may wish to discuss the issue with a consultant haematologist and obstetrician, and may even wish to seek compensation.

Should childbearing women receive Kell-negative blood?

The leading authors on the subject agree that anti-Kell isoimmunisation is mainly a result of blood transfusion of incompatible blood (Babinszki et al 1998, Bowman et al 1992, Goh et al 1993, Grant et al 2000, Leggat et al 1991, McKenna et al 1999, Redman and Lee 1995, Vaughan et al 1998). Clearly, the recommendation that Kell-compatible blood should be used for all blood transfusions in women of childbearing age should be implemented nationally (it is the current policy of the National Blood Service). If it were, 'we would expect to see the absolute number and proportion of transfusion-induced anti-Kell to decrease as the policy for the use of Kell-negative blood becomes universally acceptable and available' (Grant et al 2000). 'It would seem appropriate to check for Kell status of donor blood prior to the transfusion of blood to a Kell-negative woman who has not reached the end of her reproductive life' (Goh et al 1993). 'The best prospect of reducing morbidity due to anti-Kell is to prevent transfusion-induced sensitisation of women to the Kell antigen. All women before and during childbearing age should receive Kell-compatible blood whenever they are transfused' (Leggat at al 1991).

Julie didn't.

Difficulties

So why isn't this being done? An editorial in The Lancet explains that it is not as easy as it sounds. Cross-matching is not a precise process – haematologists get the best match they can in the time they have. There are many other antigens similar to anti-Kell such as anti-c, and 'to provide matched blood for all such mothers would be difficult to organise and could even dangerously delay transfusion' (The Lancet 1991).

Cross-matching can only detect the presence of antibodies to blood group antigens present on the surface of red cells that are about to be transfused. Thus, in a Kell-negative mother who has never been immunised with Kell-positive blood (such as Julie when she was having her first baby), no antibodies will be present and incompatibility will not be detected by cross-match. This is how Julie was immunised: her cross-match detected no previous anti-Kell antibodies, and she was transfused with Kell-positive blood.

Generally, as the numbers of babies affected by anti-Kell alloimmunisation are very small, 'such disadvantages have been thought to outweigh the infrequent severe clinical effects' (The Lancet 1991). But one of these 'severe clinical effects' could have been Julie's baby. In her case, it was not an emergency transfusion in the presence of a massive obstetric haemorrhage but a calm, restorative and unhurried one done on the postnatal ward.

Could the obstetric team liaise with the haemotologists in the blood bank to let them know the degree of urgency attached to any proposed blood transfusion? If a woman is having a massive obstetric haemorrhage, then clearly the very small risk of anti-Kell isoimmunisation is heavily outweighed by the need to stabilise the woman's circulation quickly. Equally, before consenting to a blood transfusion, particularly one of a non-urgent, therapeutic nature, any woman of childbearing age or younger should be alerted to the very small but real risks so that she can make an informed decision. Perhaps putting up with some extreme tiredness following the birth, however debilitating, might be preferable to risking the health of future children, however small that risk might be.

A lucky escape

Julie's story has a happy ending. Her partner's blood results finally came back and showed he was among the 91 per cent of the population who are Kell-negative (which confirms that Julie's antibodies had occurred as a result of the blood transfusion). Julie confirmed to the midwife in private that he was definitely the father; there was no chance that it could be anyone else's baby. Everyone breathed a sigh of relief. Julie's now harmless anti-Kell antibodies were monitored just as a precaution for the remainder of her pregnancy but never rose beyond 1 : 8. Her baby, born at home, was pink, beautiful and the picture of health.

But it could have been very different. If her partner had been Kell-positive, it could have meant a nightmare pregnancy of tertiary centre referral, blood tests, amniocentesis, serial ultrasound scans, fetal blood sampling, in utero blood transfusions and possible early delivery. It could have meant intensive neonatal care, neonatal blood transfusions and, in the worst case, fetal or neonatal death – for this baby and every baby she tried to have with the same partner thereafter.

And all from a simple postnatal blood transfusion two years before . . . Makes you stop and think, doesn't it?

REFERENCES

Babinszki A, Lapinski R H and Berkowitz R L (1998). 'Prognostic factors and management in pregnancies complicated with severe Kell alloimmunisation: experiences of the last 13 years'. American Journal of Perinatology, 15 (12): 695–701.

Bowman J M, Pollock J M, Manning F A, et al (1992). 'Maternal Kell blood group alloimmunization'. Obstetrics and Gynecology, 79 (2): 239–244.

Goh J T, Kretowicz E M, Weinstein S and Ramsden G H (1993). 'Anti-Kell in pregnancy and hydrops fetalis'. Australian and New Zealand Journal of Obstetrics and Gynaecology, 33(2): 210–211.

Grant S R, Kilby M D, Meer L, et al (2000). 'The outcome of pregnancy in Kell alloimmunisation'. BJOG: An International Journal of Obstetrics and Gynaecology, 2000, 107: 481–485.

Huntley B (2001). 'The fetus as patient'. Lancet supplement, s58, Dec 2001.

Lancet editorial (1991). 'Dangers of anti-Kell in pregnancy'. The Lancet, 337: 1319–1320.

Leggat H M, Gibson J M, Barron S L, et al (1991). 'Anti-Kell in pregnancy'. BJOG: An International Journal of Obstetrics and Gynaecology, 98: 162–165.

McKenna D S, Nagaraja H N and O'Shaughnessy R (1999). 'Management of pregnancies complicated by anti-Kell isoimmunisation'. Obstetrics and Gynecology, 93 (5), Part 1: 667–673.

Redman C M and Lee S (1995). 'The Kell blood group system'. Transfus Clin Biol, 4: 243–249.

Sweet B R (1997). Mayes' Midwifery, London: Baillière Tindall.

Vaughan J, Manning M, Warwick R, et al (1998). 'Inhibition of erythroid progenitor cells by anti-Kell antibodies in fetal allo-immune anemia'. New England Journal of Medicine, 338: 798–803.

The Practising Midwife 2004; 7(3): 12–16

Coagulation disorders (1)

Deep vein thrombosis: breaking the silence

Tracey Hodgson

Thrombo-embolic disease (TED) continues to be a major public health concern and a significant cause of maternal morbidity and leading direct cause of maternal death (RCOG 2004b). Due to hypercoagulability changes, childbirth increases the risk of TED tenfold (RCOG 2004a), with overall health status and mode of birth adding or detracting incidence. For this reason, the midwife has a vital role in prevention, early diagnosis with prompt treatment and education to enhance maternal outcome. To achieve this, a working knowledge of underlying patho-physiology, risk factors, recognition of signs and symptoms with appropriate intervention is required.

The aim of this series of articles is to enhance the comprehension of TED, and highlight the midwife's role. The first condition to be discussed is deep vein thrombosis (DVT): as the possible sequelae are pulmonary embolism (PE) and cerebral vascular accident (CVA), these will be addressed in subsequent articles.

Pathophysiology

DVT occurs when a thrombus forms in a deep vein, frequently near a valve or in a sinus. This reduces venous return and stimulation of blood coagulation (Gorman 2000), resulting in the destruction of valves in deep veins, leaving permanent malfunction. In 70 per cent of cases, long-term problems of oedema and potential ulceration occur (Bergqvist et al 1990, Girling 2004), both of which cause distress, pain and interfere with daily living. DVT usually manifests in the lower limbs, so the focus of this article will be DVT in the leg (Belcaro et al 1995).

It is often referred to as the 'silent disease' (Wallis and Autar 2001) since signs and symptoms vary (see Box 4.2.1), do not reflect the severity of condition and are absent in 50 per cent of sufferers. Accuracy of incidence is difficult in light of this: however, it is generally accepted that only one in nine episodes is accurately diagnosed (Turner and Turner 1982). Risk of DVT continues until six weeks

Box 4.2.1 Clinical signs and symptoms of DVT

- Positive Homans' sign (dorsiflexion)
- Deep calf pain
- Heaviness in leg
- Distended superficial veins
- Tender hard veins may be palpable
- Affected leg oedematous
- Heat in leg and associated colour changes

postpartum, assuming the woman has no previous underlying pathology such as thrombophilia (Girling 2004).

Primary cause of DVT remains unknown but it is hypothesised that weak venous wall with valve incompetence promotes poor venous return. Secondary causes relate to damaged epithelial lining (hypertension), obstruction (lithotomy poles) and compression (gravid uterus). Accompanied with altered clotting factors, the incidence of DVT is increased. The Virchow's Triad (Bothamley 2002) identifies key criteria, stasis of venous circulation, trauma to veins and blood coagulation factors: these are illustrated in Table 4.2.1 and applied to current midwifery practice.

Hypercoagulation is a key criteria in this triad yet is normal physiology for all pregnant women or women who have just given birth: therefore, one key criteria met, this explains why childbearing has an increased risk of DVT. Midwives are recommended to use criteria assessment to identify risk (NMC 2004b) and indicate prophylactic management: this should be repeated on each hospital admission (RCOG 2004a). When undertaking risk assessment, it is worth noting that some risk factors double due to the influence on body function – eg, extreme obesity where body mass index (BMI) is greater than 30 (RCOG 2004a).

This is influenced further by overall health status, and must be assessed on an individual basis and reviewed if circumstances change – eg, bed rest. If the woman has a

Table 4.2.1 Thrombo-embolic disorders: risks during pregnancy to puerperium

Virchow's Triad	
Blood composition	Increased platelet adhesiveness Known family history (50% have family history of TED) Thrombophilia Poor nutrition Smoking Pre-eclampsia
Blood flow	Prolonged standing Gravid uterus Venous dilatation (raised estrogen) Lithotomy poles Dehydration Surgery (including instrumental delivery) Obesity (BMI >30) Reduced mobility (bed rest) Long-distance travel (air, rail and road)
Vein wall damage	Lithotomy poles Pelvic trauma Sepsis Known vascular disease (eg, diabetes, diverticulitis) Personal history of TED Parity 4 plus Intravenous drug user Hypertension

Box 4.2.2 Contra-indications to elasticated stockings

- No stockings of correct size
- Micro-vascular disease
- Rheumatoid arthritis
- Disseminated lupus erythematosis

(Collier 1999)

family history of thrombophilia, screening is recommended and if relevant a management plan developed.

Investigations

Diagnostic tools vary according to availability, specialists' preference and health of the woman. Common and non-invasive tests used are Doppler and ultrasonography; sometimes venogram will be performed (where radiopaque dye is intravenously administered via the dorsal foot and subsequent x-rays taken to observe venous flow). Pelvic vein thrombosis is difficult to diagnose accurately. However, if the woman's condition supports transfer to another department, an MRI may be performed (de Swiet 1999).

Nowadays, the D-dimer is performed – a finger prick test which produces quick results. It measures the D-dimer level, which is raised due to fibrinolysis: however, it cannot be indicative of TED without other supportive evidence such as clinical signs or positive Doppler test, as levels are normally raised during pregnancy (McKay 2004). It is worth noting that this test is less reliable in women over the age of 40 (O'Shaughnessy and Thomas 1999) and has little clinical value during the puerperium (Bothamley 2002).

Treatment

Treatment involves obstetric-led care whereby the obstetrician liaises with relevant members of the multi-disciplinary team. Clear explanation for the woman is essential as success of long-term management relies on her comprehension and compliance with treatment. Initially, anticoagulant therapy (usually heparin) will be started as per local regime – reliant on BMI for accuracy (RCOG 2004a) – with up to five days' bed rest. When at rest the legs may be elevated but care should be taken to ensure pressure is not on the calf, and hips not above the shoulders. After 48 hours (or until fully heparinised) elasticated stockings need to be worn (there are a few contra-indications – see Box 4.2.2). Elasticated stockings protect against venous dilatation, and reduce endothelial damage and subsequent risk from post-thrombotic syndrome. They must be applied correctly, with accurate measurements, put on before rising (ensuring no wrinkles) and the tops must not be turned down.

Observations include temperature to exclude infection; if the woman is breathless, oximetry is required until settled or pulmonary embolus ruled out. Calf and thigh circumference should be measured as the condition dictates. Leg skin colour and texture changes need to be monitored, and an emollient may be required if the skin becomes dry or irritated. Leg exercises are essential, especially while on bed rest, to prevent further thrombotic development. Warm compresses can offer relief and improve circulation (Anon 2005), but the lower limb should not be massaged as there is a risk of dislodging the clot. Pain management is often codeine based, so prevention of side effects such as constipation should be considered. A plan for labour will be required and/or help with babycare until the woman is fully mobile.

Anticoagulation

Drug therapy always comes with potential complications, so careful assessment for signs of health improvement should be made and the occurrence of side effects monitored and recorded (NMC 2004b). The purpose of anticoagulants is to prevent further thrombus formation or extension of the existing clot: they inhibit prothrombin being converted to thrombin and conversion of fibrinogen to fibrin (Downie et al 1999). The kidneys are responsible for clearing heparin from the system, so women with renal problems or pre-eclampsia require accurate assessment and, if anticoagulants are used, vigilant monitoring must be undertaken (Bothamley 2002).

Anticoagulants do not work directly on an established clot, since this relies on the natural fibrinolysis process within the body. Low weight molecular heparin (LWMH) is as effective as unfractionated heparin, has a longer half-life, improved bioavailability and fixed-weight-related dose. The severity of side effects is reduced, particularly thrombocytopenia, osteoporosis (RCOG 2004a) and haemorrhage (Rodie et al 2002).

There should be careful observation of the woman's skin for necrosis, hypersensitivity and alopecia. If the woman remains on heparin once stabilised, weekly assessment of platelet count is required – most women are gradually transferred to oral anticoagulants (with a transition period of two to three days).

Warfarin crosses the placental barrier and causes intracerebral bleeding, retroplacental haemorrhage and fetal abnormalities such as chondrodysplasia punctata and diaphragmatic hernia. Therefore, use in pregnancy is not recommended and should be avoided for at least the first trimester (BNF 2004). While warfarin is the only oral anticoagulant used in obstetrics, there is a new drug being researched called Exanta (ximelagatran). Currently this is used for knee surgery, showing up to 50 per cent reduction in DVT (www.protein.org.uk/forum). There are few side effects, and a fixed dose is given with no titration or coagulation monitoring required. Future use in pregnancy is currently unlikely as alteration to liver function has occurred in some patients, but research is continuing.

Management

Discharge depends on the woman's ability to inject herself with heparin and observations remaining within normal limits. Considerable information should be offered, supported by literature. This includes:

- avoidance of standing or sitting for long periods
- wearing elasticated stockings
- continuing with calf and respiratory pump exercises
- avoiding restrictive clothing – eg, 'pop' socks
- ensuring medication is understood, administered correctly and sharps are disposed of safely
- avoiding aspirin because of the risk of haemorrhage (due to aggregation of platelets)
- importance of observing limb changes and reporting any concerns promptly to the doctor or midwife.

Future management of pregnancies with appropriate contraceptive advice is essential, and it is important to ensure that the woman has an anticoagulation card explaining the implications and containing confirmation about haematological follow-up.

A labour care plan must include discontinuation of anticoagulants and assessment of clotting factors, repeated as necessary – eg, prior to epidural. If the woman is high risk, requires surgical intervention or there is a need for lithotomy poles, elastic stockings are essential. Avoiding dehydration and encouragement of mobilisation will reduce risk and promote normal progress of labour. If regional anaesthetic is used, LWMH must be withheld for four hours (this applies to insertion and removal of epidural catheter).

Health promotion is vital to prevent vascular problems or consequential complications. If women are offered informed choice, they can directly influence prevention or prognosis of disease. The midwife as a public health carer has the ideal opportunity to educate the woman, assess her lifestyle and support decisions made (NMC 2004b).

Key issues in reducing associated mortality and morbidity are:

- inform about signs and symptoms (Reynolds 2004)
- reduce or stop smoking
- healthy eating and drinking – eg, reduce salt and fat intake, choice of cooking methods
- reduce obesity, aim for normal BMI range
- exercise – development of arterial collateral blood supply, improve venous return, increase muscle tone and posture
- importance of postnatal examination in assessing venous return, danger of time restraints or limited visiting (Reynolds 2004) reviewed
- if the woman is diagnosed with DVT once she has given birth, give appropriate contraceptive advice, preconception assessment for subsequent pregnancies and/or surgical/hospital interventions.

Since prophylactic treatment was introduced nationally (RCOG 2004b), the incidence of DVT has been reduced.

Implications for midwifery practice

- An accurate history should be reviewed as condition dictates and a BMI must be performed.
- Use risk assessment criteria to identify category risk and implement appropriate prophylactic measures (RCOG 2004a).
- Advise if the woman has a sedentary lifestyle – eg, if desk worker, about moving and posture.
- Use stockings when lithotomy poles are required. Gently move leg away from poles and encourage movement of toes to relieve pressure and enhance circulation.
- Midwives need to review local guidelines, ensuring they follow RCOG (2004a) recommendations on heparin dosage.

- Design maternity facilities to encourage ambulation – eg, communal dining area rather than eating in bed.

Prevention could have significant influence on future morbidity. Midwives often do not observe the consequences of education or outcomes of care as they practise within a limited timeframe, but they are part of a large multi-disciplinary public health team with responsibility to educate women and their families (NMC 2004a).

Conclusion

Venous thrombotic disease is a public health issue, and midwives are likely to care for increasing numbers of high-risk women. Lifestyle changes are well documented in the media: obesity, sedentary habits (accompanied with associated hypertension), more women having babies in their forties, increased LSCS rate and high proportion of teenage girls smoking.

Prevention is paramount; accurate history with BMI at booking are early detectors and can facilitate appropriate care. Encouraging mobilisation and hydration in labour can reduce the risk. The importance of postnatal examination must not be underestimated, including careful assessment of limbs. Management of TED is complex; clear guidelines and a plan of action are important to reduce the risk and enhance prophylaxis. The outcome of DVT can lead to more significant health problems, thus PE will be the focus of the next article.

REFERENCES

Anon. (2005). Cardiovascular Care Made Incredibly Easy, Lippincott Williams & Wilkins.
Belcaro G, Nicholaides A and Vellar M (1995). 'Deep vein thrombosis'. In: Venous Disorders. London: WB Saunders Company Ltd.
Bergqvist A, Bergqvist D, Lindhagen A et al (1990). 'Late symptoms after pregnancy-related DVT'. British Journal of Obstetrics and Gynaecology, 97: 338–341.
Bothamley J (2002). 'Thromboembolism in pregnancy'. In: Emergencies Around Childbirth. M Boyle (ed). Oxford: Radcliffe Medical Press.
BNF (2004). British National Formulary (Sept No 48) www.BNF.org Accessed 7 December 2004.
Collier M (1999). 'Brevet tx: anti-embolism stockings for prevention and treatment of DVT'. British Journal of Nursing, 8 (1): 44–49.
De Swiet M (1999). 'Thromboembolic disease'. In: High Risk Pregnancy (2nd edn). D James, P Steer et al (eds). London: WB Saunders.
Downie G, Mackenzie J and Williams A (1999). Pharmacology and Drug Management for Nurses. Second Edition, Edinburgh: Churchill Livingstone.
Girling J (2004). 'Thromboembolism and thrombophilia'. Current Obstetrics and Gynaecology, 14: 11–22.
McKay K (2004). 'A guide to less common antenatal blood tests'. The Practising Midwife, 7 (3): 14–26.

NMC (2004a). The NMC Code of Professional Conduct: Standards for Conduct, Performance and Ethics, London: NMC.
NMC (2004b). Midwives Rules and Standards, London: NMC.
O'Shaughnessy D and Thomas M (1999). 'Use of D-dimer test in deep vein thrombosis'. Thrombosis, Spring: 5.
RCOG. (2004a). 'Thromboprophylaxis during pregnancy, labour and after vaginal delivery'. RCOG Guideline No 37, January.
RCOG. (2004b). Confidential Enquiry into Maternal Deaths, London: RCOG.
Reynolds S (2004). 'Deep vein thrombosis: are postnatal women aware?' British Journal of Midwifery, 12 (10): 636–640.
Rodie V, Thomson A, Stewart F et al (2002). 'Low molecular weight heparin for the treatment of venous thromboembolism in pregnancy: a series'. British Journal of Obstetrics and Gynaecology, 109: 1020–1024.
Turner A and Turner J (1982). 'An unexpected killer'. Nursing Mirror, 155: 64–65.
Wallis M and Autar R (2001). 'Deep vein thrombosis: clinical nursing management'. Nursing Standard, 15:18: 47–54.

Website: www.protein.org.uk/forum

The Practising Midwife 2005; 8(3): 12–15

Coagulation disorders (2)
Pulmonary embolism

Tracey Hodgson

Introduction

Venous thromboembolism (VTE) is 10 times more common in pregnant women than in non-pregnant women (Rodger et al 2003) and the leading cause of maternal death (RCOG 2004a). Deep vein thrombosis (DVT) was the first article in this series; a serious complication of DVT is pulmonary embolism (PE), the focus of this article.

Definition

PE occurs when a blood embolus blocks the pulmonary artery or one of its branches. The original thrombosis is usually from a deep vein in the leg, but may arise from a pelvic vein thrombus or the right atrium (Rodger et al 2003).

Incidence

Massive PE is the second commonest cause of unexpected death at any age (Feied 2005); PE with DVT causes 10 per cent of all hospital deaths (Feied 2005, www.dh.gov.uk). VTE remain the commonest direct cause of maternal disease (RCOG 2004a) and one of the most challenging conditions to diagnose due to the variety of signs and symptoms (Box 4.3.1) and differential diagnosis (Box 4.3.2) (Owen and Gibson 2004, Rodger et al 2003, Thomson and Greer 2000). In the past maternal mortality report there were 26 deaths due to PE, 25 directly thromboembolic, six fewer than in the previous triennium. The reduction is during the antenatal period, but the reason for this is unclear (RCOG 2004a).

Pathophysiology

Physiological changes to respiratory, cardiovascular and haematological systems are essential to promote

---

Box 4.3.1 Signs and symptoms of pulmonary embolism

- Dyspnoea*
- Tachycardia*
- Cyanosis
- Cough
- Fever
- Chest pain
- Shoulder pain
- Pleuritic pain
- Leg pain*
- Haemoptysis
- Anxiety
- Tightness in chest
- Crackles on oscillation of chest

*Common signs and symptoms with pregnancy and PE (Thomson and Greer 2000)

(Bothamley 2002, Feied 2005, Rodger et al 2003)

Box 4.3.2 Differential diagnosis of pulmonary embolism

- Chest infection
- Pneumothorax
- Pulmonary aspiration
- Amniotic fluid embolism
- Intra-abdominal bleeding
- Septicaemia
- Intracerebral haemorrhage
- Hypoglycaemia
- Hyperglycaemia
- Aortic aneurysm
- Myocardial infarction
- Pleurisy
- Tuberculosis
- Pericarditis

(Bothamley 2002, Feied 2005)

---

maternal health and development of the baby. However, these alterations favour VTE events. During pregnancy the normal changes to the respiratory system include the flaring and lowering of the ribs, rising of the diaphragm and hyperventilation, in response to increased progesterone levels. This lowers tension in the alveolar and a PCO_2 relative to respiratory alkalosis (Gilbert and Harmon 2003). Vital capacity decreases, and tidal volume increases to accommodate these changes and facilitate oxygenation and excretion of waste products.

PE occurs when an embolus lodges in the pulmonary circulation, causing inadequate oxygen to local tissue, reduction in oxygenated blood and volume returning to the left atria. This results in pain in the chest and/or shoulder, and dyspnoea and cyanosis if the embolus is large (Bothamley 2002). Dead space is created which inhibits gaseous exchange (Gilbert and Harmon 2003), and can be single or multiple depending on the distribution of the embolus.

Risk factors

Reviewing the literature, with the exception of Stein et al (2004) reference to race is not specific although cultural influences are evident (RCOG 2004a). The main risk factors are:

- Pregnancy
- Previous thromboembolism
- Thrombophilia
- Obesity
- Over 35 years
- Prolonged immobility
- Emergency LSCS (lower segment caesarean section).

Signs and symptoms

Signs and symptoms associated with PE are numerous (Box 4.3.1) and vary in severity without always reflecting the extent of the embolus. The accuracy of history regarding current complaint/condition and the woman's personal and family history are essential to facilitate diagnosis. Many authors have offered their interpretation of sign and symptoms which, combined, confirm PE (Bothamley 2002, Conway 2003, Feied 2005, Herbert 1997, Rodger et al 2003, Thomson and Greer 2000). However, the recommendation increasingly being used nationally is from the British Thoracic Society (BTS). If a woman has breathlessness and/or tachypnoea with or without haemoptysis or pleuritic pain, these are compatible with PE if combined with any of the risk factors; and in the absence of an alternative diagnosis (Box 4.3.2) PE is the likely diagnosis and should be treated accordingly (BTS 2003).

It is clear why and how PE is misdiagnosed. However, midwives have an advantage as they care for women during the childbearing process. Therefore, if the above clinical features are evident, the fact that the woman is pregnant or has recently given birth favours the diagnosis of PE.

Diagnosis

Up to 35 per cent of women who are suspected of having a PE are misdiagnosed (Rodger et al 2003). However, the mortality and morbidity rate of PE outweighs these risks. If the woman collapses with cyanosis, tachypnoea and complains of chest pain (may be conscious), it is likely to be a PE and the midwife should treat it as an emergency call and start resuscitation. If the embolus is large, instantaneous death is likely. However, Bothamley (2002) recommends prolonged cardiac massage to break the thrombus up. If peripheral pulses and adequate oxygen are established, recovery is possible (Herbert 1997).

The diagnosis is more challenging when the symptoms are vague. However, all complaints of chest pain and lower limb pain should be thoroughly investigated (RCOG 2004a). Acute minor embolism can be a useful warning of potential collapse, so prompt and appropriate treatment is essential. For example, if a woman presents with unexplained pyrexia, cough, chest pain and breathlessness, it could be a chest infection or a PE. So, while waiting for medical assistance to arrive, the midwife should review the woman's risk factors. Administer oxygen with the woman in a supported sitting position (this may help reduce symptoms and anxiety) and gain IV access for fluid and drug management.

Management

The majority of research relating to PE is reliant on non-pregnant women who have a higher incidence of pulmonary circulating conditions – eg, asthma and cystic fibrosis (BTS 2003). This is due to relatively low numbers and the ethical and moral issues relating to research on pregnant women, although it should be remembered that the physiological changes which occur during pregnancy influence the ability to cope with disorders and disease.

Nishinura et al (1998) state that two-thirds of deaths caused by PE occur within the first hour; the other deaths usually happen in the following six hours. Prompt action is therefore essential to decrease mortality.

If the woman collapses, emergency resuscitation procedures should follow, including oxygenation, intravenous access and anticoagulant therapy (and transfer to hospital if in the community):

- Give oxygen and assess oxygen saturation levels to expedite clinical condition and exclude alternative diagnosis. A pulse oximeter is less invasive than arterial puncture, and does not carry the risk of haemorrhage (Thomson and Greer 2000). However, if arterial blood is required, the woman's position needs to be upright to keep the weight of the uterus off the major vessels (Bothamley 2002, Walsh and

Rice 1999). Normal results will follow with 10 per cent of women, but hypoxemia and primary respiratory alkalosis with no other pulmonary disease means it is likely to be PE (Bothamley 2002).

- Intravenous access is vital to facilitate resuscitation and give drug therapy as required.
- Vital signs should be observed and recorded for ongoing assessment and to guide recovery or further management. This includes pulse for rate, volume and rhythm; blood pressure and respirations for rate, depth, audibility, effort and cyanosis. (Observations of nasal flaring and use of accessory shoulder and neck muscles imply that respiratory effort is laboured and the condition is deteriorating).
- Electrocardiogram is required to monitor the woman's condition and rule out heart anomalies.
- Portable chest X-ray is routine: it demonstrates atelectasis and consolidated areas in response to infarcts and inflammation in the lungs. Regrettably, the X-ray can be normal (Girling 2004, Thomson and Greer 2000), but can exclude other diagnoses – eg, pneumothorax.
- Anticoagulants as per RCOG (2004b) guidelines, with observations and monitoring as condition dictates (Hodgson 2005). Rapid and prolonged anticoagulants are used to prevent thrombus extension and further emboli; if promptly used, mortality is reduced by 10–30 per cent (Feied 2005).
- Accurate assessment of fluid balance is achieved by central venous pressure line, indwelling urinary catheter and hourly measurements.
- A small amount of morphine (1–2 mg IV) can be administered to relieve pain and reduce anxiety (Bothamley 2002), but caution is required due to the effect on the respiratory centre (BNF 2004).

Throughout these procedures the midwife needs to explain events to the mother and her supporters, facilitate the team, undertake observations, maintain contemporaneous records (NMC 2004) and ensure the baby is cared for appropriately.

It can be seen from the above that the diagnosis of PE is difficult; while some view it as challenging, others may feel frustrated that test results are not definitive in terms of diagnosis. This is where a holistic approach to care and treatment is important to aid management.

Treatment

Heparin takes too long to lysis the embolus: recombinant tissue plasminogen activators are administered (Thomson and Greer 2000); streptokinase can be used but might worsen hypotension and cannot be given with heparin (Owen and Gibson 2004). Alteplase is preferred as it has

fewer side effects (Feied 2005): however, safety during pregnancy is not established (BNF 2004).

If DVT is diagnosed, no further investigations are warranted as they all carry risk. If DVT is not evident, then a ventilation perfusion (V/Q) scan is the investigation usually performed (De Swiet 1999, Feied 2005). This is when perfusion of intravenous injection of albumin labelled with radioactive technetium is administered. The albumin is distributed around the pulmonary circulation and areas of compromised perfusion (Rodger et al 2003). De Swiet (1999) states that the mother can be reassured as it does not harm the baby, but Rodger et al (2003) argue there is a minimal risk of childhood malignancy and congenital eye abnormalities. The risk of PE to the mother and viability of the baby need to be considered in balance to the small but evident risk. If a scan has been performed, the mother should refrain from breastfeeding for 15 hours (Thomson and Greer 2000).

Alternative tests

- Duplex ultrasound, a non-invasive method which can be repeated if required (Thomson and Greer 2000), needs to be performed within 24 hours of the event, as it reverts to normal. The scan relies on demonstrating the presence of DVT to diagnose PE, but the majority of DVTs cannot be visualised (Feied 2005). Resources are limited due to location and out-of-hours access.
- D-dimer is recommended, although unreliable; if the result is negative, it is unlikely to be a PE (McKay 2004, Owen and Gibson 2004).
- Pulmonary angiography is the preferred choice for accuracy (Feied 2005) but extremely invasive.
- Helical Computed Tomographic Angiography is a relatively new procedure that is less invasive and becoming more widely used (O'Neill et al 2004).
- Pulmonary embolectomy is extreme and only undertaken for pregnant women when thrombolytic therapy has failed (Feied 2005).

Midwives' role

Understanding alterations in pulmonary physiology during pregnancy can help the midwife anticipate problems and prevent adverse events (Gilbert and Harmon 2003). Breathlessness, malaise and leg pain are often associated with pregnancy and easily dismissed as musculoskeletal, anxiety or cramp. Careful exploration of history and observations are required.

If the woman presents with suspected PE the midwife needs to summon appropriate assistance (NMC 2004) whilst remaining calm. The woman is likely to be frightened as she struggles to breathe and/or cope with acute pain; a calm, controlled environment is therefore essential to reduce anxiety and support the woman who may undergo invasive and unpleasant investigations while diagnosis is confirmed.

Midwives need to work effectively within a multidisciplinary team (NMC 2004) as this challenging situation requires prompt treatment and use of large-dose anticoagulants which in themselves carry risk.

Postnatally, the immediate needs of the mother and baby should be met and reassessed as recovery occurs. The mother may require time to discuss and debrief her experiences and to understand diagnosis and future risk. She will require follow-up at the haematology clinic and need to carry an anticoagulant card in case of accident or other health intervention. Support in administrating medication and knowledge of side-effects takes time and should not be a one-off event – this promotes compliance and reduces accidents. Advice on contraception choices and information to reduce further VTE events is necessary for good health.

Potential complications for the woman surviving PE include added risk of recurrent PE, development of pulmonary hypotension, chronic corpulmonale (Feied 2005) and those associated with DVT (Hodgson 2005).

Conclusion

The incidence of PE during the childbearing process has fallen dramatically over the past 30 years (RCOG 2004b). The midwife has a key role in assessing risk, health education and use of prophylactic measures (Hodgson 2005).

Resources within the NHS are constantly stretched, and while it is ideal for a woman with PE to be cared for in ITU a bed might not be available. If this is the case, the woman will remain in the maternity unit – the midwife is likely to be a key carer and should facilitate the team in managing the situation.

Key points

- To continue reducing VTE events by obtaining comprehensive history, accompanied by accurate assessment, is essential.
- Health education regarding risk factors and taking precautions – eg, wearing of elasticised stockings, leg exercises and taking breaks during long-distance travelling by air, train or car.
- Weighing women during pregnancy had become unfashionable, but there is now clear evidence of its importance. Calculating and recording the BMI helps assess risk and achieve therapeutic medication, so failing to do so is substandard care.

- If there is a VTE risk, screening for thrombophilia and prophylactic measures should be taken.
- A pregnant woman with chest pain should be assumed to have a PE unless another cause can be proved.
- Interprofessional learning is essential so that those working in emergency departments, gynaecology and intensive care appreciate the significance of these symptoms in pregnancy and puerperium.
- Policies must be kept up to date to reflect current guidelines and recommendations.

REFERENCES

BNF (2004). British National Formulary, September, No 48. www.BNF.org

Bothamley J (2002). 'Thromboembolism in pregnancy'. In: M. Boyle (ed), Emergencies Around Childbirth, Oxford: Radcliffe Medical Press, pages 23–40.

British Thoracic Society (2003). 'British Thoracic Society guidelines for the management of suspected acute pulmonary embolism'. Thoracic, 58: 470–475.

Conway A (2003). 'Pulmonary embolism'. Nurse2Nurse, 3 (6): 32–33.

De Swiet (1999). 'Thromboembolic disease'. In: D James et al (eds), High Risk Pregnancy, 2nd edition, London: W B Saunders, pages 901–909.

Feied C (2005). 'Pulmonary embolism'. http://www.eMedicine.com/EMERG/topic490.htm

Gilbert E and Harmon J (2003). Manual of High Risk Pregnancy and Delivery (3rd edition), USA: Mosby.

Girling J (2004). 'Thromboembolism and thrombophilia'. Current Obstetrics and Gynaecology, 14: 11–22.

Herbert L (1997). Caring for the Vascular Patient, Edinburgh: Churchill Livingstone.

Hodgson T (2005). 'Deep vein thrombosis: breaking the silence'. The Practising Midwife, 8 (3): 28–31.

McKay K (2004). 'A guide to less common antenatal blood tests'. The Practising Midwife, 7 (3): 14–26.

Nishinura K, Kawaguchi M, Shimokawa M, Kitaguchi K and Furuya H (1998). 'Treatment of pulmonary embolism during caesarean section with recombinant plasminogen activator'. Anesthesiol, 89: 1027–1028.

NMC (2004). Midwives' Rules and Standards, London: NMC.

O'Neill J, Wright L and Murchison J (2004). 'Helical CTPA in the investigation of pulmonary embolism: a 6 year review'. Clinical Radiology, 59: 819–825.

Owen A and Gibson M (2004). 'Pulmonary embolism: advances in diagnosis & treatment'. Care of the Critically Ill, 20 (3): 79–83.

RCOG (2004a). Confidential Enquiry into Maternal Deaths, London: RCOG.

RCOG (2004b). 'Thromboprophylaxis during pregnancy, labour and after vaginal delivery'. RCOG guideline No 37, January.

Rodger M, Walker M and Wells P (2003). 'Diagnosis and treatment of venous thromboembolism in pregnancy'. Best Practice and Research Clinical Haematology, 16 (2): 279–296.

Stein P, Kayali F and Olson R (2004). 'Incidence of venous thrombosis in infants and children: data from the national hospital discharge survey'. The Journal of Pediatrics, October: 563–565.

Thomson A and Greer I (2000). 'Non-haemorrhagic obstetric shock'. Clinical Obstetrics and Gynaecology, 14 (1): 19–41.

Walsh M and Rice K (1999). 'Venous thrombosis and pulmonary embolism', in V Fahey (ed), Vascular Nursing, 3rd edition, London: W B Saunders.

The Practising Midwife 2005; 8(6): 34–37

An early warning system for pre-eclampsia

PRECOG/Action on Pre-eclampsia[1]

This article introduces the pre-eclampsia community guideline, published by the PRECOG development group under the auspices of Action on Pre-eclampsia.

Midwives and PRECOG

Helen Crafter

Community midwives and GPs have long wondered what to do with pregnant women they see at home or in a community clinic when they give a personal or family history of pregnancy-induced hypertension, or present with mild, sometimes non-specific, symptoms of pre-eclampsia. Many will increase visits to such women in the community on a regular basis; many will refer a woman to hospital (with a day assessment unit if they are lucky), perhaps feeling that they might just be wasting everybody's time.

The PRECOG document is a short, concise, easily portable, practice-based paper which puts all the evidence together in simple-to-read tables so health professionals can feel that the information they have at their fingertips provides them with high-quality evidence. It also provides the opportunity for midwives to read and discuss the guideline with women so that together they can decide 'best practice' and the best course of action. It enables midwives and GPs to escape from defensive practice 'just in case', and it provides a communication tool so both hospital and community staff have a clear rationale about the quality of, and approach to, antenatal care all pregnant women should be offered.

It is hoped that the PRECOG guideline, with widespread and consistent use especially by midwives, will reduce the maternal and perinatal morbidity and mortality rates significantly over the next few years.

PRECOG: the user's story

Fiona Milne

There are nearly a thousand of us who are members of the charity Action on Pre-eclampsia. Hundreds more contact the helpline while thousands access the website daily. Most of us first contact the charity because we want information about pre-eclampsia, to understand what is happening or has happened to us and whether the same will occur again if we are brave enough to risk another pregnancy.

As well as general information and emotional support, Action on Pre-eclampsia offers women expert referral for post-pre-eclampsia counselling. As part of this process, past history and pregnancies are examined, further investigations are carried out where necessary, and the end result for the woman is an understanding of the way her body works in pregnancy and advice that she can take to her healthcare professional at the start of her next pregnancy.

Until PRECOG, to get this level of evidence-based and individual support you would have to have gone through the trauma of pre-eclampsia, been lucky enough to be told about the charity, and lucky enough to live near enough to travel for the expert advice.

Importantly, the guideline reveals that previous pre-eclampsia is only one of the risk factors that make someone more likely to develop the condition. To me, PRECOG, if and when it is adopted by all trusts across the country, will provide this evidence-based understanding for all pregnant women and their healthcare professionals and will provide it before pre-eclampsia develops.

---

[1]Contact Action on Pre-eclampsia: 020 8863 3271; mikerich@apec.org.uk; www.apec.org.uk. Expert speakers can visit locally, and further training is available at six-monthly pre-eclampsia health seminars.

Definitions and terminology

Term	Definition used in the guideline
Fetal compromise	Reduced fetal movements, small for gestational age infant
Hypertension	A diastolic blood pressure of 90mmHg or more
New hypertension	Hypertension at or after 20 weeks' gestation in a woman with a diastolic blood pressure of less than 90mmHg before 20 weeks
Pre-existing hypertension	A diastolic blood pressure pre-pregnancy or at booking (before 20 weeks) of 90mmHg or more
New proteinuria	The presence of proteinuria as shown by 1+(0.3g/l) or more on proteinuria dipstick testing, a protein/creatinine ratio of 30mg/mmol or more on a random sample or a urine protein excretion of 300mg or more per 24 hours
Significant proteinuria	Urine protein excretion = 300mg per 24 hours
Pre-eclampsia	New hypertension and significant proteinuria at or after 20 weeks of pregnancy, confirmed if it resolves after birth
Superimposed pre-eclampsia	The development of features of pre-eclampsia in the context of pre-existing hypertension, pre-existing proteinuria or both

The guideline

Recommendation 1

Identify the presence of any of the factors in Table 4.4.1 that predispose a woman in a given pregnancy to pre-eclampsia (grade B/C).

Recommendation 2

Offer pregnant women with the predisposing factors for pre-eclampsia shown in Table 4.4.2 referral early in pregnancy for specialist input to their antenatal care plan (grade D/good practice point). The factors indicate an underlying pathology, concomitant condition or otherwise high level of obstetric risk related to pre-eclampsia, which would benefit from specialist input: this may be for further specialist investigation, for clarification of risk

Table 4.4.1 Factors that can be measured early in pregnancy that increase the likelihood of pre-eclampsia developing in any given pregnancy

Factor	PRECOG grade
First pregnancy	B
Multiparous with: • pre-eclampsia in any previous pregnancy • ten years or more since last baby	 B B
Age 40 years or more	B
Body mass index of 35 or more	B
Family history of pre-eclampsia (in mother or sister)	B
Booking diastolic blood pressure of 80mmHg or more	B
Booking proteinuria (of ≥1+ on more than one occasion or quantified at ≥0.3g/24 hours)	C
Multiple pregnancy	B
Certain underlying medical conditions: • pre-existing hypertension • pre-existing renal disease • pre-existing diabetes • antiphospholipid antibodies	B

Table 4.4.2 Factors for referral in early pregnancy for specialist input to care

Factor	PRECOG grade
Multiple pregnancy	D
Underlying medical conditions: • pre-existing hypertension or booking diastolic BP ≥90mmHg	 D
• pre-existing renal disease or booking proteinuria (≥1+ on more than one occasion or quantified at ≥0.3g/24 hours)	D
• pre-existing diabetes	D
• antiphospholipid antibodies	D
Pre-eclampsia in any previous pregnancy	D
Any two other predisposing factors from Table 4.4.1: ie, first pregnancy, age 40 years or more, BMI ≥35, family history, booking diastolic BP ≥80mmHg <90mmHg	GPP*

*Note that the effect of two predisposing factors on the overall likelihood of developing pre-eclampsia has yet not been studied, so there is no evidence. Therefore, the recommendation that these women would benefit from specialist input to assess their obstetric risk is the opinion of the pre-eclampsia specialists in the PRECOG group.

or to advise on early intervention or pharmacological treatment.

It is not within the remit of this guideline to prescribe specialist-led care or to exclude GP- or midwife-led care. It is recognised that all women benefit from continuity of care and need midwifery care as part of their individual antenatal care plan, whatever their obstetric risk.

Table 4.4.3 Frequency of community monitoring after 20 weeks for indications of pre-eclampsia*

Frequency level	Women who qualify**	Frequency interval	
		24 to 32 weeks' gestation	**32 weeks' gestation to birth**
Level 1	None of the predisposing factors listed in Recommendation 1	As per local protocols/NICE antenatal guideline for low-risk multiparous women	As per local protocols/NICE antenatal guideline for low-risk multiparous women
Level 2	One predisposing factor listed in Recommendation 1. No factor that requires referral in early pregnancy (Recommendation 2)	Minimum standard no more than three-week interval between assessments, adjusted to individual needs and any changes during pregnancy***	Minimum standard no more than two-week interval between assessments, adjusted to individual needs and any changes during pregnancy***

*By definition, pre-eclampsia cannot be diagnosed before 20 weeks' gestation

**Note that women who have been referred early in pregnancy (see Recommendation 2) do not qualify for level 1 or level 2 of midwife- or GP-led PRECOG community monitoring

***Interval corresponds to NICE antenatal guideline for primiparous women

Recommendation 3a

Offer pregnant women one of two levels of midwife-/GP-led community monitoring after 20 weeks* (see Table 4.4.3) for indications of pre-eclampsia, according to their level of risk of developing pre-eclampsia (grade B).

Recommendation 3b

All pregnant women should be aware that after 20 weeks' gestation pre-eclampsia may develop between antenatal assessments, and that it is appropriate for them to self-refer at any time (grade B).

Recommendation 4

At every PRECOG assessment the healthcare provider and pregnant woman should identify the presence of any one of the five significant signs and symptoms of the onset of pre-eclampsia shown in Table 4.4.4 and act according to recommendation 5 (grades B and C).

Description of symptoms (GPP): As there are limited data from studies, the following are descriptions and comments from the pre-eclampsia specialists in the PRECOG group and from CEMD (good practice points).

Table 4.4.4 Community monitoring: content

Signs and significant symptoms	PRECOG grade
New hypertension	B
New and/or significant proteinuria	B
Maternal symptoms of headache and/or visual disturbance	C
Epigastric pain and/or vomiting	C
Reduced fetal movements, small for gestational age infant	B

Headache and visual disturbances
- Severe pounding headache, partial loss of visual acuity, bright/flashing visual disturbances. Migraines can continue during pregnancy, and any migraine can be excruciating without being life-threatening or associated with signs of pre-eclampsia.
- A headache of sufficient severity to seek medical advice (CEMD).

Epigastric pain
- Epigastric pain, especially if severe or associated with vomiting. The most sinister epigastric pain is described by the sufferer as severe and is associated with definite tenderness to deep epigastric palpation (the woman winces).
- New epigastric pain (CEMD).

Recommendation 5

See Table 4.4.5.

Recommendation 6

Reducing errors in blood pressure measurement
- Use accurate equipment – mercury sphygmomanometer or validated alternative method (grade C).
- Use sitting or semi-reclining position so that the arm to be used is at the level of the heart (GPP).
- Do not take the blood pressure in the upper arm with the woman on her side as this will give falsely lower readings (grade D).
- Use appropriate size of cuff: a standard size (13 × 23cm) for an arm circumference of up to 33cm, a large size (33 × 15 cm) for an arm circumference between 33 and 41cm, and a thigh cuff (18 × 36cm)

Table 4.4.5 Community monitoring: thresholds for further action

Description	Definition	Action by midwife/GP	PRECOG grade
New hypertension without proteinuria after 20 weeks	Diastolic BP ≥90 and <100mmHg	Refer for hospital step-up assessment within 48 hours	C
	Diastolic BP ≥90 and <100mmHg with significant symptoms*	Refer for same-day hospital step-up assessment	C
	Systolic BP ≥160mmHg	Refer for same-day hospital step-up assessment	C
	Diastolic BP ≥100mmHg	Refer for same-day hospital step-up assessment	C
New hypertension and proteinuria after 20 weeks	Diastolic BP ≥90mmHg and new proteinuria ≥1+ on dipstick	Refer for same-day hospital step-up assessment	A
	Diastolic BP ≥110mmHg and new proteinuria ≥1+ on dipstick	**Arrange immediate admission**	A
	Systolic BP ≥170mmHg and new proteinuria ≥1+ on dipstick	**Arrange immediate admission**	A
	Diastolic BP ≥90mmHg and new proteinuria ≥1+ on dipstick and significant symptoms*	**Arrange immediate admission**	A
New proteinuria without hypertension after 20 weeks	1+ on dipstick	Repeat pre-eclampsia assessment in community within 1 week	C
	2+ or more on dipstick	Refer for hospital step-up assessment within 48 hours	C
	≥1+ on dipstick with significant symptoms*	Refer for same-day hospital step-up assessment	C
Maternal symptoms or fetal signs and symptoms without new hypertension or proteinuria	Headache and/or visual disturbances with diastolic BP less than 90mmHg and a trace or no protein	Follow local protocols for investigation. Consider reducing interval before next PRECOG assessment	C
	Epigastric pain with diastolic BP less than 90mmHg and a trace or no protein	Refer for same-day hospital step-up assessment	C
	Reduced movements or small for gestational age infant with diastolic BP less than 90mmHg and a trace or no protein	Follow local protocols for investigation of fetal compromise. Consider reducing interval before next full pre-eclampsia assessment	C

*Epigastric pain, vomiting, headache, visual disturbances, reduced fetal movements, small for gestational age infant

for an arm circumference of 41cm or more. There is less error introduced by using too large a cuff than by too small a cuff (grade C).

- Deflate the cuff slowly, at a rate of 2mmHg to 3mmHg per second, taking at least 30 seconds to complete the whole deflation (grade D).
- Use Korotkoff V (disappearance of heart sounds) for measurement of diastolic pressure, as this is subject to less intra-observer and inter-observer variation than Korotkoff IV (muffling of heart sounds) and seems to correlate best with intra-arterial pressure in pregnancy (grade A); in the 15 per cent of pregnant women whose diastolic pressure falls to zero before the last sound is heard, both phase IV and phase V readings should be recorded – eg, 148/84/0mmHg (GPP).
- Measure to the nearest 2mmHg to avoid digit preference (grade D).

- Obtain an estimated systolic pressure by palpation to avoid auscultatory gap (grade D).
- If two readings are necessary, use the average of the readings and not just the lowest reading. This will minimise threshold avoidance – the tendency to repeat a reading until one that is below a known threshold is recorded that requires no action (GPP).

Recommendation 7

The performance of a semi-quantitative dipstick is dependent on many variables, including how the dipstick is read (by all-comers to a clinic, staff at a routine clinic, trained research observers or a machine) and the urine concentration of the sample. The performance of quantitative methods of measuring protein is also dependent on a number of factors, such as the adequate collection of a 24-hour sample and the method used to measure protein.

Improving reliability of proteinuria estimate using dipstick testing

- Reduce false positive results by training the reader of the dipstick to use the correct methodology to read the dipstick tests – the manufacturer's recommendations should be followed (grade C).
- Automated dipstick readers reduce reader error (grade C).
- Do not repeat a test on a second sample as this does not improve the predictive value of result for significant proteinuria (grade D).
- Use a 24-hour urine collection to quantify excreted protein. The use of a protein/creatinine ratio instead of a 24-hour urinary protein requires local confirmation of performance, as the method of measuring proteinuria has been shown to modify the results (grade C).
- Reduce concentration-related errors by assessing specific gravity or urine creatinine simultaneously with the protein dip result (grade C).
- When required, confirm a 1+ result from a dipstick test for proteinuria by measuring protein excretion in a 24-hour urine collection (grade C).

Clinical illustrations

Risk assessment

Case 1

Ms AB is age 28, currently nine weeks pregnant in her third pregnancy. In her first pregnancy five years ago, before she came to this area, she developed high blood pressure and protein in her urine at about 32 weeks. She gave birth to a boy weighing 2.2kg by elective caesarean at 36 weeks' gestation. Her second pregnancy was uncomplicated, her BP remained normal, and a daughter weighing 3.1kg was born via normal vaginal birth at 39 weeks.

Action: Ms AB's last pregnancy was normal, but she does have a predisposing factor: her previous history of pre-eclampsia and pre-term birth (see Table 4.4.1). According to Recommendation 2 (Table 4.4.2), she should be offered an early consultation with an obstetrician to discuss her previous pre-eclampsia and other relevant history.

The obstetrician will be able to help clarify her obstetric risk in the current pregnancy and provide useful input into her individual antenatal care plan. As she has a factor from Recommendation 2, she does not qualify for level 1 or 2 of community monitoring (Table 4.4.3).

Case 2

Ms CD is 32 years old and in her second pregnancy at 11 weeks' gestation. She had a normal pregnancy and birth three years ago, but she now tells you that her sister in New Zealand had bad pre-eclampsia last year.

Her booking blood pressure is 116/80. She is keen on normal antenatal shared care and vaginal birth.

Action: According to Recommendation 2 Ms CD should be offered a referral in early pregnancy for specialist input, as she has two predisposing factors: her booking diastolic BP and her family history of pre-eclampsia. You explain pre-eclampsia to her and offer her an information leaflet about the condition.

After spending time discussing it with her partner and mother, she decides that she would like more information from a specialist obstetrician. After you have both obtained the obstetrician's opinion, Ms CD may still have the antenatal care and birth she originally hoped for.

How community monitoring works

Case 3

Miss EF, age 26, is 24 weeks pregnant in her first pregnancy. Following Recommendation 3a (Table 4.4.3), she has started the level 2 frequency of community monitoring as she has one risk factor. That means that from 24 to 32 weeks' gestation there should be no more than three weeks between her assessments, and from 32 weeks to birth no more than two weeks between her assessments.

Miss EF's BP at booking was normal but now, at 24 weeks, it is 128/90. She is well and has recently started feeling fetal movements. The fundal height is compatible with her due date. On dipstick testing, she has no proteinuria. She is anxious to get back to the office this afternoon, and not at all keen on any course of action that could lead to more time off work.

Action: She has new hypertension until proved otherwise, but there is nothing so far to suggest fetal compromise. She has no headache, visual disturbance, epigastric pain or vomiting. According to Recommendation 5, she should be referred for hospital step-up assessment within 48 hours (see Table 4.4.5). An explanation of the potential seriousness of pre-eclampsia helps her to understand the logic behind your advice, and she is happy to be assessed at the hospital the next day. (Had her diastolic blood pressure been 100 or more, you would have explained how quickly pre-eclampsia can progress, and encouraged her to go to hospital for step-up assessment the same day.)

Case 4

Mrs GH is 39 years old and in her third pregnancy, at 28 weeks' gestation. She is well but tired (her twins are only two years old and the eldest is four). She is getting a lot of fetal movements at night. Her fundus corresponds to her dates. Her BP is 114/72, but on dipstick testing she has 1+ of protein. She has no pyrexia.

Action: Mrs GH has new proteinuria without hypertension. As it is only 1+, you ask to see her again in one week, in accordance with Recommendation 5 (Table 4.4.5). She asks if she could test her own urine with a dipstick instead of returning to the surgery, but you encourage her to attend in person. You check the specific gravity of the sample in case it is highly concentrated, which may have given a false positive result. She asks if she will be checked for a urinary infection, but as she has no symptoms and only 1+ proteinuria, you explain that an infection is unlikely.

The following week, she is well. In addition to testing her urine again, you also check her BP once more and enquire about any symptoms and about fetal movements (see Recommendation 4). She has no proteinuria or other significant signs or symptoms, and her BP is still normal. She therefore returns to the routine schedule of antenatal care.

Case 5

Ms IJ is 29. She, too, is 28 weeks pregnant and in her third pregnancy. She had been feeling very well indeed until late yesterday when she developed epigastric pain. In fact, she is beginning to wonder if it was something she ate, but she has never had pain quite like this.

She has no headache or visual disturbance. Today her BP is 118/86 and she has no proteinuria on testing with a dipstick in the surgery. She reports that the baby is kicking just as much as ever, and she has no other symptoms. She has no liver tenderness on palpation or signs or symptoms of placental abruption.

Action: Ms IJ has developed symptoms without hypertension or proteinuria. At this stage you are not sure how significant her symptoms will turn out to be but, according to Recommendation 5, you refer her the same day for hospital step-up assessment. What happens there is the subject of a follow-on guideline.

Grading of recommendations and evidence

Grade A	Directly based on category I evidence
Grade B	Directly based on category II evidence or extrapolated recommendation from category I evidence
Grade C	Directly based on category III evidence or extrapolated recommendation from category I or II evidence
Grade D	Directly based on category IV evidence or extrapolated recommendation from category I, II or III evidence

Good practice point: the view of the guideline development group.

Comments from validation procedure

'Guidance highly commended.'
Royal College of Obstetricians and Gynaecologists

'If the recommendations in this guideline are followed, pregnant women will be alerted to the possibility of developing pre-eclampsia during pregnancy, the symptoms to look out for and the care they may need. The NCT welcomes this development and the opportunity of better team-working to ensure that all women are appropriately referred for specialist care when it is needed.'
National Childbirth Trust

'The guidelines have been positively received by the RCM. The RCM is supportive of work being done in piloting the [PRECOG] guidelines and will support the future processes of implementation and wider dissemination.'
Royal College of Midwives

'The RCGP is happy to support this work.'
Royal College of General Practitioners

The Practising Midwife 2005; 8(9): 17–23

Topics for further reflection

- The concept of risk has become a key issue in midwifery. How do you address this concept with women in practice? Do you talk about the concept of risk in a general sense, or focus on specific risks in particular areas? Has your attitude towards the concept of risk changed since you became a midwife and, if so, in what ways?
- Tricia Anderson's article highlights one area which is not well known, and raises questions about the risks of certain medical procedures. When you talk to women, do you tend to focus more on the risks of having medical tests and treatments, on the risks of not having them, or on both? What do you feel are the key issues in this area?

Labour and Birth

SECTION CONTENTS

Births that taught me important lessons

Pamela Hunt

Birthings are like snowflakes, all unique in their own way. This is one of the things that makes birth so delightful and interesting. Every birth, every woman and baby I attend presents an important lesson, something new to learn, some new information buried in the fabric of that particular event alone. You already know that we are all a bit different. Every baby that is born is also different, and the circumstances around each birth change every time. Any mother will tell you that it doesn't matter how many children she's had, each birth will be as different as each child.

Because of this, we as midwives cannot take birth for granted at any time. Each birth and the circumstances around it are distinctive, which means that we must pay good attention all the time. In the lab of our clinic we have a little sign that our lab technician posted on the wall years ago. It says:

Pay
Attention

The 'P' and the 'A' are very large and the other letters are very small so when you see the 'PA' you have to walk up close to see the rest of the words. The point is made. It may be the little things that tip you off that something is amiss, or that this baby or mother will need help of some kind. Every birth presents infinite possibilities and our thoughts and actions may make a difference to the outcome. The key to safe home birth is to acknowledge and recognize all the signs that are telling you something.

To be able to pay attention at this level, one must have an open, clear mind, good knowledge of the birth process, solid training, and critical thinking skills. Experience also helps.

When I come to a woman to help her with her labour and birth, that woman and that delivery has to be the most important thing on my mind. To be able to be telepathic with this woman and her baby, all other events and happenings in my life at the time need to be put in a special place in my mind that I can come back to after the birth. The birthing women and their babies are of prime importance during the birth. Furthermore, I cannot be practising with ego or some pre-conceived notion of how a birth should go. Hopefully, I have had the time with this woman to build up a heart connection and a trust between the two of us to establish a good relationship.

I want to relate the following birth tales. I learned something significant at each one. (For privacy concerns, all names and dates have been changed.)

Annie's unusual birth

Annie is an Amish woman who contacted me when she was pregnant with her 14th baby. The Amish granny midwives had helped her with her other 13 babies, all girls by the way. She had never had any significant problems but this time she felt that she wanted a midwife. She was a healthy 41-year-old woman, about 5 feet 4 inches and fully pregnant at about 170 lb. She had long dark hair combed back into a bun and covered with a white cotton cap with tiny pleats in it. Annie was outspoken and direct with her comments and she didn't spare words. She ran an organized home, teaching the girls how to cook, clean, sew, garden, and take care of the little ones when a new baby had arrived. Since all the children so far were girls, the girls also took turns helping their father with the big draft horses in the fields. These were very capable young women and teenage girls. The younger children helped with the house and the farm too. It was not unusual to walk into Annie's house and see the 7- and 9-year-olds doing the dishes.

Annie contacted me when she was 8 months pregnant. I was able to squeeze in four prenatal visits with her before she went into labour. She was due around the beginning of January.

On New Years Eve at around 9.00 p.m. Annie's neighbour called and said that Annie needed me. Amish don't have telephones so they always ask a neighbour to call. I usually don't get a lot of information from Amish neighbours but I know when they call it is time to go. Everything was already packed in my car. It wasn't very cold for the end of December, maybe around 50°F.

I drove the 12 miles over the countryside to their farm. As I drove up, their house had the soft glow of the kerosene lamps shining through the cracks in the curtains and one lamp had been put outside on the porch so I could see my way in. Once inside, I found Annie up walking around, stopping, and leaning on a kitchen chair to 'rush'. The girls had all been sent out to a neighbour's house, and the only people there were Annie, her husband and both grandmothers. She was having strong rushes every 3–4 minutes, was being quite verbal in German, and the grandmothers wanted me to check her right away. Annie moved into the bedroom, lay down and pulled her dark blue skirt up. Upon examination, I found a very bulgy water bag, a dilation of 8 cm and an engaged head that was still high at −3. Annie asked me to break the water bag and we all expected the baby to move right down. It did a little but not much. I could tell that the head was un-flexed and that this was an 'occiput posterior' baby. I gently tried to manoeuvre the head to a flexed position over the next several rushes both externally and eternally. Annie worked over the next 2 hours. She opened up to 10 cm and moved the baby down to a −2 station, still pretty high and still un-flexed. We had a good heartbeat on the baby. She squatted, she walked, and she got on hands and knees and moved her hips back and forth. She pushed. She had given birth to 13 other children so she knew how to do this dance of labour. She usually had 2–5 minute second stages and normally gently grunted her babies out. She couldn't figure out why the baby wasn't coming and neither could the grandmothers who had each attended no less than 50 deliveries of their other daughters and daughters-in-laws. One of the grandmothers exclaimed, 'it looks like there is plenty of room for it to come on down'.

Several more times, I tried to turn and manoeuvre the head to a flexed position with no luck. Annie did some more walking, squatting, and pulling on a rope that one of the grandmothers had hung from a rafter, Annie talking all the time, sometimes in English and sometimes in German. I believe she used some strong words at one point. I couldn't understand them but the grandmothers both said, 'Now Annie, don't use those words'. I did understand that.

Annie finally said, 'I don't think it's going to come, let's go to the hospital'. 'OK,' I answered, 'but let me check you once more. Maybe the last couple of rushes moved the baby down'. This time while inside her I felt that I was able to move the baby head just the tiniest bit by putting some pressure with two of my fingers on the baby's forehead and turning gently. Maybe that would do it. She felt it too. She had five or six more rushes and still no movement down and she was tired. 'I'm ready to go', she said. 'All right', I responded, thinking she had been pushing at full dilation for a few hours now and was getting pretty tired. The hospital wasn't far and I hoped we would make it there. When an Amish mother wants to transport to the hospital I usually honour that wish.

So we packed up the car with Annie, her husband and one grandmother in the back seat, and one grandmother in the front seat. I started to drive. By now it was 11.30 p.m. We had to drive about 12 miles to get to the hospital over winding, bumpy roads. I drove slowly so as not to make either of the grandmothers car sick, which they both had warned me happened if they went around curves too fast. Annie quietly continued to rush every 3–4 minutes.

We came into town and were about 2 miles from the hospital when Annie said, 'I think it's coming'. 'You've got to be kidding', I thought, but I started to look for a place to pull off the road. 'We'll be at the hospital in a few minutes, Annie, can you wait?' I am sure she was now thinking, 'You've got to be kidding!' There was a place in my mind where I thought we would have another 5 or 10 minutes before the baby would actually birth. The baby hadn't moved down so far with all we had done, and I didn't see how much could have changed it in the last 10 minutes. Foolish me! Then Annie said, 'Here comes the head!'

I pulled into the nearest parking lot which was a Taco Bell restaurant, stopped the car and ran around to her side of the car, opened the door and there was the little blonde baby head between her thighs. There was a shoulder dystocia, which I resolved quickly by reaching for the posterior shoulder, and Annie pushed out a healthy baby girl.

We wrapped the baby in warm blankets, which we had had the foresight to bring with us, put her in Annie's arms, turned around and drove home. I called the hospital and said we had had the baby on the way there, everything was fine, and we wouldn't be coming in. The nurse said, 'I hope your car seats didn't get wet' and 'Congratulations!'

We had a beautiful baby and a very happy family, with Annie talking constantly. She was a delightful woman to work with, exciting, creative and unforgettable.

The lesson Annie's delivery taught me was that, if you are in a situation with a 'posterior arrest' baby and an unflexed head, and you manage to move the baby's head even a tiny bit, give it some time and a couple more tries. Make sure the baby's heart is good, then try again to turn the baby's head. There is a really good chance that the little bit you manoeuvred the head will help the baby to resolve itself into a good position and it will be born. The last time I checked Annie, I did manage to move the baby's head ever so slightly. I should have trusted that movement and tried again. The baby's heart was good and though Annie was tired, she was healthy and strong.

Lesson two with this birth: If a mother says the baby is coming, believe her!

Real peace

Life is so simple here at Lizzy and Dan's home in the country. The clock ticks on the wall, 2.10 a.m. Amish time (an hour slower than our time during the summer). The concept of slow time, which is how they refer to it, has a calming effect on life.

The lamp on the tall oak dresser is casting shadows on the hardwood floor from the rocker and the other two chairs in the room. Lizzy is about 7.5 cm dilated and progressing right along, however very quietly. I notice when the rushes are getting strong and help her with some breathing techniques to relieve some of the tension. She is softly using slow deep breathing to ease the rushes. It's 3.00 a.m.

Her mother, Dora, has gone back to bed for a while. We can hear her snoring in the other room. The snoring, the creak of the rocking chair, and the tick of the clock are the only sounds in the house. At 4.00 a.m. I go in and check Lizzy and sit with her for a while. The baby's heart is 140 bpm and Lizzy is doing well. She smiles when I come in to help her. Dan is with her all the time, holding her hand, and putting some gentle pressure on her lower back.

It's 4.30 a.m. and the roosters are starting to crow. There is a goat outside Lizzy's window, munching on the grass. Lizzy is 9.5 cm dilated and I can tell when she has a rush now because she wrinkles her forehead in a way that one eyebrow goes higher than the other. She is also squeezing on Dan's hand during rushes until her knuckles turn white.

It's hot and humid tonight and we pull back the dark blue curtains to let in the cool fresh air. Lizzy said, 'feels good'. She talks in German to Dan, slow quiet sweet sounding words. The sky is just starting to lighten and at 4.45 a.m. Lizzy begins to push.

I go and wake up Dora and tell her it won't be long. I have everything set up. I give my hands a good scrubbing with Betadine and a hand brush then bring some boiled water in a stainless steel bowl to wash Lizzy with. She is having good pushing pains now. Her face turns a rosy pink as she pulls on her knees to pull herself up into a good pushing position during a rush. The rushes come with nice rests of 3 or 4 minutes between them. By 5.20

a.m. the baby is crowning and at 5.23 a.m. the head is born. The little one opens her eyes and cries before her slippery plump body comes out about 45 seconds later. It's a healthy baby girl with Apgars of 10 and 10.

I put the baby on Lizzy's belly and she touches her head covered with dark hair, and holds her tiny hands. A few minutes pass but it feels timeless. In due course, I cut and clamp the cord and Grandma Dora takes the baby to dress her over on the cedar chest. I check Lizzy's vagina for any tears (no tear) and deliver the placenta. Dan brings me some fresh warm water to wash Lizzy.

Seeing Lizzy all settled with clean sheets under her, I go where Grandma Dora is caring for the baby. We weigh her in at 7 lb 1 oz. She has a pink colour and a strong heart. Her head is 35.7 cm round and she is 19.5 inches long. Her eyes are bright and she looks around, blinking in the lamplight. It's still early morning and we haven't blown the lamps out yet. Grandma Dora looks at me and says, 'This is as good a start to a day that we could have, and look, the sky is turning all pink outside'.

I have taught students for years that the Amish have an easier time at birthing. We see fewer problems, shorter labours and less bleeding. We still have to pay very close attention to all aspects of pregnancy and birth and can never take normalcy for granted but it is what we expect when we help this community of women.

The above birth is just an example. Their country-based life is simple, conscientious and honest. They don't watch television. They are not rich but they are secure. They know they will be with their partners for the rest of their lives and that both families will be supportive. They know all their neighbours and have a good relationship with them. They have no fear of the birth process or of life itself. Birth is natural and usually non-problematic.

Kittens, kids, mama goats and baby

Janie played beautiful music in her bedroom, the light was coming in the windows in a special way and at times it felt like a cathedral.

A month before her birthing, Janie's cat had kittens and then disappeared so Janie was raising a litter of kittens including bottle feeding them every so many hours as well as growing her own baby. Her other two children, an 8- and a 10-year-old would help. A couple of weeks before her birthing, all the little children in the neighbourhood would gravitate to the sandbox in Janie's yard. So there were kittens and kids, and, even two mother goats out in the yard playing, eating and having fun. It all felt like waiting for something special and felt very mellow. The kids were playing well and were helpful with the kittens.

Janie's labour was one that progressed steadily but slowly. During the first part of her labour, the rushes were strong enough to wake her up every 6 to 8 minutes. I had seen her in the afternoon and told her to sleep as much as she could between rushes, then I went home to get dinner for my family and get some sleep too. Janie's sister, Alice, was going to call me when the labour was more regular and rushes closer together.

I got the call at about 4.00 a.m. and went down the gravel road to her house, only a hundred yards from our house. Janie was rushing every 3 to 5 minutes but was only 5 cm dilated. She was tired and wondering why this wasn't going as fast as her previous labours had. There was a whole household full of friends who had come over to be helpful. They had been massaging her and helping her through each rush. There was a hubbub of activity in the house, good food and a friendly atmosphere.

The problem was obvious. She needed some quiet and maybe some sleep more than she needed a household full of well-meaning friends. She was happy her friends were there, but what she really needed and wanted was low lights and some quietness. So I suggested that everyone go to bed and give Janie a little quiet time. Her sister telepathically stayed and sat next to her and rubbed her back for the next hour. Once everyone left except for Alice, Janie's rushes came a little further apart but stronger. In an hour and a half she had opened up to 8 cm, dozing off between each rush.

She continued this throughout the rest of her labour; waking up for a rush then sleeping 4 or 5 minutes, then waking up for another rush. It was beautiful and peaceful to witness and finally she felt some pushing urges. She gently breathed and pushed the baby down. This was her third child and the baby was big with a large round head, and it took her almost an hour of grunting and pushing to get the baby out. He came out strong and crying and was a beautiful baby boy.

The lesson in this birth? Well-meaning family and friends can be helpful and fun to have around; however when a mother is birthing she needs to have some quiet and introspective time, some time to rest and sleep, some time to go back into her mind and soul and feel her strength, and some undisturbed time to communicate with her baby. This is a very spiritual time for the mother, and her family and everyone around the birthing environment need to respect that.

Fast birth

Patty was pregnant for the fifth time in 6.5 years. She had been to see a doctor for her prenatal care. Everything was normal and the baby's head was down. In her 8th month she came to our clinic and asked if I would attend her delivery. When I checked her she was in her 34th week of gestation, dilated 5 cm and the baby's head was very low. This was due to a weakened pelvic floor from having her previous babies close together. Her cervix, while dilated, was still thick and she was not having any labour yet.

Patty and I have known each other for several years prior to this pregnancy. I had helped her with three of her other babies and she had always had 5–6 hour labours. We made an agreement that she would call me as soon as any signs of labour started. I went to visit her the following week; her blood pressure was normal, the baby's heart rate was normal and nothing had changed with her dilation or the baby's position and station.

I ended up doing two more visits with her, with everything looking good each time. The only unusual thing was how low the baby was, but her cervix seemed to be holding.

Then at 10.50 p.m. one Saturday evening, I received a call from her neighbour: 'Come right away, Patty had a baby boy.' The following is Patty's account.

'At 10.35 p.m. my water bag broke and I sent my husband to the neighbour's house to call you and to get my mother to help. Five minutes after he left to call, I had one pain and the head came out. Five minutes later I had another pain and the baby's body came. I noticed he was a boy. I sat up and wrapped him in a blanket from my bed to keep him warm. He started to cry right away. Shortly afterwards, my husband came back, tied and cut the cord and helped me put our baby in my arms. All 9 lb 14 oz of him.' She smiled.

When I got to Patty's house, her mother had arrived and everything looked fine. Patty looked vibrant. I checked her uterus, which was firm and low, and she hadn't torn. I checked the baby; weighed and measured him and bundled him in a blue blanket and gave him to Patty who put him right to breast. Mother and baby were doing great. By this time the father had also relaxed some and the grandmother joked about training him for midwifery.

Patty started exercises the week after she had her baby in order to get her muscle tone back. She had six children after this and each following labour was at least 5 hours long.

I feel this is a reminder to always teach pelvic floor exercises and remind the mother often about the importance of doing them. After this birth Patty did pelvic floor exercises every day and with her subsequent deliveries she did not have precipitous deliveries. I also advised her to stay off her feet during her future pregnancies. She did walk but she had help for her house chores.

The clue was silence

Rose Lakota, was born to David and Shasta with Apgar scores of 9 and 10 and weighing 9 lb 6 oz. She was born at 2.25 a.m. after 2 hours of labour.

Shasta called me at 12.45 a.m. saying she was having some light rushes. She stopped talking for a minute, and then went on saying, 'You don't have to come right away but I just wanted to let you know my labour was starting and I might have my baby later this morning'. I asked her how far apart the rushes were. She said, 'Oh, pretty far, about 6 minutes'. Then she stopped talking again. Silence . . .

'Was that a rush that made you pause?' I asked. I had only been on the phone to her for about 3 minutes. She said, 'Yes but you really don't need to worry, they're really not strong'. I wasn't worried but I knew Shasta would have this baby quickly and also knew that she tended to make light of some things. I had known her for many years.

I said I'd see her soon, hung up the phone, got dressed and went straight to her house. When I got there she was 6 cm dilated and opening quickly. I called up Ina May, and Deborah and got things set up. By 2.25 a.m. she had delivered a healthy 9 lb 6 oz girl. This was a very sweet healthy girl. The placenta came 10 minutes later.

Every midwife misses a delivery once in a while. Usually everything turns out fine, and sometimes this can't be helped, as in Patty's story; however when a mother calls and says she is starting labour, it's good to wake up and go and check the mother. She did call, after all, because something got her attention. A visit won't hurt anyone and you can get baseline blood pressures and fetal heart tones. If things are going slow, you can always drive home, or if she lives some distance away you can sleep in the back bedroom. Some labours will go slow, but some will surprise you and the baby will come quickly.

Unlocking the potential for normality

Sarah J. Buckley

Birth is a normal life event, happening every day for around a quarter of a million mothers and babies worldwide (UNFPA 1999). Birth is also a singular and extraordinary event, occurring only a few times during a woman's life, and having a powerful influence on her subsequent health and well-being. A woman's memories and perceptions of childbirth remain vivid and deeply felt, even decades later (Simkin 1991).

Birth is also the culmination of pregnancy and our initiation into motherhood. Our experiences of birth will significantly shape our mothering and our relationship with our children. The joy and satisfaction of a normal birth lay a foundation for ease and pleasure in mothering. Conversely, as research is increasingly showing us, a difficult birth can disrupt self-esteem (Fisher et al 1997) as well as early mother-baby relationships (Rowe-Murray and Fisher 2001), with potentially serious consequences. These include less positive attitudes to the baby after the birth; more difficulty with breastfeeding and greater fatigue (DiMatteo et al 1996); higher rates of postnatal depression (Astbury et al 1994, Boyce and Todd 1992); more sexual problems (Brown and Lumley 1998); differences in the experience of motherhood (Green et al 1990) and in the ongoing mother-child relationship (de Chateau and Wiberg 1984, Wiberg et al 1989).

Our growing understanding of the psychoneuroendocrinology (the psyche-brain-hormones) of birth gives us further insights into the impact of a difficult and/or very medicalised birth. This perspective, which I have written about elsewhere (Buckley 2003), emphasises the complex yet delicate hormonal orchestration of labour and birth – and illustrates both the superb design of our female bodies for birth, and the consequences of medicalised disturbance in labour, birth and the early post-natal time.

From this perspective, birth is a normal life event because its processes are genetically encoded in our female bodies. When the time is right, these processes will unfold in a precise sequence, with exquisite and exact orchestration. What is required for normal birth are the conditions that will allow this genetic imprint to unfold most easily for the individual birthing woman. This is, for me, the crux of normal birth, as well as the core of midwifery knowledge.

Optimal conditions for birth

What are the conditions that will help a birthing woman's genetic imprint to unfold most easily? I believe that the most basic requirement for human birth is the same as for all our mammalian cousins – 'a perception of safety and avoidance of disturbance during parturition' (Naakteborgen 1989).

As well as feeling safe and undisturbed, the birthing female of every mammalian species has a need for privacy. For some species, such as domestic cats, privacy means giving birth in absolute solitude. For other species, including dolphins and elephants, privacy means being supported and protected by group members (Naakteborgen 1989). Human females also vary in their need for privacy, with some women labouring more effectively when left alone and other women preferring to have helpers around them to support and protect their privacy.

We can also learn about the optimal conditions for normal birth by studying human sexual activity, which involves very similar patterns of hormonal release. Both processes involve increasing levels of the hormones of love (oxytocin), pleasure (beta-endorphin) and excitement (adrenaline/noradrenaline); at the culmination of both events, climactic levels of all of these hormones engender feelings of love, pleasure, excitement and mutuality, or bonding. In our culture, we recognise the need to feel safe, private and unobserved during sexual activity, yet we have not realised that a labouring woman is equally sensitive to her surroundings. How would it be to attempt to make love in the conditions under which we expect women to give birth?

When we provide optimal conditions for normal birth, we benefit the mother and the baby, who has his/her own genetically encoded imprint for birth. For example, during labour the baby produces increasing levels of catecholamines (adrenaline/noradrenaline), which redistribute cardiac output and so protect the heart and brain from the inevitable hypoxia that occurs with each contraction (Lagercrantz 1986).

Close to the time of birth, the baby has a marked surge in catecholamine hormones, particularly noradrenaline, which is thought to be caused by pressure on the head as the baby descends (Lagercrantz 1986). This catecholamine surge enhances adaptation to extra-utero life by: increasing the absorption of amniotic fluid from the lungs and stimulating surfactant release (Irestedt et al 1984); increasing cardiac contractility; increasing blood levels of glucose and free fatty acids (Hagnevik et al 1984); and enhancing responsiveness and tone in the newborn (Irestedt et al 1984). Babies born by caesarean miss out on the catecholamine surge, and have poorer lung compliance (Lagercrantz 1986). Babies born after epidural analgesia in labour have lower catecholamine levels than undrugged babies, although no significant differences in lung or cardiac function have been documented thus far (Hirsimaki et al 1992, Jones et al 1985).

Normal birth has evolved, over millennia, to ensure maximum survival for mother and baby. Maximum survival obviously begins with survival at birth, but also includes factors that will enhance longer-term outcome for both, such as responsiveness of the new baby, ease of breastfeeding, maternal devotion and protectiveness, and ongoing maternal well-being. These factors are built into normal birth, being optimised by maternal and newborn hormones (Buckley 2003).

Medicalised birth is again likely to counteract these benefits. Drugs and interventions used in labour and birth can disrupt hormonal release in birth and so create difficulties with later mothering (Buckley 2003). For example, caesarean mothers have different patterns of hormonal release during breastfeeding two days after birth, with no rise in prolactin and absent oxytocin pulses, compared with women who have given birth vaginally (Nissen et al 1996). This may explain why caesarean mothers transfer less milk to their babies in the first five days, and why their babies gain less weight in the first week of life (Evans et al 2003). Caesarean babies are also less likely to be successfully breastfed (DiMatteo 1996), which puts both mothers and babies at risk of poorer long-term outcomes, as below.

Breastfeeding and normal birth have other parallels. Decades ago, women were told that formula feeding was at least as good as – and probably better than – breastfeeding. Now we are discovering the amazing properties of breast milk, and the long-term detriments of formula feeding. These may include some of our society's most prevalent health issues, such as diabetes, obesity, asthma, allergies, osteoporosis and breast cancer. (See www.promom.org/101 for references and a comprehensive lists of the advantages of breastfeeding.)

Currently, medical professionals are telling women that medicalised birth is a safe substitute for normal birth – perhaps even safer. Yet the short-term studies do not back up this assertion, and the scant long-term research that has been done suggests that exposure to drugs and obstetric procedures around the time of birth could have serious consequences for our offspring. These may include some of our society's most worrying social issues, such as drug addiction (Jacobson et al 1990, Nyberg et al 2000), youth suicide (Jacobson and Bygdeman 1998, Jacobson et al 1987, Salk et al 1985) and violent criminality (Raine et al 1997).

Normal birth is the birthday gift that Mother Nature intends for all of us. Normal birth is a gift that keeps on giving, and I believe that, in modern times, we need its assistance more than ever. My hope is that we will, as carers and as a culture, come to appreciate the value of normal birth, and reclaim the knowledge and power of its unfolding for ourselves, and for all mothers and babies.

Acknowledgment

This article is based on 'Undisturbed birth – nature's Hormonal Blueprint for Safety, Ease and Ecstasy' published in MIDIRS Midwifery Digest (Buckley 2003).

REFERENCES

Astbury J, Brown S, Lumley J and Small R (1994). 'Birth events, birth experiences and social differences in postnatal depression'. Australian Journal of Public Health, 18 (2): 176–184.

Boyce P M and Todd A L (1992). 'Increased risk of postnatal depression after emergency caesarean section'. Medical Journal of Australia, 157 (3): 172–174.

Brown S and Lumley J (1998). 'Maternal health after childbirth: results of an Australian population based survey'. British Journal of Obstetrics and Gynaecology, 105 (2): 156–161.

Buckley S (2003). 'Undisturbed birth: nature's blueprint for ease and ecstasy'. Journal of Prenatal and Perinatal Psychology and Health, 17 (4): 261–288. Reprinted as: Buckley S (2004) 'Undisturbed birth: nature's hormonal blueprint for safety, ease and ecstasy'. MIDIRS, 14 (2): 203–209, and Buckley S (2004) 'What disturbs birth?' MIDIRS, 14 (3): 353–359.

de Chateau P and Wiberg B (1984). 'Long-term effect on mother-infant behaviour of extra contact during the first hour post partum, III, follow-up at one year'. Scandanavian Journal of Social Medicine, 12 (2): 91–103.

DiMatteo M R, Morton S, Lepper H S et al (1996). 'Cesarean childbirth and psychosocial outcomes: a meta-analysis'. Health Psychology, 15 (4): 303–314.

Evans K C, Evans R G, Royal R et al (2003). 'Effect of caesarean section on breast milk transfer to the normal term newborn over the first week of life'. Archives of Disease in Childhood, Fetal and Neonatal Edition, 88 (5): F380–382.

Fisher J, Astbury J and Smith A (1997). 'Adverse psychological impact of operative obstetric interventions: a prospective longitudinal study'. Australia New Zealand Journal of Psychiatry, 31: 728–738.

Green J M, Coupland V A and Kitzinger J V (1990). 'Expectations, experiences, and psychological outcomes of childbirth: a prospective study of 825 women'. Birth, 17 (1):15–24.

Hagnevik, K, Faxelius, G, Irestedt I et al (1984). 'Catecholamine surge and metabolic adaptation in the newborn after vaginal delivery and caesarean section'. Acta Paediatrica, Scandinavica, 73 (5):602–609.

Hirsimaki H, Kero P, Ekblad H et al (1992). 'Mode of delivery, plasma catecholamines and Doppler-derived cardiac output in healthy term newborn infants'. Biology of the Neonate, 61 (5): 285–293.

Irestedt L, Lagercrantz H and Belfrage P (1984). 'Causes and consequences of maternal and fetal sympathoadrenal activation during parturition'. Acta Obstetrica et Gynecologica Scandinavica, Supplement 1, 18: 111–115.

Jacobson B, Eklund G, Hamberger L et al (1987). 'Perinatal origin of adult self-destructive behavior'. Acta Psychiatrica Scandinavica, 76 (4): 364–371.

Jacobson B, Nyberg K, Gronbladh L et al (1990). 'Opiate addiction in adult offspring through possible imprinting after obstetric treatment'. British Medical Journal, 301: 1067–1070.

Jacobson B and Bygdeman M (1998). 'Obstetric care and proneness of offspring to suicide as adults: case-control study'. British Medical Journal, 317 (7169): 1346–1349.

Jones C R, McCullouch J, Butters L et al (1985). 'Plasma catecholamines and modes of delivery: the relation between catecholamine levels and in-vitro platelet aggregation and adrenoreceptor radioligand binding characteristics'. British Journal of Obstetrics and Gynaecology, 92 (6): 593–599.

Lagercrantz H (1986). 'The stress of being born'. Scientific American, 254 (4): 100–107.

Naakteborgen C (1989). 'The biology of childbirth'. In: Effective care in pregnancy and childbirth, Vol 2, Oxford: OUP.

Nissen E, Uvnas-Moberg K, Svensson K et al (1996). 'Different patterns of oxytocin, prolactin but not cortisol release during breastfeeding in women delivered by caesarean section or by the vaginal route'. Early Human Development, 45:103–118.

Nyberg K, Buka S L and Lipsitt L P (2000). 'Perinatal medication as a potential risk factor for adult drug abuse in a North American cohort'. Epidemiology, 11 (6): 715–716.

Raine A, Brennan P and Mednick S A (1997). 'Interaction between birth complications and early maternal rejection in predisposing individuals to adult violence: specificity to serious, early-onset violence'. American Journal of Psychiatry, 154 (9):1265–1271.

Rowe-Murray H J and Fisher J R W (2001). 'Operative intervention in delivery is associated with compromised early mother-infant interaction'. British Journal of Obstetrics and Gynaecology, 108 (10): 1068–1075.

Salk L, Lipsitt L P, Sturner W Q et al (1985). 'Relationship of maternal and perinatal conditions to eventual adolescent suicide'. American Journal of Psychiatry, 154(9): 1265–1271.

Simkin P (1991). 'Just another day in a woman's life? – women's long-term perceptions of their first birth experience'. Birth, 18 (4): 203–210.

UNFPA (1999). The state of the world population report. http://www.unfpa.org/swp/1999/newsfeature1.htm

Wiberg B, Humble K and de Chateau P (1989). 'Long-term effect on mother-infant behaviour of extra contact during the first hour post partum. V. Follow-up at three years'. Scand J Soc Med, 17 (2):181–191.

The Practising Midwife 2004; 7(6); 15–17

Lambs to the slaughter

Virginia Howes, Kay Hardie

Thousands of women in this country with normal pregnancies and healthy babies are being put at risk every day in maternity units across the country. Like lambs to the slaughter, they pack up their bags and head for the hospital in the belief that the doctors who instigate the barbaric treatment they are about to undergo are saving their babies' lives. Many of them then spend the next few days in excruciating pain over and above what is experienced in normal labour in an effort to drag their unready and unwilling bodies into labour. Their bodies are filled with drugs that may compromise their long-term health. So they begin the spiralling cascade of interventions that all too often culminates in entry through the theatre doors.

The women and their families thank the doctors and hospital guidelines for saving them from the problems they had, problems that are often iatrogenic in origin. And so the myth, that their bodies are failing them in the one thing women are best at – procuring a future generation – is perpetuated. To add insult to injury, my colleagues, midwives – who, by definition of their title, should be the protectors of women and babies – help daily to continue this unnecessary practice.

Socially acceptable

Induction of labour (IOL) for no medical reason has become a socially acceptable procedure. The NICE (National Institute for Clinical Excellence 2001) guidelines (the 'gold seal') have been adopted with open arms; they are now governing practice in maternity units throughout the country (NICE 2001). Induction of labour is one such guideline, and recently instigated a rather heated conversation between a hospital antenatal clinic midwife and myself.

Her role as head of the clinic involved speaking to many women who were booked for induction, and there-fore she was in a very responsible position to give true and unbiased information about IOL to large numbers of women. I had telephoned the clinic to arrange an ultrasound scan for a client who was 42 weeks' pregnant with her second baby. The pregnancy was normal. The client was very well informed and, despite knowing there was no evidence to support fetal surveillance, had decided on a scan to check the well-being of her baby. Social pressure had made her feel that she needed to 'do something', and this course of action, she felt, at least appeased her family, friends and neighbours. What she did emphasise to me was that she did not want to be put under any pressure by anyone to be induced, and this I clearly explained to the midwife I conversed with. I asked her to pass that information on to the midwife in charge; an appointment was made for two days hence.

The following morning I received a letter from the midwife in charge. The letter informed me that a review of the hospital notes made the client's dates 'wrong', and stated: 'In accordance with NICE guidelines on post maturity, no woman should go over 42 weeks'. After reading the letter, my client, feeling that this was just the sort of pressure she did not want to subject herself to, lost all faith in the maternity unit. She understandably felt that she would not be given the respect to make her own decisions, especially as, without meeting her, judgement had been passed on her by the professionals from whom she had requested help. Also, she must be a stupid woman after all if she did not know when she got pregnant! She cancelled the appointment.

Personal interpretation

The guidelines, of course, do not say what the midwife had stated. The letter left me in no doubt that this head of antenatal clinic not only had failed to read the guidelines but also, more worryingly, had put her own interpretation on them. If this is but one example of how they are being used to manipulate and lie to women, what hope do women and society have of knowing the truth and making an informed choice?

Following the publication, in Canada (Hannah 1992), of the largest randomised controlled trial (RCT) to date concerning induction of labour and further meta-analysis of other RCTs, the Royal College of Obstetricians and Gynaecologists (RCOG) adopted the policy of offering induction at 41 weeks. This is now the recommendation contained in what is regarded as the gold standard NICE guidelines.

However, what is not widely known by obstetricians and midwives alike is that all the studies used to govern today's practice are based on eight babies – in the case of induction of labour, on the number of babies who died following their mothers being induced versus the numbers of babies who died following their mothers having been left to proceed with pregnancy beyond 41 weeks. There were approximately 3,000 women in the IOL group, and 3,000 in the expectant management group. One baby died in the IOL group, and seven died in the expectant management group. Hey presto, it is obvious that many babies' lives will be saved if we offer to induce every woman over 41 weeks!

The wider picture

Does anyone care about looking at the wider picture? I was taught to read critically research that is more than 10 years old. Yet to govern and recommend practice affecting thousands of women and babies, many of the RCTs in the meta-analysis used to compile the NICE guidelines are more than 20 years out of date – some are 40 years old.

While the way women grow and birth babies has not altered in millions of years, the ways in which our health as a nation has changed, and maternity care is delivered and received, certainly have – never more so than in the last 40 years. We now have testing and screening so that abnormalities can be detected earlier; fetal surveillance is available for 'at risk' babies; and the appropriate care is free and accessible to all women.

If we do indeed look at the wider picture, we see a whole new one emerging. Of the seven babies who died, two were born in the 1960s. One had a suspected diabetic mother – hardly a good inclusion criterion in a controlled trial by today's standards. One baby had pneumonia. One was from a Chinese study, in which the baby had meconium aspiration following refusal of induction of labour by its mother after a positive amnioscopy. Another had meconium aspiration at 43+3 weeks, which would not have any bearing on induction at 41 weeks. One was from a placental abruption, which could occur at any time. One was a baby of 2.6 kg and clearly growth retarded, and the mother had received no antenatal care (Menticoglou and Hall 2002).

Hard evidence required

Based on these findings, where is the evidence that there is an increased risk of unexplained stillbirth at 41 weeks?

How are the benefits to the 20–25 per cent of women and babies induced daily being demonstrated?

How are we as professionals informing women of the risks of induction of labour versus continuing the pregnancy? Are women given the information in a true and unbiased manner? I doubt it. In the same way, women are told the 'risks' about birth only when they are planning a home birth, but are conveniently not told the many more risks associated with going into hospital. A woman screened for having a Down's Syndrome baby is informed that if she has a risk factor of less than 1 : 250 she is low risk and further action is not recommended. Yet, at 41 weeks' gestation she is offered (if, indeed, it is an offer) IOL because the (very dubious) risk of increased stillbirth is 1 : 1,000.

In a detailed review of the literature, Menticoglou and Hall (2002) also highlighted details of a woman who died in hospital awaiting treatment for what appeared to be fulminating eclampsia. She was waiting because the wards were full and busy. As many midwives know, on many occasions the wards are full to capacity, often due to the number of routine inductions of labour going on at any one time. Where do women and babies such as these two who died feature in the calculation of risk?

Other than the Hannah trial, no further studies were looked at in depth when devising the NICE guidelines. There are other good retrospective studies looking at this subject, many of which show a substantial increase in the caesarean section rate for routine induction of labour – and no significant difference in neonatal outcomes for women and babies left alone to continue with healthy pregnancies.

The cost to the maternity services must be phenomenal. This is money that could be put to far better use improving services so that midwives come back into the profession. Then women and babies who are at risk from ongoing pregnancies might well be highlighted appropriately through good antenatal care instead of a hurried 10 minutes at each antenatal visit and routine induction for all!

We also must not forget the baby in the whole process; it, too, plays its part in the instigation of labour. The baby is not a passive receiver of the labour process; and, induced early, may not have the readiness for labour itself. The biggest reason of all (22 per cent) given for surgical intervention in the National Sentinel Caesarean Section Audit (RCOG 2001) was fetal distress. Even given the many wrong diagnoses of fetal distress that exist, how many of these babies were induced before they were ready to be born?

Routine induction of labour has become the socially acceptable norm. It is time we professionals – we who are the instigators of what, over time, becomes 'normal' in women's and society's eyes – stopped this barbaric treatment and gave back to women the respect they and nature deserve.

REFERENCES

Hannah M et al (1992). 'Induction of labour as compared with serial antenatal monitoring in post-term pregnancy'. New England Journal of Medicine, 326 (24): 1587–1592.

Menticoglou S and Hall P (2002). 'Routine induction of labour at 41 weeks gestation: nonsensus consensus'. BJOG an International Journal of Obstetrics and Gynaecology, PII: S1470–0328(02) 01004–2.

NICE (2001). Induction of Labour: Inherited Clinical Guideline D. London: NICE.

RCOG (2001). The National Sentinel Caesarean Section Audit Report. London: RCOG.

The Practising Midwife 2004; 7(7): 45–46

Water: what are we afraid of?

Ethel Burns

The majority of maternity units in the UK now have a birthing pool facility. The extent to which it is used, however, varies greatly. Pool use is inevitably influenced by the degree of support and enthusiasm displayed by midwives in a given centre, as most women in labour take their cue from caregivers. This extends even to mothers who may have written a wish to consider pool use in their birth plan.

I am undertaking an international audit of the use of pools during labour and/or birth, and notice wide variation across different units, even in the same country. In the UK, NHS finances are wasted when pool rooms are established but used infrequently. Women are told they have choice, but in reality are often denied the option. Reasons given for them not being able to use the pool include, 'We're too busy at the moment', 'There is no midwife "trained" to "do" waterbirth' and 'Cannot guarantee a second midwife will be able to attend the birth, and that is in our protocol'.

Such obfuscation may belie underlying concerns the midwife has because she does not feel supported by peers/managers. This relates to the complex issue of power and control. Kirkham (1999) explored the NHS culture and noted a key emergent theme of service and sacrifice, in which midwives felt disempowered as women, presenting a dilemma when expected to empower women in their care.

Whatever the situation, midwives are expected to undertake evidence-based practice. So what do we know about bathing during labour/birth? In 2002, I conducted a systematic review to investigate the effects of labour and/or birth in water, which I shall now summarise, including further studies that have since been published.

Collectively, comparative observational studies evaluating the effects of waterbirth provide data on 5,077 mothers and babies. Several of these report a significant reduction in the uptake of pharmacological pain relief and the incidence of perineal trauma compared with normal birth on land (Aird et al 1997, Burke and Kilfoyle 1995, Burns and Lloyd 2001, Eldering 1995, Garland and Jones 1994, Geissbuhler and Eberhard 2000, Moneta et al 2001, Otigbah et al 2000). It might be argued that, because the women in these studies chose water immersion rather than being randomly allocated, they were less likely to opt for pharmacological pain relief. However, as we know, a woman's wishes antenatally may change when she experiences the reality of labour. Perineal trauma can occur whatever a woman's wishes, and any reduction is to be welcomed given that it can have long-term physical and psychological effects.

Labouring in water

Randomised controlled trials (RCTs)

Cluett et al (2004a) examined the impact of water immersion on nulliparae in the event of labour dystocia (defined as cervical dilatation of <1cm/hr). The group randomised to water had 19 per cent fewer epidurals, 25 per cent less augmentation and 9 per cent fewer incidences of artificial rupture of the membranes. There was no difference in the operative delivery rate.

The same study noted an increased transfer rate to the neonatal intensive care unit (NICU) for the water group (6/49 v 0/50), although there were no differences in the incidence of infection rate, umbilical pH or Apgar scores. Three babies were transferred to the NICU with low temperature. Eckert et al (2001) reported an increased incidence of neonatal resuscitation for the water group, although this finding has reduced reliability because the result was presented as a combination of three distinct outcome measures.

Rush et al (1996) found a reduction in the epidural rate. Another RCT showed that women in water had less pain and felt more relaxed, with 88.8 per cent (48/54) of the sample saying they would like to bathe during a subsequent labour (Cammu at el 1994). A fourth RCT of water immersion during the first stage of labour revealed fewer deflexed fetal positions among bathers (Ohlsson et al 2001). Women experience greater pain and often longer labours when the fetus is in a deflexed position. So if water immersion facilitates flexion, it is of benefit.

Waterbirth

To date, no waterbirth study has found any increase in the incidence of maternal infection or postpartum haemorrhage when compared with spontaneous birth on land.

Up to this point, there has been one RCT that investigated the effects of water immersion during the second stage (Nikodem 1999, cited in Cluett et al 2004b); this reported an increased maternal satisfaction with pushing for the water group.

There has been a recent RCT pilot study, which also included waterbirth (Woodward and Kelly 2004). The design of this feasibility study incorporated a preference arm; i.e. women could choose to opt for water or land, and data were collected in the same way as for the randomised group. The researchers reported an increased incidence of lower umbilical arterial PCO_2 for the water group, although they acknowledge the sample was underpowered, and only 10 women actually had a waterbirth. Cord pH at time of birth is, of itself, a poor predictor of adverse long-term outcome. This pilot study did not note any difference in maternal satisfaction levels for either the randomised or preference arm, which is encouraging for future trial recruitment.

Comparative observational studies also report a significantly shorter labour length associated with waterbirth (Aird et al 1997, Moneta et al 2001, Otigbah et al 2000).

There is evidence that waterbirth, when compared with land birth, is associated with greater maternal satisfaction (Burns and Lloyd 2001, Geissbuhler and Eberhard 2000, Grodzka et al 2001). A qualitative study reported that women felt a greater sense of control when labouring in water (Hall and Holloway 1998). Maternal choice, control and satisfaction have been highlighted as key recommendations in maternity care provision in the UK (Department of Health 1993, House of Commons Select Committee 2003). This acknowledges the fact that maternal physical and psychological well-being are important determinants of future health and can also have a crucial influence on maternal infant attachment.

Waterbirth studies failed to detect differences in the incidence of neonatal morbidity or mortality between water and land birth. Gilbert and Tookey (1999) conducted a national survey of 4,032 waterbirth babies born in England and Wales. The authors found that perinatal mortality was 1–2/1,000 (95 per cent confidence interval (CI): 0.4–2.9) live births. Comparison with women at low risk of complication failed to detect a statistically significant difference in perinatal death – relative risk 0.9 (99 per cent CI: 0.2; 3.6) (Gilbert and Tookey 1999).

The survey detailed five perinatal deaths. Two were stillbirths: one following an unattended birth at home with a concealed pregnancy, and a known intrauterine death in which the woman chose to have a waterbirth. Three neonatal deaths 'were associated with abnormal pathological findings', namely hypoplastic lungs, neonatal herpes infection and intracranial haemorrhage (Gilbert and Tookey 1999: 484). The survey reported an incidence of five snapped umbilical cords. There was no comparable data presented for land births. Snapped umbilical cord is not an event unique to waterbirth. Nguyen et al (2002) describe four case studies of babies admitted to hospital with respiratory problems following waterbirth. Unfortunately, potentially useful information regarding details about the labour and birth for each baby was not available.

Rosser (1994) cites a case of an unattended waterbirth in Austria when the parents did not lift their baby out of the water: the baby was still under water 25 minutes following birth when a midwife arrived. There are two reports of neonatal death following waterbirth. One occurred in Sweden following a straightforward labour in which the midwife did not auscultate any fetal distress (Rosser 1994). The author mentions that the paediatrician in charge attributed this tragedy to 'the 20 per cent of babies born severely asphyxiated in whom there are no detectable problems with the heart rate in labour' (Rosser 1994: 5). The comment is made, however, that resuscitation was more difficult because of the water-filled lungs. The second neonatal death followed a normal labour with no discernible fetal distress, but the baby suffered severe blood loss from a vasa praevia and died at four days, despite prompt resuscitation (Burns and Lloyd 2001).

Conclusion

While death and other adverse events have occurred following waterbirth, these are rare, and mainly reported as case studies. Causality cannot be inferred. We need to appraise the evidence objectively, and consider the most appropriate study design for future study. One possibility is a randomised controlled trial with preference arms, such as the pilot study by Woodward and Kelly (2004), as this option would not affect maternal choice. In the meantime, the collection of audit information is vitally important.

Given the evidence, I suggest that we should feel sufficiently comfortable to proactively support mothers in choosing a pool wherever one is available.

REFERENCES

Aird IA, Luckas JM, Buckett WM and Bousfield P (1997). 'Effects of intrapartum hydrotherapy on labour related parameters'. The Australian & New Zealand Journal of Obstertrics & Gynaecology, 37 (2): 137–142.

Burke E and Kilfoyle A (1995). 'A comparative study: waterbirth and bedbirth'. Midwives, 108: 327.

Burns E and Lloyd A (2001). 'Waterbirth'. MIDIRS Midwifery Digest (September), 11 (3), Supplement 2.

Cammu H, Clasen K, Van Wettere L and Derde MP (1994). ' "To bathe or not to bathe" during the first stage of labor'. Acta Obstetricia et Gynecologica Scandinavica, 73: 468–467.

Cluett ER, Pickering R, Getliffe K and Saunders N (2004a). 'Randomised controlled trial of labouring in water compared with standard of augmentation for management of dystocia in first stage of labour'. BMJ (7 February); 328: 314.

Cluett ER, Nikodem VC, McCandlish RE and Burns EE (2004b) 'Immersion in water in pregnancy, labour and birth (Cochrane Review)'. In: The Cochrane Library, Issue 2, 2004. Chichester, UK: John Wiley & Sons, Ltd.

Department of Health (1993). Changing Childbirth. Report of the Expert Maternity Group, London: HMSO.

Eckert K, Turnbull D and MacLennan A (2001). 'Immersion in Water in the First Stage of Labor: A Randomized Controlled Trial'. Birth, 28 (2): 84–93.

Eldering G (1995). 'Water birth – a possible mode of delivery?', in BAL Beech (ed), Water Birth Unplugged. Proceeding of the First International Water Birth Conference, Books for Midwives Press.

Garland D and Jones K (1994). 'Waterbirth, "first-stage" immersion or non-immersion?' British Journal of Midwifery, 2 (3): 113–119.

Geissbuhler V and Eberhard J (2000). 'Waterbirths: a comparative study. A prospective study on more than 2000 waterbirths'. Fetal Diagnosis and Therapy, 15: 291–300.

Gilbert RE and Tookey PA (1999). 'Perinatal mortatility and morbidity among babies delivered in water: surveillance study and postal survey'. BMJ, 319: 483–487.

Grodzka M, Makowska P, Wielgos M et al (2001). 'Water birth in the parturient's estimation'. Ginekol Pol, 72: 1025–1030.

Hall SM and Holloway IM (1998). 'Staying in control: women's experiences of labour'. Midwifery, 14 (1): 30–36.

House of Commons Select Committee (2003). Choice in Maternity Services, London: HMSO.

Kirkham M (1999). 'The culture of midwifery in the National Health Service in England'. Journal of Advanced Nursing, 30 (3): 732–739.

Moneta J, Okinninska A and Wielgos et al (2001). 'The influence of water immersion on the course of labor'. Ginekol Pol, 72 (12): 1031–1036.

Nguyen S, Kuschel C, Teele R and Spooner C (2002). 'Water birth – a near-drowning experience'. Pediatrics, 110 (2): 411–413.

Ohlsson G, Bucchave P, Leandersson U et al (2001). 'Warm tub bathing during labor: maternal and neonatal effects'. Acta Obstet Gynecol Scand, 80 (4): 311–314.

Otigbah CM, Dhanjal MK, Harmsworth G and Chard T (2000). 'A retrospective comparison of water births and conventional vaginal deliveries'. European Journal of Obstetrics & Gynecology & Reproductive Biology, 91 (1): 15–20.

Rosser J (1994). 'Is water birth safe? The facts behind the controversy'. MIDIRS, 4 (1): 4–6.

Rush J, Burlock S, Lambert K et al (1996). 'The effects of whirlpool baths in labor: a randomized, controlled trial'. Birth, 23 (3): 136–143.

Woodward J and Kelly S (2004). 'A pilot study for a randomised controlled trial of waterbirth versus land birth'. British Journal of Obstetrics & Gynaecology, 111 (6): 537–545.

The Practising Midwife 2004; 7(10): 17–19

Routine cord blood gas analysis: an overreaction?

Siew Quek

Cord blood gas analysis on all babies at birth is increasingly common in many maternity units. However, the practice is not evidence-based and could influence how parents view their well baby. I believe that a blanket approach to cord blood gas analysis is not in the best interests of women or the midwifery professional since it has compromised the midwife's efforts to use clinical judgement and accountability in her/his practice. Furthermore, the approach could be used to audit a midwife's practice in relation to normal birth, and one could argue that a low result of cord blood gas analysis could be used to question competence.

This article aims to discover:

- why cord blood gas analysis is currently performed on all babies
- what research evidence supports this practice
- when analysis should be performed
- the legal and ethical aspects of routine sampling.

The case for routine testing

Monitoring the well-being of the fetus during labour has been one of the key areas of concern for maternity units over the past three decades. Continuous intrapartum electronic fetal monitoring was introduced in an attempt to provide a screening test to predict the development of asphyxia in the fetus, with subsequent hypoxic ischemic encephalopathy, long-term neurology damage or sudden death (Edington et al 1975, Johnstone et al 1978, Shenker et al 1975). Evaluation of changes in fetal heart rate (FHR) patterns was expected to identify fetuses at risk of asphyxia, and allow early and appropriate intervention before the development of intrapartum asphyxia.

The term asphyxia is defined experimentally as impaired respiratory gas exchange accompanied by the development of metabolic acidosis. This is usually reserved for experimental situations where these changes can be accurately established. In the clinical context, fetal asphyxia is progressive hypoxemia and hypercapnia with a significant metabolic acidaemia (Greene and Rosen 1995). In practice, MacLennan (1999) argues that the timing of the onset and progression of these changes can be difficult to ascertain when they occur during the antenatal, intrapartum or neonatal period. The term 'perinatal asphyxia' can be used when the timing is uncertain.

The fourth report of the Confidential Enquiries into Stillbirths and Deaths in Infancy (CESDI) (1997) highlights the difficulties encountered with intrapartum surveillance. More than 50 per cent of 1,300 intrapartum deaths were attributed to the failure to recognise the abnormality in the cardiotocograph (CTG) tracing or failure to take timely action (CESDI 1997). In 1998, nearly £200m paid out for medical litigation was related to obstetrics claims, largely 'birth asphyxia'. Allegations of causation of cerebral palsy in clinical negligence claims usually centre on care in the intrapartum period (Sloan et al 1997, Towbin 1986). To minimise liability, various strategies were incorporated into labour ward guidelines, clinical audit and monthly feedback meetings. In addition, mandatory training sessions were organised on intrapartum CTG interpretation. A significant increase in routine sampling of cord blood for gas analysis to assess oxygen reserves in newborn infants was subsequently observed in obstetric/midwifery practice (Young et al 2001).

The 26th Royal College of Obstetricians and Gynaecologists Study Group on Intrapartum Fetal Surveillance (1993) recommended measurement of umbilical artery and vein cord blood gases analysis after birth to measure the fetal response to labour. Although most studies have used the combination of low pH and Apgar scores for identifying abnormal neurological outcome, most studies suggest that pathologic fetal acidaemia be defined as an arterial pH (Gilstrap et al 1989, Goldaber et al 1991, Goodwin et al 1992, Winkler et al 1991, van den Berg et al 1996). According to Thorp and Rushing (1999), cord blood gases analysis may exclude the diagnosis of birth asphyxia in approximately 80 per cent of 'fetal distress' at term. Pathological fetal acidaemia (pH <7.0 and base deficit ≥12mmol/l) may be correlated with an increased risk of neurological deficit (Goldaber et al 1991).

The Royal College of Obstetricians and Gynaecologists and the Royal College of Midwives (1999) have jointly recommended that routine measurement of cord blood gas is essential for all caesarean sections or instrumental vaginal births performed because of fetal distress. They also recommend that it should be considered for all vaginal births to exclude hypoxia as a cause of brain damage because of the medico-legal implications. By implementing this policy, normal cord blood gas results can be used as evidence to eliminate any suggestion of a damaging intrapartum hypoxic event as a cause of cerebral palsy diagnosed in later childhood (MacLennan 1999).

If routine cord blood gas analysis significantly reduces the chances of litigation for damaging intrapartum events as a cause of cerebral palsy, it is difficult to understand why only 13 per cent of units in the UK perform cord blood gas analysis for all births, and 68 per cent for all caesarean sections or instrumental births (CESDI 2001).

While routine cord blood gas analysis aims to reduce the cost of litigation, one could argue that the implementation of this routine practice actually imposes an additional financial burden on cash-strapped hospitals when cost-savings have not been demonstrated.

What does the research say?

Cerebral palsy is characterised by non-progressive, abnormal control of movement or posture, which is not usually diagnosed until months or years after birth. It usually presents with excessive muscular tonus, spasticity with increased stretch reflexes, and hyperactive tendon reflexes as a result of damage to the upper motor neurons of the brain (Badawi et al 1998). Cerebral palsy is associated with developmental and metabolic abnormalities, autoimmune and coagulation disorders, infections, and trauma and hypoxia (asphyxia) in the fetus and newborn (MacLennan 1999).

A common assumption is that perinatal asphyxia is the usual cause of cerebral palsy in term babies (Nelson et al 1996). However, the epidemiological studies indicate that only about 10 per cent of cases were caused by intrapartum asphyxia (Blair and Stanley 1988, Gaffney et al 1994, MacLennan 1999). These studies show that a large proportion of cerebral palsy cases are associated with maternal and antenatal factors such as prematurity (limited essential fatty acids for brain growth in preterm infants), intrauterine growth restriction, intrauterine infection,

fetal coagulation disorders, multiple pregnancy, antepartum haemorrhage, breech presentation, and chromosomal or congenital anomalies (Blair and Stanley 1990, Crowford 1992, Duncan et al 2002, Grether and Nelson 1997, Pharoah 1995, Pharoah et al 1987).

According to Crowford's thesis (1992), poor maternal nutrition prior to conception results in fetal malnourishment and affects fetal cell division. Additionally, poor maternal nutrition results in fragile membranes with the limited essential fatty acids in the preterm infant and cannot be replaced by an external feeding regime. Therefore, Crowford (1992) argues that cerebral palsy in premature or low-birthweight infants may not be due to obstetric or paediatric mismanagement but to poor preparation for life.

Cerebral palsy in term babies is thought to be caused exclusively by asphyxia at birth, and is preventable if detected early (MacLachlan et al 1992, Spencer et al 1997). This assumption has been an important factor in the development and widespread use of electronic fetal monitoring and other forms of antenatal and intrapartum surveillance, and has influenced the rate of caesarean section delivery (Clark and Hankins 2003).

In spite of these changes in obstetric management and a fivefold increase in the caesarean section delivery over the past 30 years (Parer and King 2000, Freeman, 2002), the rate of cerebral palsy in term infants has not declined (Hagberg et al 1996, Pharoah et al 1996). Approximately one in every 1,500 term infants born has disabling cerebral palsy (Cummins et al 1993). Neonatal survival rates have improved during this period. These observations have led to the hypothesis that increased survival of premature, neurologically impaired infants may have masked an actual reduction in cerebral palsy among term babies as a result of the use of electronic monitoring and the avoidance of intrapartum asphyxia (Clark and Hankins 2003).

Assessment of the contribution of asphyxial events to cerebral palsy is complicated by the fact that there is no generally available tool for direct measurement of birth asphyxia. In the absence of a validated means for its recognition, birth asphyxia is commonly diagnosed on the basis of abnormalities on electronic fetal monitoring, low Apgar scores, need for respiratory support, neonatal encephalopathy, and evidence of metabolic acidosis which is confirmed by cord blood gas analysis at birth (MacLennan 1999). Metabolic acidaemia is defined as pH <7.00 and a base deficit of >16mmols. These are the criteria agreed by the Royal College of Obstetricians and Gynaecologists, the American College of Obstetricians and Gynecologists, and the Society of Obstetricians and Gynaecologists of Canada (MacLennan 1999).

Metabolic acidaemia at birth is comparatively common (2 per cent of all births) but the vast majority of such infants do not develop cerebral palsy (Goodlin et al 1994). According to Casey et al (2001), cord blood gas analysis should be repeated within two hours of birth if the cord pH was low in order to exclude chronic hypoxia. Therefore, there remains a need for better markers of acute intrapartum injury (Greenwood et al 2003). Neonatal nucleated red blood cells and lymphocyte counts have been shown to be raised in asphyxiated infants, but the rise is seen both in definite intrapartum events and in those that started antenatally (Phelan et al 1998). Other acute inflammatory markers might be more useful in the future (Nelson and Willoughby 2000).

Westgate et al (1994) and Harris et al (1996) have highlighted the problem associated with cord blood sampling. In order to identify whether hypoxia or asphyxia was an acute or chronic event during labour, the records of both arterial and venous umbilical cord gases need to be reviewed. If records of both exist, then a difference in partial pressure of carbon dioxide of >25 mm Hg suggests an acute rather than chronic acidosis (Westgate et al 1994). However, the technique for measuring arterial versus venous gases is critical. Individual partial pressures of oxygen are not helpful in this context as they correlate poorly with fetal acidosis (Harris et al 1996). Therefore, the cord blood gas analysis will be valuable only if the samples are correctly taken, correctly measured and the results correctly interpreted (Westgate et al 1994). In terms of validity and reliability, this test needs to be undertaken by a trained technician and interpreted by a paediatrician.

Consideration is also needed for women who have a water birth and/or physiological third stage when cord blood sampling is delayed because the cord is not clamped until it stops pulsating. Available evidence has not explored the effects of delayed cord clamping with the result of cord blood gas analysis.

Performing cord blood gas analysis at birth may predict short-term neonatal complications (Gilstrap et al 1989, Low et al 1995, van den Berg et al 1996), but the predictive value of cord blood pH on long-term handicap is limited (Low et al 1988, Ruth and Raivio 1988, Socol et al 1994). Goodlin et al (1994) argue that there is no evidence that cord blood gas analysis at birth is of benefit to mother and baby, or can specifically rule out or identify when damage to a baby occurred.

Within the five years of the study of West Midlands Perinatal Audit (1996), the proportions of babies with low Apgar scores and low cord pH have not changed. Neither are any fewer being admitted for neonatal intensive care, even with better intrapartum care. This report has shown that better fetal monitoring and earlier intervention to caesarean section are unlikely to reduce cerebral palsy, and there is no evidence to suggest that it reduced litigation (West Midlands Perinatal Audit 1996).

Regardless of proper surveillance and new insights, in most cases of cerebral palsy there will be nothing or nobody to blame. Focus should therefore be on providing optimal care for affected infants and their families.

When is analysis appropriate?

Most of the literature available has shown the inconsistencies and imponderables associated with introducing cord blood gas analysis as a routine procedure at all births. Cord blood gas analysis at birth offers objective data on fetal status at birth, and it may be useful for evaluation of perinatal care. Therefore, it is valuable if carried out in high-risk births and whenever non-reassuring fetal heart tracing occurs and fetal blood sampling has been performed (Thorp and Rushing 1999).

National Institute for Clinical Excellence (NICE) guidelines (2001) state that cord blood gas analysis should be performed after:

- an emergency caesarean section
- an instrumental vaginal birth
- a fetal blood sample has been performed in labour
- birth, if the baby's condition is poor.

To operate on the basis of current best evidence, cord blood gas analysis should be performed on selective cases and not as a routine procedure (NICE 2001).

Legal and ethical aspects

All studies failed to consider informing parents about performing routine cord blood sampling for gas analysis. However, the Human Rights Act (1998) has stated that consent needs to be sought from patient or client before any treatment or procedure takes place. Vision 2000 (RCM 2000) and the client-focussed section from Delivering the NHS Plan (DoH 2002) has an emphasis on woman-centred care, which means that women should be involved prior to all care or procedures. In addition, The Bristol Royal Infirmary Inquiry (2001) recommended that patients should be given an explanation of what is going to happen before embarking on any procedure, and should also have the opportunity to review what has happened.

It is not ethically acceptable to perform cord blood sampling without informing parents and gaining their informed consent. Research has shown that women often require more realistic information than is provided (Hillan 1992, McKay et al 1990).

To enable parents to give informed consent, they must be fully informed about the procedure and the benefits of the test for them and their baby. Before performing cord blood sampling, written consent should be obtained.

The midwives' Code of Professional Conduct firmly states that: 'As a registered midwife you must obtain consent before you give any treatment or care' (NMC 2002: 9).

In the light of litigation, investigations and defensive practice have increased. This has serious implications for standards of care, as people are no longer treated as individuals (Symon 2000). Kirkham and Stapleton (2001) also found that fear of litigation influences the way in which information is presented to, or withheld from, patients.

Performing cord blood sampling without informing parents contradicts some of the recommendations of Delivering Choice (DoH 1994), and shows obvious lack of respect for parents as individuals. At present, parents are not told initially when routine cord blood sampling is done – they may later be made aware of the result if the test was sub-optimal despite the baby appearing well.

According to the study of Lavender et al (1999), it was evident that many women felt reassured that practices were based on evidence. As the literature on cord blood gas analysis is rife with inconsistencies, it is not possible for midwives in the unit to reassure the woman about this screening test. Further work needs to be done to look critically at the value and reliability of this screening test.

Conclusion

Much well-known evidence has already called into question the value of electronic fetal heart rate monitoring and 'timing intervention' of caesarean section to prevent cerebral palsy. Even if cerebral palsy is intrapartum in origin, this need not necessarily imply negligence; neither does an antenatal aetiology exclude negligence (Greenwood et al 2003). Therefore, the ability of measurement of cord blood gas at birth to reduce litigation is questionable. On the basis of current best evidence, cord blood gas analysis for all births has no scientific basis and is not justified on ethical or professional grounds.

REFERENCES

Badawi N, Kurinczuk J J, Keogh J M, et al (1998). 'Intrapartum risk factors for newborn encephalopathy: the Western Australian Case Control Study'. British Medical Journal, 317: 1554–1558.

Blair E and Stanley F (1988). 'Intrapartum asphyxia: a rare cause of cerebral palsy'. Journal of Paediatrics, 112 (4): 515–519.

Blair E and Stanley F (1990). 'Intrapartum growth and spastic cerebral palsy: association with birth weight for gestational age'. American Journal of Obstetrics and Gynecology, 162 (1): 229–237.

Bristol Royal Infirmary Inquiry (2001). Learning from Bristol: the Report of the Public Inquiry into Children's Heart Surgery at the Bristol Royal Infirmary, 1984–1995, command paper CM5207, July, www.bristol-inquiry.org.uk

Casey B, Goldaber K G, McIntire D D et al (2001). 'Outcome among term infants when two-hour postnatal pH is compared with pH at delivery'. American Journal of Obstetrics and Gynecology 2, 184 (3): 447–450.

Clark S L and Hankins G D V (2003). 'Temporal and demographic trends in cerebral palsy – fact and fiction'. American Journal of Obstetrics and Gynecology, 188 (3): 628–633.

Confidential Enquiry Into Stillbirths And Deaths In Infancy (CESDI) (1997). CESDI 4th Annual Report. Concentrating on Intrapartum Related Deaths 1994–1995, London: Maternal and Child Health Research Consortium.

Confidential Enquiry Into Stillbirths And Deaths In Infancy (CESDI) (2001). CESDI 8th Annual Report, London: Maternal and Child Health Research Consortium.

Crowford M A (1992). 'Essential fatty acid and neurodevelopment disorder'. In: Neurobiology of Essential Fatty Acids, Bazan et al (ed), New York: Plenum Press.

Cummins S K, Nelson K B, Grether J K et al (1993). 'Cerebral palsy in four northern California counties, births 1983 through 1985'. Journal of Paediatrics, 123: 230–237.

Department of Health (DoH) (1994). Delivery Choice Midwife and General Practitioner-led Maternity: Report of the Northern Ireland Maternity Units Study Group, Belfast: Department of Health and Social Services.

Department of Health (DoH) (2002). Delivering the NHS Plan: Next Steps on Investment, Next Steps on Reform, www.doh.gov.uk/deliveringthenhsplan/index.htm

Duncan J C, Cock M L, Scheerlinck J P et al (2002). 'White matter injury after repeated endotoxin exposure in the preterm ovine fetus'. Paediatric Research, 52 (6): 941–949.

Edington P T, Sibanda J and Beard R W (1975). 'Influence on clinical practice of routine intrapartum fetal monitoring'. British Medical Journal, 3: 341–343.

Freeman R K (2002). 'Problems with intrapartum fetal heart rate monitoring interpretation and patient management'. Obstetrics and Gynaecology, 100 (4): 813–825.

Gaffney G, Flavell V, Johnson A et al (1994). 'Cerebral palsy and neonatal encephalopathy'. Arch Disable Child, 70: F195–F200.

Gilstrap L C III, Leveno K J, Burris J et al (1989). 'Diagnosis of birth asphyxia on the basis of fetal pH, Apgar score, and newborn cerebral dysfunction'. American Journal Obstetrics and Gynecology, 161 (3): 825–830.

Goldaber K G, Gilstrap L C, Leveno K J et al (1991). 'Pathologic fetal acidemia'. Obstetrics and Gynecology, 78 (6): 1103–1106.

Goodlin R C, Freeman W L, McFee J G et al (1994). 'The neonatal with unexpected acidemia'. Journal of Reproductive Medicine, 39: 97–100.

Goodwin T M, Belai I, Hernandez P et al (1992). 'Asphyxia complications in the term newborn with severe umbilical artery acidemia'. American Journal of Obstetrics and Gynecology, 167 (6): 1506–1512.

Greene K R and Rosen K G (1995). 'Intrapartum asphyxia'. In: M L Levene and R J Lilford (eds), Fetal and Neonatal Neurology and Neurosurgery, 2nd edn, Edinburgh: Churchill Livingstone.

Greenwood C, Newman L I and Johnson A (2003). 'Cerebral palsy and clinical negligence litigation: a cohort study'. British Journal of Obstetrics and Gynaecology, 110 (1): 6–11.

Grether J K and Nelson K B (1997). 'Maternal infections and cerebral palsy in infants of normal birth weight'. JAMA, 278 (3): 207–211.

Hagberg B, Hagberg G, Olow I et al (1996). 'The changing panorama of cerebral palsy in Sweden, VII: prevalence and origin in the birth year period 1987–90'. Acta Paediatrics, 85: 954–960.

Harris M, Beckley S L, Garibaldi R D K et al (1996). 'Umbilical cord blood analysis at the time of delivery'. Midwifery, 12: 146–150.

Hillan E (1992). 'Issues in the delivery of midwifery care'. Journal of Advanced Nursing, 17 (3): 274–278.

Human Rights Act (1998). http://www.doh.gov.uk/ consent/refguide. htm

Johnstone F D, Campbell D M and Hughes G J (1978). 'Antenatal care: has continuous intrapartum monitoring made any impact on fetal outcome?'. Lancet, 1: 298–300.

Kirkham M and Stapleton H (2001). Informed Choice in Maternity Care: an Evaluation of Evidence-based Leaflets, University of York: NHS Centre for Reviews and Dissemination.

Lavender T, Walton I and Walkinshaw S (1999). 'Which factors contribute to a positive birth experience? A prospective study of women's views'. Midwifery, 15: 40–46.

Low J A, Galbraith R S, Muir D W et al (1988). 'Motor and cognitive deficits after intrapartum asphyxia in the mature fetus'. American Journal of Obstetrics and Gynecology, 158 (2): 356–361.

Low J A, Panagiotopoulos C and Derrick E J (1995). 'Newborn complications after intrapartum asphyxia with metabolic acidosis in the preterm fetus'. American Journal of Obstetrics and Gynecology, 172: 1152–1157.

MacLachlan N, Spencer J A D, Harding K et al (1992). 'Fetal acidaemia, the cardiotocograph and the VQRS ratio of the feta ECG in labour'. British Journal of Obstetrics and Gynaecology, 99: 26–31.

MacLennan A (1999). 'A template for defining a causal relationship between acute intrapartum events and cerebral palsy: international consensus statement'. British Medical Journal, 319: 1054–1059.

McKay S, Barrows T and Roberts J (1990). 'Women's views of second stage labour as assessed by interviews and videotapes'. Birth, 17 (4): 192–198.

National Institute for Clinical Effectiveness (NICE) (2001). The Use of Electronic Fetal Monitoring: the Use and Interpretation of Cardiotocography in Intrapartum Fetal Surveillance, London: NICE Publications.

Nelson K B, Dambrosia J M, Ting T Y et al (1996). 'Uncertain value of electronic fetal monitoring in predicting cerebral palsy'. New England Journal of Medicine, 334 (10): 613–618.

Nelson K B and Willoughby R E (2000). 'Infection, inflammation and the risk of cerebral palsy'. Current Opinion Neurology, 13 (2): 133–139.

Nursing Midwifery Council (2002). Code of Professional Conduct, London: NMC.

Parer J T and King T (2000). 'Fetal heart rate monitoring: is it salvageable?'. American Journal of Obstetrics and Gynecology, 182: 982–989.

Pharoah P O D (1995). 'Cerebral palsy and perinatal care'. British Journal of Obstetrics and Gynaecology, 102 (5): 356–358.

Pharoah P O D, Cooke T, Rosenbloom I et al (1987). 'Trends in birth prevalence of cerebral palsy'. Archives of Disease in Childhood, 62 (4): 379–384.

Pharoah P O D, Platt M J and Cooke T (1996). 'The changing panorama of cerebral palsy'. Archives of Disease in Childhood, 75: F169–173.

Phelan J P, Korst L M, Ahn M O et al (1998). 'Neonatal nucleated red blood cell and lymphocyte counts in fetal brain injury'. Obstetrics and Gynaecology, 91 (4): 485–489.

Royal College of Midwives (RCM) (2000). Vision 2000 RCM, London: RCM.

Royal College of Obstetricians and Gynaecologists (RCOG) (1993). 'Recommendations arising from the 26th RCOG Study Group: intrapartum fetal surveillance'. In: J A D Spencer and R H T Ward (eds), Intrapartum Fetal Surveillance, London: Royal College of Obstetricians and Gynaecologists Press: 392.

Royal College of Obstetricians and Gynaecologists (RCOG) and Royal College of Midwives (RCM) (1999). Towards Safer Childbirth: Minimum Standards for the Organisation of Labour Ward, London: Royal College of Obstetricians and Gynaecologists Press.

Ruth V J and Raivio K O (1988). 'Perinatal brain damage: predictive value of metabolic acidosis and the Apgar score'. British Medical Journal, 297: 991–999.

Shenker L, Post R C and Seiler J S (1975). 'Routine electronic monitoring of fetal heart and uterine activity during labour'. Obstetrics and Gynaecology, 46: 185–189.

Sloan F A, Whetten-Goldstien K, Stout E M et al (1997). 'No fault system of compensation for obstetric injury and subsequent cerebral palsy: medicolegal issues'. Paediatrics, 99 (6): 851–859.

Socol M L, Garcia P M and Riter S (1994). 'Depressed Apgar scores, acid-base status, and neurological outcome'. American Journal of Obstetrics and Gynecology, 170: 991–998.

Spencer J A D, Badawi N, Burton P et al (1997). 'The intrapartum CTG prior to neonatal encephalopathy at term: a case-control study'. British Journal of Obstetrics and Gynaecology, 104 (1): 25–28.

Symon A (2000). 'Litigation and changes in professional behaviour: a qualitative appraisal'. Midwifery, 16 (1): 15–21.

Thorp J A and Rushing R S (1999). 'Umbilical cord blood gas analysis'. Obstetrics and Gynaecology Clinical North American 12, 26 (4): 695–709.

Towbin A (1986). 'Obstetric malpractice litigation: the pathologist's view'. American Journal of Obstetrics and Gynecology, 155 (5): 927–935.

van den Berg P P, Nelen W L D M, Jonsma H W et al (1996). 'Neonatal complications in newborns with an umbilical artery pH less than 7.00'. American Journal of Obstetrics and Gynecology, 175: 1152–1157.

West Midlands Perinatal Audit (1996). Stillbirth and Neonatal Death 1991–1994. Report of National, Regional, District and Unit Mortality Rates, Keele: West Midlands Perinatal Audit.

Westgate J, Garibaldi J M and Greene K R (1994). 'Umbilical cord blood gas analysis at delivery: a time for quality data'. British Journal of Obstetrics and Gynaecology, 101 (12): 1054–1063.

Winkler C L, Hauth J C, Tucker J M et al (1991). 'Neonatal complications at term as related to the degree of umbilical artery acidemia'. American Journal of Obstetrics and Gynecology, 164 (2): 637–641.

Young P, Hamilton R, Hodgett S et al (2001). 'Reducing risk by improving standards of intrapartum fetal care'. Journal of the Royal Society of Medicine 5, 94 (5): 226–231

The Practising Midwife 2004; 7(10): 20–23

Need to know: vaginal birth after caesarean (Part 1)

Rosemary Mander

Although some would argue that it doesn't make a difference as long as the mother and baby are well, the way in which a woman gives birth does matter. There is an increasing body of research that shows her disappointment when her birth experience does not match up to her aspirations and expectations. Some suggest that this negative reaction may be especially marked if her baby is surgically removed from her, as in the caesarean operation, rather than if she is able actively to assist her baby's entry into the world (Ryding et al 1998). On the other hand, it may be that caesarean is coming to be regarded as little more than an optional way to give birth (Mutryn 1993).

In the short term, the way that a woman gives birth is becoming more significant for a number of reasons: one is the increasing frequency of the caesarean operation (Warwick 2001). In the long term, though, there may be an even more serious implication: the confidence of women in their ability to give birth spontaneously may be under threat.

Because of the increasing incidence of caesarean, vaginal birth after caesarean (VBAC) is necessarily of increasing significance. VBAC matters to the individual woman because, among other factors, she may feel that a caesarean has deprived her of the satisfaction and achievement that actively giving birth brings with it.

As well as a range of personal aspects, the VBAC issue also has serious implications for the woman's relationship with those who provide her maternity care. The traditional assumption of 'once a caesarean, always a caesarean' explicitly reduces the woman's freedom of choice in the way in which she gives birth. As a result, her control over her birth experience has been effectively removed from her and assumed by those who are, supposedly, providing her care. Although this traditional diktat is currently widely rejected, its influence may still be evident in the concept of the 'repeat caesarean'. This influence manifests itself in the words that appear all too frequently in women's maternity notes, 'Previous CS'. Thus, the VBAC issue matters to women in general because it represents a form of 'one size fits all' policy-making that serves to deny the woman the individualised maternity care to which she is entitled.

In these two articles I outline the information that the midwife is able to provide for the woman who is contemplating VBAC. The material in this, the first part, seeks to address some of the background to the caesarean operation, including issues relating to rupture of the uterus and research more generally. This leads to the concept of VBAC. The research evidence relating to VBAC is examined in the second article. I then consider some of the factors that have been shown to influence the likelihood of VBAC being successful. On the basis of this material I draw certain conclusions.

1. The context

The caesarean operation has a long history, but it is only since the latter half of the 20th century that its incidence has increased exponentially (Curtin et al 2000). This increase may be associated with a wide range of factors, including convenience, fashion, litigation anxiety, declining medical skills, changing anaesthetic practice, increased use of continuous electronic fetal monitoring or a combination of all of these (Dodd et al 2004, Lowdon and Derrick 2002).

In spite of these changing circumstances, the caesarean operation is defined in terms of a surgical incision into the woman's uterus or womb in order to remove the baby (or babies) through the abdominal wall. The processes of the decision and operation, though, have varied and continue to vary according to the circumstances and the medical practitioner's predilection. Consideration of these details is likely to be helpful in understanding the debates that arise out of the relevant research.

The decision to undertake the caesarean may be made prior to the woman going into labour. In this situation the surgery would be elective – if the woman's pelvis was seriously damaged due to rickets, for example. Alternatively, circumstances may arise during the labour, such as serious uterine haemorrhage, that suggest that a caesarean would be appropriate; in these circumstances this intrapartum operation would be regarded as an urgent or emergency procedure. In a small number of women, a condition may arise during pregnancy that means an emergency caesarean is indicated.

Irrespective of the position of the skin incision on the abdominal wall, a horizontal incision into the lower part (or segment) of the uterus is the currently preferred practice. This is because the blood supply and uterine activity are less in this lower part; supposedly, the risk of haemorrhage is limited and healing is facilitated. Occasionally, a classical or vertical incision into the upper segment of the uterus may be employed. Although this form of incision may carry certain benefits, there are also additional risks.

Following the birth of the baby or babies and the placenta, the incisions into the uterus and superficial tissues are sutured. The repair may be made separately, in two or more layers, or in a single layer. The materials and techniques used vary according to a number of factors (discussed in Part 2).

If a woman has not experienced a caesarean operation previously, it is referred to as a primary caesarean; if she has, the term is secondary or repeat caesarean. Although 'secondary' describes more precisely the nature of the subsequent operation, the term 'repeat' is more widely used in the literature. For this reason, I will use the term 'repeat caesarean' here. The major risks of caesarean for the mother are associated with the actual surgery, the administration of the anaesthetic and the postoperative recovery period. These risks have been shown to increase with the number of caesareans an individual woman undergoes (Dodd et al 2004).

(a) Research and other literature

In considering the issue of VBAC, it is necessary to bear in mind that the term itself and much of the literature originated in North America. This is partly because of major concerns, particularly in the US, about the escalating costs of healthcare (Harer 2002). Of course, these costs are aggravated by the relatively frequent use of caesarean there. Further, the relative novelty of VBAC in North America means that it attracts far more attention there than in Europe (Flamm 2001). Thus, in interpreting this literature, it is necessary to bear in mind the different cultures and healthcare systems in the countries from which much of the research and other literature originates. It may be necessary to question its relevance to women in the UK.

(b) The woman's experience

As mentioned already, some women may encounter negative feelings following a caesarean. These feelings may be sufficiently severe to be regarded as constituting an illness and being classified as maternal morbidity. These negative feelings may include depression, guilt, loss of self-esteem, grief reactions, feelings of violation, dissatisfaction with care and resentment towards care providers (Small et al 2000). As a consumer representative, Bainbridge identifies the range of these feelings as varying from slight disappointment in their mildest form, to post-traumatic stress disorder (PTSD) in their most severe (2002). She goes on to mention the likelihood of the woman feeling frightened and confused at experiencing such negative feelings. This confusion may be aggravated by the woman's conviction that she should really be grateful that the operation and the people who performed it have given her a live, healthy baby.

A research project undertaken in Sweden (Ryding et al 1998, Wijma et al 2002) demonstrated that there is one group of women particularly vulnerable to these negative reactions – those who undergo an emergency caesarean. The researchers interviewed a sample of these women two days after the operation using a research instrument that diagnoses PTSD in disaster situations. The researchers were able to trace the woman's change from being self-confident on entry into the labour room to being intensely fearful as the need for the operation became apparent. The twin focus of the woman's fear was split equally between her own survival and that of her baby.

While the women generally showed a good understanding of the reason for the caesarean, a quarter still held themselves responsible for this 'adverse' outcome to their labour. These researchers consider that such negative feelings may eventually come to dominate the woman's recollection of her experience of giving birth. In this way, anxiety about this scenario recurring would feature prominently if she were ever to become pregnant again.

(c) Body processes

Following a caesarean, as with any form of bodily hurt, healing occurs in the damaged tissues. This is of immense importance in the uterine wound, as the effectiveness of this healing is thought to affect subsequent events. In general terms, the adequacy of healing has been shown to be affected by factors such as age, hydration, cleanliness, freedom from infection, certain medications, tissue oxygenation and nutrition (RCSE 2003). Clearly, in a childbearing woman these factors will ordinarily function healthily to ensure that her wound heals optimally.

The healing of the uterine wound (as with any wound) involves a healthy, localised inflammatory reaction. Platelets and thrombin in the wound form a network with collagen fibres. Cells such as macrophages are carried to the wound site, and fibroblasts develop to facilitate healing and the formation of a scar (Ganong 1997). In this way, the integrity or wholeness of the uterus is re-established.

Under certain circumstances, though, the edges of a wound that was thought to have healed may begin to separate or undergo 'dehiscence'. These circumstances may include 'marked distension' (Brunner and Suddarth 1992). In the present context, this separation may happen in a subsequent pregnancy or labour and is known as rupture of the uterus. This obstetric accident may carry serious risks for the baby and for the mother. In this event, the baby's oxygen supply could be severely compromised or might totally cease. This would result in damage to the baby or possibly death. In the event of rupture of the uterus, the mother might die due to haemorrhage or other complications, or she might sustain such serious damage to her uterus that it warrants being removed surgically by hysterectomy.

Rupture of the uterus may occur in first-time mothers, in women who have previously given birth spontaneously and in women who have previously given birth by caesarean (Lewis 1998, Shaw 2001).

The major issues in the debate about VBAC revolve around the conditions that affect the likelihood of the uterus undergoing a rupture. The research literature that informs this debate is addressed in Part 2.

(d) Trial of labour

Vaginal birth is generally regarded as the optimal outcome for a woman who has previously given birth by caesarean.

This subsequent birth may, however, be recommended to happen under the conditions of a 'trial of labour' (TOL). This has been defined as 'a purposeful attempt to permit active labour development with progression to vaginal delivery' (Harer 2002). Because it is the strength or integrity of the uterine scar that is effectively 'on trial', this labour may sometimes be known as a 'trial of scar' (Flamm 2001, Lowdon and Derrick 2002).

A trial of labour is usually conducted only in the presence of certain criteria, such as the baby being in a cephalic presentation (head first), the scar being transverse in the lower segment of the uterus, and the estimated weight of the baby being less than four kilos. These criteria, however, have been criticised – in an appropriately scathing manner (Lowdon and Derrick 2002) – for limiting the woman's choice. The trial of labour involves close observation of the progress of labour along with similar observation for any signs that the scar may be threatening to rupture. American figures show that 34.5 per cent of women who have had a previous caesarean achieve a VBAC (Curtin et al 2000). Of the remaining women, a small majority will have had an elective repeat caesarean. The other small number of women will have had a trial of labour that ended with a caesarean, because incidental problems such as fetal distress have supervened.

The terminology relating to this labour and the associated intensive monitoring are likely to engender anxiety and resentment in the woman and those near to her (Robinson 2001). Thus, we should consider the possibility of a trial of labour being counterproductive, in that anxiety may jeopardise the healthy progress of labour (Lowdon and Derrick 2002). Further, if the trial of labour is ended by a caesarean, the operation would be an emergency. As well as the after-effects of the labour, the anaesthetic and the surgery, this form of birth would carry with it the negative outcomes mentioned already in the context of the Swedish study (Ryding et al 1998, Wijma et al 2002).

The importance of the woman being given a full account of the risks and benefits of a trial of labour are emphasised in the literature (Harer 2002). Such an account would also include information about the risks inherent in a further caesarean. This information would allow the woman to make a knowledgeable decision about whether to go ahead with this form of labour.

2. Research matters

In the field of healthcare, the randomised controlled trial (RCT) started to become, in the latter part of the 20th century, a major research tool in finding out what forms of care are effective and safe. The RCT is, probably appropriately, regarded as the 'gold standard' in providing rigorous information or evidence to assist decisions about the form of care to be offered. In the context of birth following caesarean, an RCT large enough to permit calculations of statistical significance would provide answers to the outstanding questions about the relative costs and benefits of VBAC and elective repeat caesarean.

Dodd et al (2004) outline their plans for a systematic review of such RCTs.

My MEDLINE (1966–2003) search, though, suggests that these reviewers are likely to encounter difficulty.

Using the search terms (1) 'VBAC' or 'Vaginal birth after caesarean' and (2) 'Trial of labour', my search produced 601 and 536 hits respectively. However, when 'RCT' was added to each of these search terms, there were no hits for either. Thus, using an authoritative database, I have been unable to identify any RCTs focusing on vaginal birth after caesarean.

It is not hard to imagine why this should be. In order to undertake such an RCT, it would be necessary to recruit a suitable sample of women. This would involve pregnant women being given complete information about the issues, including the possible risks, of each type of birth. On the basis of this information, each woman would be asked to consent to being randomised into one type of birth group or the other – elective repeat caesarean or trial of labour with a view to VBAC. It is likely that, even if such a study were to be given ethical and managerial approval, the women themselves would have serious misgivings about being randomised.

This lack of relevant RCTs is, I suggest, likely to persist in spite of the optimism of Dodd and her colleagues. In the absence of more rigorous research findings, it is necessary to examine meticulously the research that exists. I begin this examination, though, with an overview of any other potential problems that have been identified in relation to the research methods.

A methodological problem encountered in scrutinising this research is the one experienced by Bujold et al (2002). These Canadian researchers sought to examine the effect of different suturing or wound closure techniques on the incidence of rupture of the uterus in a subsequent pregnancy. In order to do this, they examined the medical and nursing notes and operation reports of more than 2,000 women who had undergone a trial of labour in one maternity unit during the previous 12 years.

These researchers obviously had to rely on retrospective data, which is fraught with difficulty – in part, with the interpretation of data collected at a time when practices and attitudes would have been different. Thus, a historical bias would be present. It is for this reason that, in another project, Boulvain et al (1997) used only ongoing or prospective studies for their meta-analysis of trial of labour in sub-Saharan Africa. The differences in practices and attitudes can only have been aggravated by the fact that the Canadian data would have been collected for some purpose other than this research. These criticisms are among the issues raised by Flamm in his mercilessly withering critique (2001) of the study by Lydon-Rochelle et al (2001) – see next article – and his even harsher condemnation of the supporting editorial by Greene (2001).

It is possible that Flamm's criticisms may apply equally to other research in this area.

A further research problem identified by Flamm (2001) relates to the lack of definition of the severity of rupture of the uterus. This matters because rupture of the uterus varies immensely in its seriousness. The rupture may comprise a very slight degree of separation, sometimes known as 'scar dehiscence', which causes a little pain to the woman and no other problems. On the other hand, a severe rupture carries an immediate threat to the life of both the woman and her baby. Flamm criticises researchers for not clarifying the gravity of the condition they label 'rupture of the uterus'.

Although Flamm does not use the term, this phenomenon whereby the researcher may surreptitiously 'enhance' the research findings to suit his agenda has been dubbed 'massaging the data'. This activity, which has also been entitled 'spin doctoring' (Goer 2003), is clearly unethical as it denies the reader the opportunity to make a sensible judgement on the basis of unambiguous research findings. Goer (2003) effectively levels this accusation at the work of McMahon et al (1996). McMahon's manipulation of the data during analysis involved the categorisation of wound infections and haemorrhage (sufficient to need blood transfusion) as 'minor' complications. In this way, these researchers were able to suggest that elective repeat caesarean is the safer way of giving birth.

In the same paper, Goer (2003) similarly criticises Mozurkewich and Hutton (2000) for their relaxed interpretation of statistical significance and their innovative classification of perinatal deaths. Her paper continues by showing how Smith et al (2002) chose to magnify the number of babies dying as a result of VBAC. This was achieved by regarding any emergency caesarean, such as those for problems as serious as abruptio placenta or eclampsia, after 37 weeks' gestation as simply a trial of labour.

By the use of techniques and tactics such as these, medical researchers studying this area have been in a position to present VBAC as an infinitely more dangerous alternative to elective repeat caesarean. As a result of such 'research', the opportunities for rational decision-making available to the childbearing woman have been seriously curtailed.

Acknowledgement

I would like to acknowledge the help of the AIMS Committee in the development of these articles.

REFERENCES

Bainbridge J (2002). 'A consumer viewpoint: choices after cesarean'. Birth, 29 (3): 203–206.

Boulvain M, Fraser W D, Brisson-Carroll G et al (1997). 'Trial of labour after caesarean section in sub-Saharan Africa: a meta-analysis'. British Journal of Obstetrics & Gynaecology, 104 (12): 1385–1390.

Brunner L S and Suddarth D S (1992). The Textbook of Adult Nursing, London: Chapman & Hall.

Bujold E, Bujold C, Hamilton E F et al (2002). 'The impact of a single-layer or double-layer closure on uterine rupture'. American Journal of Obstetrics & Gynecology, 186 (6): 1326–1330.

Curtin S C, Kozak L J and Gregory K D (2000). 'US cesarean and VBAC rates stalled in the mid-1990s'. Birth, 27 (1): 54–57.

Dodd J, Crowther C A and Huertas E (2004). 'Planned elective repeat caesarean section versus planned vaginal birth for women with a previous caesarean birth (Protocol for a Cochrane Review)'. In: The Cochrane Library, Issue 3, Oxford: Update Software.

Flamm B L (2001). 'In the literature: vaginal birth after cesarean and the New England Journal of Medicine – a strange controversy'. Birth, 28 (4): 276–279.

Ganong W F (1997). Review of Medical Physiology, 18th edition, Stamford, Conn: Appleton & Lange.

Goer H (2003). 'A consumer viewpoint: "spin doctoring," the research'. Birth, 30 (2): 124–129.

Greene M F (2001). 'Vaginal delivery after cesarean section – is the risk acceptable?'. New England Journal of Medicine, 345 (1): 54–55.

Harer W B Jr (2002). 'Vaginal birth after cesarean delivery: current status'. Journal of American Medical Association, 287 (20): 2627–2630.

Lewis G (1998). Why Mothers Die 1994–1996, London: The Stationery Office.

Lowdon G and Derrick D C (2002). 'VBAC – on whose terms?' AIMS Quarterly Journal, 14 (1): 5–7.

Lydon-Rochelle M, Holt V L, Easterling T R and Martin D P (2001). 'Risk of uterine rupture during labor among women with a prior cesarean delivery'. New England Journal of Medicine, 345 (1): 3–8.

McMahon M J, Luther E R, Bowes W A and Olshan A F (1996). 'Comparison of a trial of labor with an elective second cesarean section'. New England Journal of Medicine, 335: 689–695.

Mozurkewich E L and Hutton E K (2000). 'Elective repeat cesarean delivery versus trial of labor: a meta-analysis of the literature from 1989 to 1999'. American Journal of Obstetrics & Gynecology, 183 (5): 1187–1197.

Mutryn C S (1993). 'Psychosocial impact of cesarean section on the family: a literature review'. Social Science & Medicine, 37 (10): 1271–1281.

RCSE (2003). 'Factors affecting wound healing'. http://www.edu.rcsed.ac.uk/Wound%20Management/Factors%20Affecting%20Wound%20Healing.htm

Robinson J (2001). 'Research round-up: vaginal birth after caesarean'. AIMS Quarterly Journal, 13 (4): 16–17.

Ryding E L, Wijma K and Wijma B (1998). 'Experiences of emergency cesarean section: a phenomenological study of 53 women'. Birth, 25 (4): 246–251.

Shaw R (2001). 'Other direct deaths'. In: G Lewis (ed), Why Mothers Die 1997–1999, London: RCOG Press.

Small R, Lumley J, Donohue L et al (2000). 'Randomised controlled trial of midwife-led debriefing to reduce maternal depression after operative childbirth'. British Medical Journal, 321 (7268): 1043–1047.

Smith G, Pell J P, Cameron A D and Dobbie R (2002). 'Risk of perinatal death associated with labor after previous cesarean delivery in uncomplicated term pregnancies'. Journal of American Medical Association, 287: 2684–2690.

Warwick C (2001). 'A midwifery perception of the rising caesarean rate'. MIDIRS Midwifery Digest, 11 (2): 152–156.

Wijma K, Ryding E L and Wijma B (2002). 'Predicting psychological well-being after emergency caesarean section: a preliminary study'. Journal of Reproductive & Infant Psychology, 20 (1): 25–36.

The Practising Midwife 2004: 7(10): 12–15

Need to know: vaginal birth after caesarean (Part 2)

Rosemary Mander

In this, the second of two articles, I examine the research evidence and the factors that have been shown to influence the likelihood of vaginal birth after caesarean (VBAC) being successful. This examination allows certain conclusions to be drawn about the woman's experience and her ability to learn from it.

(a) Background factors

There are a number of phenomena that have been shown by research to be linked with the different forms of birth following a caesarean. Some of these relate to events around the time of the previous caesarean, some relate more generally to the woman's childbearing experience, and some relate to her own personal characteristics.

(i) Factors associated with previous caesarean(s)

Scar on uterus

As may seem obvious, the scar from the previous caesarean has been linked with the subsequent birth outcome. This applies particularly to the 'classical' vertical incision into the upper part or segment of the uterus (fundus). This operation is used rarely now, because greater activity in the upper segment is thought to interfere with optimal healing. This is supposed to be associated with an increased risk of rupture of the uterus in a subsequent pregnancy. Rosen et al (1991) found a 12 per cent risk of rupture of classical scars, which may be compared with the standard figure of 0.5–1 per cent mentioned already (see Part 1, p. 180). Thus, a previous classical caesarean is likely to be a contraindication to VBAC.

Method of suturing the wound in the uterus

The technique used to suture the wound in the uterus has attracted some research attention. This is because the 'traditional' technique has been to repair the wound in layers. This has involved, first, a single continuous interlocking suture, rather like a blanket stitch. The second, similar, layer of suturing effectively 'buries' the first layer. An innovative technique, involving only the first layer in a single layer, was introduced in North America because of short-term benefits and cost savings due to reduced time in the operating theatre (O'Brien-Abel 2003). Bujold et al (2002) sought to evaluate the effects of this innovative technique, using rupture of the uterus as the criterion for evaluation. In order to assess the birth outcomes following repair using these two techniques, these researchers undertook a retrospective survey of women's medical notes for the previous 12 years.

Bujold and colleagues found that rupture of the uterus happened in eight (0.54 per cent) of the 1,491 women in whom the traditional double layer technique had been used. This incidence corresponds closely with the standard figure mentioned already (see Part 1, p. 180). For the women in whom the innovative single layer technique had been used, however, the risk of rupture of the uterus was significantly higher at 3.1 per cent (15 out of 489 women). Thus, these researchers consider that, in the long term, single layer closure is significantly riskier than the traditional technique. Bujold and colleagues admit that they are not certain why this should be. It may be that the increased strength of the scar resulting from a repair in two layers is due to the better approximation of the tissues, the more adequate blood supply or the greater thickness of the scar.

Suture material

Dodd et al (2004: 5) suggest that the nature of the suture material that is used to repair the caesarean wound may affect its healing. While this suggestion is eminently reasonable, I have not been able to locate any research supporting these researchers' suggestion.

Mother's health after caesarean

The healing process mentioned in Part 1 (pp. 178–179) is crucial in re-establishing the integrity of the woman's uterus. It has been suggested that the healing process might be impaired if the mother experiences some form of ill health (Dodd et al 2004). An example of such an illness, fever in the mother, has been found to be associated with an increased incidence of rupture of the uterus in the next pregnancy (Shipp et al 2003). These American researchers undertook a retrospective study of the case notes of women who, in the previous 12 years, had experienced a painful rupture of the uterus. There were 21 such 'cases'. Each case was matched with four women controls with a similar history in every respect other than not having had a rupture of the uterus. Eight out of the 21 case women (38.1 per cent) were found to have experienced a moderate rise in temperature (to above 38°C). Among the control group, however, only 13 out of the 84 (15.5 per cent) had had such a high temperature.

While this association appears very logical, in that the woman's general condition is likely to affect healing in specific parts of her body, there may be problems with this study. First, the data used were retrospective. Second, the authors do not indicate how temperatures were measured. Glass thermometers are notoriously slow, and underestimation of the temperature was likely before electronic thermometers were introduced (Brown 1990). Third, regional analgesia such as epidural is associated with a rise in the maternal temperature, so the significance of maternal pyrexia may be reduced.

(ii) Previous childbearing

The woman's previous experience of childbearing has been shown to affect the likelihood of a rupture of the uterus.

Having given birth vaginally

An example of this previous experience is that if a woman has given birth vaginally in a pregnancy prior to the caesarean, the risk of rupture of the uterus is considerably lower. Blanchette et al (2001) found that 91.3 per cent of women with a previous vaginal birth and a caesarean succeeded in giving birth vaginally. In the study by Rosen et al (1991), the figure had been found to be only slightly lower at 84 per cent.

Reason for caesarean

Similarly, the reason for the previous caesarean appears to affect the likelihood of successful VBAC. Rosen et al (1991) found that women whose previous caesarean was for breech presentation were far more likely to be successful in their VBAC (85 per cent success) than their sisters whose caesareans were for either 'failure to progress' or 'cephalopelvic disproportion' (67 per cent success). It may be that changes happen in the circulation of the uterus during such 'non-progressive' labours, which later impede the healing of a caesarean wound (Bujold et al 2002).

Birth spacing

The spacing between the births is another factor that may affect wound healing and, hence, the risk of rupture of the uterus. Bujold et al (2002) found that women in whom 24 or more months had elapsed since the caesarean had the smallest chance of rupture of the uterus. This supports other researchers' earlier findings. It may be suggested that this is because the scar on the uterus does not heal maximally and reach its optimal strength until it is two years old.

Number of previous caesareans

The large study by Miller et al (1994) established the link between the number of previous caesareans and the likelihood of rupture of the uterus. As had been suggested before that date by a number of smaller studies, the risk of rupture increases markedly with the increasing number of previous caesareans. Miller et al found an incidence of rupture of the uterus of 1.7 per cent in women who had undergone two or more caesareans. This may be compared with an incidence of 0.6 per cent in women with only one previous caesarean. Again, it is necessary to question whether repeated surgery diminishes the healing ability of this relatively small area of the body, perhaps by reducing the crucially important circulation of blood to the area.

(iii) Mother's age

There is a general assumption that healing is less straightforward among people who are older. It may, therefore, be assumed to be the case in the context of women with a previous caesarean. If correct, this would result in a higher incidence of rupture of the uterus among older women. These assumptions have been difficult to verify by research. In a paper published in 2003, though, Shipp et al report findings supporting these assumptions. These researchers found that the incidence of rupture of the uterus among women under 30 was near to the standard rate at 0.5 per cent. The rate for an otherwise comparable sample of women of 30 or older, however, was significantly higher at 1.4 per cent.

Thus, it appears that there are a number of factors in the woman's childbearing and more general background that are likely to affect the likelihood of rupture of the uterus and, hence, the success of VBAC. Many of these factors appear to be attributable to the healing of the wound in the uterus.

(b) Current labour

Clearly, many factors relating to the labour affect the likelihood of the woman's success in achieving a VBAC. Some of these relate to the onset of the labour, in terms of the mode of onset or its timing. Other factors, however, relate to phenomena that may occur, perhaps expectedly or unpredictably, during labour.

Timing of birth

In Blanchette et al's study (2001) of the safety of vaginal birth after caesarean, the gestation at which the labour occurred was found to be associated with its success in achieving a VBAC. These researchers found that the mean gestation for successful VBAC was 39.5 weeks. On the other hand, the women whose labour ended in an emergency caesarean had a gestation of 39.6 weeks. Obviously, such a small difference carries no significance. It is, however, associated with a difference in the baby's size, which may have affected the progress of labour. In this US study, the mean weight for babies born vaginally was 7.7lb (3.374kg), whereas the mean weight for those born by emergency caesarean was significantly larger at 8lb (3.629kg).

Induction/augmentation

The association between interventions to end the pregnancy or speed up the labour and rupture of the uterus have long been recognised. The Fifth Annual CESDI Report (1998) published data from 1996 that scrutinised the circumstances of perinatal deaths. These included the deaths of 42 babies in association with rupture of the uterus. Approximately half of these babies were born to women who had had a previous caesarean and who were having labour induced.

A publication that highlighted this issue in the US, and which may have attracted more attention than it really deserves, concerns the work of Lydon-Rochelle et al (2001). Their study comprised a longitudinal retrospective analysis of the subsequent birth experience of more than 20,000 women in Washington State who gave birth between 1987 and 1996 by caesarean. The focus was on the risk of rupture of the uterus in relation to the mode of onset of labour (spontaneous or induced) or elective repeat caesarean.

As mentioned previously, Flamm (2001) has criticised this study, but a point that he does not mention is the problem of terminology. By this, I mean that these researchers discuss the implications of induction of labour (a cluster of interventions to start the labour before it begins naturally), but they do not mention the effects of augmentation of labour (interventions to speed up a labour deemed ineffective). This distinction matters, because the term 'induction' is frequently, albeit casually, used to describe either type of intervention. This is probably unsurprising in view of the similarity of the techniques (Cartwright 1979). It might be argued, though, that

because augmentation is ongoing throughout the labour, it is of greater relevance in this context than induction.

Lydon-Rochelle et al identified a hierarchy of risk of rupture of the uterus. In their study, women having an elective repeat caesarean faced a risk of 0.16 per cent (11 women). Those whose labour began spontaneously encountered near the standard rate of rupture at 0.52 per cent (56 women). Induction without prostaglandin drugs increased the risk to 0.77 per cent (15 women). The use of prostaglandin drugs, however, escalated the risk to 24.5 per cent (nine women).

These data have aroused considerable anxiety, which may not be totally justified if the context of changing practice is taken into consideration. The Cochrane reviews of the relevant prostaglandin (misoprostol) are generally reassuring (Alfirevic 2003, Hofmeyr and Gülmezoglu 2003). They do warn, however, that oral regimens are under-researched and may be associated with excessively high stimulation of contractions. These contractions may lead to rupture of the uterus in women both with and without a previous caesarean. Interestingly, despite the usual assumptions mentioned above, among the women with a previous classical incision (272 women) Lydon-Rochelle et al report that there were no ruptures of the uterus.

A factor that Blanchette et al (2001) highlight in their study on the safety of VBAC is the effect of regional anaesthesia for pain control in labour. These researchers found that all the women in their sample who experienced a rupture of the uterus had had an epidural analgesia administered. This may or may not matter, as it is likely that a majority of women in Massachusetts, where the study was completed, use epidural as a form of pain control in labour.

(c) Current postnatal recovery

Having examined the research on the factors that influence the way in which the woman gives birth, I move on now to consider some of the implications of the mode of the birth.

After the birth of her baby, irrespective of the mode of the birth, the woman has a considerable amount of work and adjustment. These activities will include her recovery from the birth. While many research studies have addressed the woman's physical recovery after a caesarean, material is lacking on her emotional and psychological recovery.

Unfortunately, though, many of the studies on physical state have involved numbers that are too small to be conclusive. In order to make better use of all of these small studies, the technique known as meta-analysis may be employed. This seeks to combine the results of a number of studies addressing a single question. If the results from all of the relevant studies are combined, then the findings may become more meaningful. It is necessary, though, to be very cautious in interpretation as they are not likely to have collected data in identical ways. In spite of this, as the meta-analysis will include more data, the overall conclusions may be more powerful than those from individual studies. The work on the woman's postnatal recovery after a birth subsequent to a caesarean draws heavily on meta-analysis.

A rise in the mother's temperature may be considered to be a trivial matter after the birth of the baby. This may be the case, even if the mother is feeling slightly 'off-colour'. The consequences, however, may be more serious. These include a regime of investigations, specimen-taking and, possibly, antibiotic drug treatment 'just in case' she has an infection. Such a regimen would be likely to require the woman to remain in the maternity unit longer than she would have expected, with the attendant unhappiness, inconvenience and potential risks for the woman and her baby (Hook et al 1997).

In their meta-analysis, Rosen et al (1991) found that women who gave birth following a trial of labour were significantly less likely to develop a high temperature. Mozurkewich and Hutton (2000) identified a similar picture, but their findings did not reach the level of significance.

A blood transfusion may be recommended postnatally if the woman loses a considerable amount of blood by haemorrhage around the time of the birth. This problem would be aggravated if she had been anaemic previously. This is not without risks. In their meta-analysis, Mozurkewich and Hutton (2000) found that the woman who has had a trial of labour is markedly less likely to receive a blood transfusion than a woman who has had an elective repeat caesarean. This finding implies that the blood loss or haemorrhage associated with birth following a trial of labour is of a smaller quantity.

(d) The baby's condition

Most of the VBAC debate has focused on the risk of rupture of the uterus. This may be a dreadful event, which may carry an immediate threat to the life of the woman and the baby. However, little research attention has been given to the less dramatic problems that may affect only the baby directly. For this reason, it is necessary to consider the implications of the mode of birth after a previous caesarean for the baby or babies.

The condition of the baby at birth is ordinarily assessed by using the Apgar scoring system, thought to reflect the baby's oxygenation. The research data agree on the relative benefits of VBAC and elective repeat caesarean in this respect. Two meta-analyses (Mozurkewich and Hutton 2000, Rosen et al 1991) have found that babies born fol-

lowing a trial of labour are more likely to have a low Apgar score at five minutes. Hook et al (1997), however, found that, although the babies born following a trial of labour needed more active resuscitation in the birthing room, their Apgar scores at five minutes did not differ. The meaning of the Apgar scores is uncertain, as assessment is highly subjective and the predictive value is questionable. This problem may have been made worse by the categorisation used by Smith et al (2002). This means that serious problems in the mother that threaten the baby's health, such as abruptio placenta, are able to be classified as trial of labour. In this way, the findings may give the impression that the situation is worse than it actually is.

In Cleveland, Ohio, Hook et al (1997) undertook a prospective study of the health of newborn babies who were born after a previous caesarean. This study had the advantage that data were collected for the purpose of this research and so there was no possibility of a historical bias. Additionally, these researchers collected data from a control group, so they were able to make comparisons with the health of babies whose mothers had never had a caesarean. Although randomisation was not attempted, this three-group study appears to be as rigorous as a non-randomised study can be. The sample comprised 497 women who chose an elective repeat caesarean, 492 who chose a trial of labour and 989 women who had never had a caesarean. Obviously, data were collected for the babies of each woman recruited. None of the women in the trial of labour group experienced any symptoms of rupture of the uterus.

The data on the health of the newborn babies present a mixed picture. The babies born by elective repeat caesarean were significantly more likely to encounter breathing difficulties than those born following a trial of labour (6 per cent and 3 per cent respectively). Additionally, two babies in the elective repeat caesarean group developed the severe respiratory problems known as 'respiratory distress syndrome'. This condition means that the baby is likely to require ventilation, following admission to a neonatal intensive care unit.

The health of the 336 babies whose mothers achieved a VBAC was optimal and comparable with the 'no caesarean' group. Babies whose mothers underwent an emergency caesarean following trial of labour fared least well. Suspected and diagnosed infections were significantly more common in babies born following a trial of labour. These babies required a longer stay in the maternity unit, but this figure may have been inflated by the proportion whose mothers were recovering from an emergency caesarean.

The incidence of respiratory problems was greater in the babies born by an emergency caesarean (8 per cent), compared with those (4 per cent) whose mothers achieved a VBAC. The incidence of hypoglycaemia was significantly higher in the emergency caesarean group of babies, carrying with it a regimen of frequent blood tests and interruption to breastfeeding.

In interpreting the data on diagnoses and investigations, it is necessary to bear in mind that researchers were unable to 'blind' neonatal paediatric staff to the group to which each baby belonged. This means that concerns about trial of labour may have been reflected in observations and investigations to which these babies were submitted.

This study by Hook et al suggests that the babies who were born vaginally following a trial of labour had the best neonatal outcomes. The other two groups – babies born by elective repeat caesarean or emergency caesarean – encountered problems that may be comparable in their severity. Thus, a successful trial of labour is clearly to the benefit of the baby, and an unsuccessful one may be no worse than an elective repeat caesarean.

As well as the baby's neonatal condition, however, we should contemplate the long-term health of the baby born following a previous caesarean.

(e) Factors/issues for consideration

There are certain issues that a woman who has previously undergone a caesarean, and contemplating the birth of her baby, should consider. These are issues that she would be well advised to discuss with those near to her and with her midwife.

The woman's experience of her previous caesarean is likely to influence her choice of how to give birth if and when she has another pregnancy. For a large majority of such women, the previous caesarean is likely to have been an emergency in labour. Scottish figures show that in 72 per cent of first-time mothers undergoing a caesarean, the reason will be either 'fetal distress' or 'failure to progress' in labour (McIlwaine et al 1998). On the basis of her work with women after the birth, Kitzinger (1998) argues that it is the experience of an unsatisfactory labour followed by an emergency caesarean that deters women from embarking on a trial of labour in any subsequent birth.

Kitzinger vividly describes the picture of the woman's first labour. A typically medicalised labour removes from the woman any vestige of control over what is happening to her, her body and her baby. The 'cascade of intervention' is frequently encountered in the form of epidural/spinal analgesia, followed by a Syntocinon infusion to speed up the slowed contractions, to which the baby responds by becoming hypoxic, which is recognised as fetal distress. This scenario requires that the baby should be removed from her potentially hostile environment immediately. This results in a rapid decision to perform an emergency caesarean and the frantic preparations for the operating theatre. Inevitably, the major concern is for the condition of the baby, and the woman is likely to miss out on the supportive care that she deserves and needs at this emotionally and physically challenging time. As Kitzinger reminds us:

> It is understandable that women who have been through an experience like that prefer with their next baby to have an elective caesarean . . . (Kitzinger 1998: 58)

Thus, the woman may subsequently be keen to avoid a repetition of her experience of her first birth. Additionally, she may seek to take control of her birth experience, when it had been previously removed. This wish to assume control may manifest itself in the choice of an elective repeat caesarean. Alternatively, the woman may choose to find more information in order to plan realistically for a more satisfying birth experience in a subsequent labour.

Discussion and conclusion

A woman's decision about whether to seek VBAC is shaped by the assumption that the pattern of her labour is likely to repeat itself. Thus, a woman having a caesarean for 'failure to progress' in her first labour will anticipate that the second will be a re-run of the first. This may be because she assumes that the factors that determine the outcome of labour are physical, unaltered and unalterable. Unfortunately, the medical profession has not sought to disabuse women of this assumption.

In the VBAC debate, almost no attention is paid to the effects of the woman's learning and experience – this means the wealth of knowledge about herself and her body that she acquires from her experience of labour and birth, and from her experience of caring for a baby. It may be that this increased self-knowledge is able to change the woman and her subsequent childbearing experience – probably to make the labour more effective and the birth outcome more satisfactory.

Acknowledgement

I would like to acknowledge the help of the AIMS Committee in the development of these articles.

REFERENCES

Alfirevic Z (2003). 'Oral misoprostol for induction of labour (Cochrane Review')'. In: The Cochrane Library, Issue 4, Chichester, UK: John Wiley & Sons, Ltd.

Blanchette H, Blanchette M, McCabe J et al (2001). 'Is vaginal birth after cesarean safe? Experience at a community hospital'. American Journal of Obstetrics and Gynecology, 184 (7): 1478–1487.

Brown S (1990). 'Temperature taking – getting it right'. Nursing Standard, 5 (12): Tissue Viability Suppl, 4–5.

Bujold E, Bujold C, Hamilton E F et al (2002). 'The impact of a single-layer or double-layer closure on uterine rupture'. American Journal of Obstetrics & Gynecology, 186 (6): 1326–1330.

Cartwright A (1979). The Dignity of Labour?: a Study of Childbearing and Induction, London: Tavistock Publications.

CESDI (1998). Fifth Annual Report: Confidential Enquiry into Stillbirth and Death in Infancy, London: Maternal & Child Health Research Consortium.

Dodd J, Crowther C A and Huertas E (2004). 'Planned elective repeat caesarean section versus planned vaginal birth for women with a previous caesarean birth (Protocol for a Cochrane Review)'. In: The Cochrane Library, Issue 3, Oxford: Update Software.

Flamm B L (2001). 'In the literature. Vaginal birth after cesarean and the New England Journal of Medicine: a strange controversy'. Birth, 28 (4): 276–279.

Hofmeyr G J and Gülmezoglu A M (2003). 'Vaginal misoprostol for cervical ripening and induction of labour'. In: The Cochrane Library, Issue 4, Chichester, UK: John Wiley & Sons.

Hook B, Kiwi R, Amini S B et al (1997). 'Neonatal morbidity after elective repeat cesarean section and trial of labor'. Pediatrics, 100 (3 Pt 1): 348–353.

Kitzinger S (1998). 'The cesarean epidemic in Great Britain'. Birth, 25 (1): 56.

Lydon-Rochelle M, Holt V L, Easterling T R and Martin D P (2001). 'Risk of uterine rupture during labor among women with a prior cesarean delivery'. New England Journal of Medicine, 345 (1): 3–8.

McIlwaine G, Boulton-Jones C, Cole S et al (1998). Caesarean Section in Scotland 1994/5: a National Audit, Edinburgh: SPECRH.

Miller D A, Diaz F G and Paul R H (1994). 'Vaginal birth after cesarean: a 10-year experience'. Obstetrics & Gynecology, 84 (2): 255–258.

Mozurkewich E L and Hutton E K (2000). 'Elective repeat cesarean delivery versus trial of labor: a meta-analysis of the literature from 1989 to 1999'. American Journal of Obstetrics & Gynecology, 183 (5): 1187–1197.

O'Brien-Abel N (2003). 'Uterine rupture during VBAC trial of labour: risk factors and fetal response'. Journal of Midwifery and Women's Health Online, July/Aug 48 (4). 249.

Rosen M G, Dickinson J C and Westhoff C L (1991). 'Vaginal birth after cesarean: a meta-analysis of morbidity and mortality'. Obstetrics & Gynecology, 77 (3): 465–470.

Shipp T D, Zelop C, Cohen A et al (2003). 'Post-cesarean delivery fever and uterine rupture in a subsequent trial of labor'. Obstetrics & Gynecology, 101 (1): 1136–1139.

Smith G, Pell J P, Cameron A D et al (2002). 'Risk of perinatal death associated with labor after previous cesarean delivery in uncomplicated term pregnancies'. Journal of American Medical Association, 287 (20): 2684–2690.

The Practising Midwife 2004; 7(11): 31–35

Does pethidine relieve pain?

Claire Wood, Hora Soltani

Pethidine, also known as meperidine, is familiar to midwives as an analgesic option for women in labour. Before the purpose of this review is presented, a brief introduction of possible maternal, fetal and neonatal effects of the drug are discussed, as are related professional and consumer views.

Following presentation of the findings from randomised controlled trials, relevant systematic reviews are examined and the effect of various dosages of pethidine compared. This leads to conclusions and consideration of midwifery practice in light of the evidence.

Maternal effects

Pethidine is an opioid, a preparation that acts on the body's opioid receptors, which normally respond to endorphins and enkephalins. Many sites of the central nervous system are affected by opioids including the spinal cord, medulla, midbrain and cerebral cortex. Nerve and smooth muscle activity is inhibited, leading to the following possible side effects in the mother: sedation, reduction of anxiety, euphoria, respiratory depression, nausea and vomiting, bradycardia and hypotension, prolonged labour, urinary retention and dysuria, gastric stasis and constipation, and hallucinations (Jordan 2002).

Given intramuscularly, pethidine has an onset time of 10 minutes and a peak response of 30 to 50 minutes, with duration of effect from two to four hours (personal communication with hospital pharmacist using Thompson Micromedex Health Care Series database 1974–2003).

Fetal and neonatal effects

Pethidine rapidly crosses the placenta and is metabolised to the active norpethidine (also known as normeperidine). Kuhnert et al (1985a) suggest that the previously accepted three- to seven-hour half life for pethidine in the mother may be an underestimate and also that norpethi-dine has a mean half life of more than 20 hours. They further suggest a half life of pethidine in the neonate of 11 to 17 hours and a half life of norpethidine of 29 to 85 hours.

Neonatal effects of maternal pethidine use have been shown to include reduced Apgar scores and increased respiratory depression (Brice et al 1979), reduced early neonatal neurobehavioural scores (Hodgkinson et al 1978), reduced early sucking behaviour (Righard and Alade 1990, Riordan et al 2000), increased heart rate (Brice et al 1979, Rooth et al 1983) and reduced crying times (Rooth et al 1983).

Adverse effects are less likely to be exhibited if the baby is born within one hour of pethidine administration (Morrison et al 1973, Rooth et al 1983). It is suggested that because fetal tissue uptake of pethidine reaches a peak approximately two to three hours post maternal injection, the infant born within one hour of a single injection would be less exposed to the rising pethidine level (Kuhnert et al 1979).

In relation to long-term effects, Nyberg et al (2000) also found that in-utero exposure to high-dose medication has been associated with a four- to fivefold increase in the odds of adult drug abuse and/or dependence. One of the drugs included in this study was pethidine.

Rates of pethidine use

Pethidine is well established as an analgesic option, with Chamberlain et al (1993) reporting 37 per cent usage in labour. Fairlie et al (1999) reported a personal communication claiming that 84 per cent of 63 units in England and Wales were offering pethidine as the standard opioid in 1997.

In order to gain a perspective of local practice related to the national picture, an audit of pethidine administration in the authors' local maternity unit was undertaken (Wood 2003). Pethidine uptake was found to be 43 per

Table 5.8.1 Percentage of women receiving various dosages of pethidine (first administration)

Dosage of pethidine	% of women receiving specified dosage at first administration
150mg	73%
100mg	25%
50mg	2%

Based on data from 1,048 births during three separate months in 2002/2003, Derby Hospitals NHS Foundation Trust, Derby City General Hospital (Wood 2003, unpublished data)

cent of all births in this unit. Although the protocol allowed for flexibility, it can be seen in Table 5.8.1 that the higher dosages were more commonly used.

Professional and consumer views

Despite the extensive use of pethidine, its administration has been challenged by midwives, medical staff and women themselves.

Midwives' unease with pethidine in regard to related maternal, fetal and neonatal complications is well documented (Downe 1997, Heelbeck 1999, Hunt 2002, Mander 1997, Priest and Rosser 1991). Heelbeck (1999) proposes the use of a pain assessment tool, in conjunction with an alteration of the dose, route and frequency of the drug, in order to increase analgesia and reduce side effects. It has also been suggested that if pethidine were newly available today, the United Kingdom Central Council (now the Nursing and Midwifery Council) would be unlikely to approve its use (Priest and Rosser 1991).

Practice related to pethidine administration may, however, vary between individual midwives and/or between low and high intervention birth environments. Indeed, Leap (2000) refers to midwives who described 'two distinct approaches to pain in labour'. One belief system apparently demanded action to relieve pain, while the other had developed a rationale for not offering pain relief and for 'working with pain'. This acknowledges that midwives cannot necessarily be considered as a group acting with uniform views and approaches to labour and analgesia.

Medical staff have long debated the merits or otherwise of opioids, particularly versus epidural anaesthesia (Aly and Shilling 2000). Oloffson et al (1996), in relation to intravenous pethidine, concluded: 'It seems unethical and medically incorrect to meet parturients' requests for pain relief by giving them sedation'. The ensuing debate (Kingdom and Woods 1997, Liston 1997, Littler et al 1997, Reynolds and Crowhurst 1997, Twycross 1997) focused readers' minds on the unsatisfactory aspects of both opioid administration and epidural anaesthesia when attempting to reduce a woman's labour pain.

Pethidine's low cost was noted (Reynolds and Crowhurst 1997) and a link made between the ability of midwives to administer it 'unsupervised' and its extensive use (Low and Tordoff 2000, Reynolds and Crowhurst 1997). Low and Tordoff (2000) concluded, 'We do not think that it is the doctors who need convincing about the need for change. In the age of evidence-based medicine this is a prime example of information without education'.

The Association for Improvement in the Maternity Services (AIMS) represents women's views on issues related to maternity services offered. Lawrence Beech (1998), as a consumer, questions the effectiveness and side effects of pethidine in an AIMS journal article titled 'Pethidine – a little shot of something not so nice'.

Although pethidine is widely used, there is evidently concern among consumer groups and professionals, especially midwives, regarding its effectiveness as an analgesic in labour. Systematic reviews of pain relief in labour are available (Bricker and Lavender 2002, Elbourne and Wiseman 2003) which provide extensive information regarding pethidine, but they may not enhance the practical knowledge of midwives. This may be due to their wide scope, which includes many other opiates given by various routes.

Therefore, it was felt that there was a need for a critical evaluation of the evidence with a particular focus on the effect of intramuscular pethidine.

Purpose of the review

The aim of this review was specifically to focus on the pain-relieving effect of intramuscular pethidine in the first stage of labour, with particular attention related to dosage. As midwives are themselves responsible for administration of the drug via the intramuscular route only, this mode of administration was the route examined.

Search strategy

The following databases from 1966 to November 2003 were searched: MEDLINE, EMBASE, CINAHL, MIDIRS, DARE and Cochrane Library.

The keywords included: pethidine or meperidine and labour or labor (MIDIRS provided a standard literature search on pethidine, with updates added as they became available).

Selection criteria

The analysis and data synthesis were undertaken by the first author and double-checked by the senior research midwife.

Types of studies

Randomised controlled trials (RCTs) and systematic reviews in English language were sought with regard to the effect of intramuscular pethidine on reduction of first-stage labour pain. In addition, reference lists from those papers were searched. The intention was not to document the outcomes of the analgesics used in comparison with pethidine but specifically to explore the outcomes of the pethidine component of the trial.

Studies were considered if they compared pethidine to placebo, one dosage of pethidine to another, pethidine to other analgesics (not only via intramuscular route) and to epidural. Trials were included if data was provided for pain assessments in labour made by the labouring women themselves (as far as could be ascertained from the text) at 60 minutes after the first pethidine injection.

Types of participants

Any woman in first stage of labour receiving pethidine intramuscularly for pain relief was included.

Findings

Two systematic reviews and 16 RCTs were identified that compared pethidine with alternative methods of pain relief. The results are discussed critically below.

Randomised controlled trials

No RCT was found that focused on intramuscular pethidine versus placebo per se. The trials included a wide range of objectives, and the effectiveness of pethidine was often not the central question. Therefore, for the purposes of this review, the information relating to analgesic effectiveness of pethidine was extracted and presented using the following three assessment categories:

1. Visual Analogue Scale pain scores – changes in score from pre-injection to 60 minutes post-injection.
2. Pain relief – reported at 60 minutes following injection.
3. Level of pain – changes reported from pre-injection to 60 minutes post-injection.

No RCTs were found that compared intramuscular pethidine to epidural (using the above pain assessment categories). One trial (Jensen et al 1984) compared pethidine to submucous paracervical blockade, but the remaining trials all compared intramuscular pethidine to other intramuscular or intravenous preparations.

Confounding factors affecting RCT results

The included RCTs had limitations with regard to application to practice, because extensive confounding factors did not easily allow direct comparison of results. These included variations in: dosage and frequency of pethidine administration; pain assessments tools and terminology within tools; co-drug administration; distribution of nulliparous and multiparous women within groups; management of labour (including fetal monitoring practices); data regarding induction/augmentation; settings; and participants' ethnic origins. There was also a lack of information on the philosophy of care towards the participants, and therefore on other aspects of care such as mobilisation, position and non-pharmaceutical interventions (eg, massage).

These confounding factors must necessarily affect the reported results, potentially to a considerable degree. Results have been presented as transparently as possible. The full details of each trial have not, however, been included in each table of results as this would have been confusing. This must be borne in mind when viewing the findings. A full table of results and related confounding factors may be obtained from the authors.

1. Visual analogue scale pain scores (VAS)

This technique entails the subject indicating on a 10cm-long unmarked line how much pain she is experiencing. 0cm represents no pain, and 10cm represents excruciating pain (Hicks 1996). If, for example, a woman indicates a point at 7.6cm, this is translated to a score of 76 (out of 100). This score was taken at time of injection and at 60 minutes post-injection.

Eleven groups were studied within six trials that used this method of pain assessment (Thurlow et al 2002, Fairlie et al 1999, Isenor and Penny-MacGillivray 1993, Morrison et al 1987, Vella et al 1985, McAuley et al 1982). The results are presented in Table 5.8.2.

Two groups reported an increase in VAS pain scores, five groups reported a decrease of less than 10, and four groups reported a decrease of more than 10. The greatest decrease in VAS pain score from an individual group pre- and post-pethidine injection was 18 points (McAuley et al 1982, Vella et al 1985), and the greatest increase was 8 points (Fairlie et al 1999).

2. Pain relief scores

Participants were asked at 60 minutes post-injection to indicate, on a verbal rating scale, the extent of their pain relief. In the studies examined, at the extreme ends of the pain relief ratings – eg, 'no relief' or 'complete relief' – the results were clear. In the middle range of ratings, however, the terminology representing the degree of pain relief could be open to varied interpretation. It might, for example, be difficult relatively to rate 'moderate relief' with 'acceptable', 'sufficient' and 'partial'. In order to reduce misinterpretation, the authors used the assessments reporting 'no relief' and 'slight relief'.

Table 5.8.2 Mean VAS pain scores pre-pethidine and 60 minutes post-pethidine administration

Study	No. of participants	Dosage	Parity of group	Anti-emetic co-drug	Pre-inj. VAS score (mean)	Post-inj VAS score (mean)*
Thurlow et al 2002**	18	100mg	72% primiparous	Promethazine 25mg or Prochlorperazine 12.5mg	68	72
Fairlie et al 1999	a) 35	a) 150mg	a) 100% primiparous	Prochlorperazine 12.5mg	a) 67	a) 62
	b) 33	b) 100mg	b) 100% multiparous		b) 63	b) 71
Isenor and Penny-MacGillivray 1993	20	50–100mg	70% primiparous	None	73	70
Morrison et al 1987	a) 230	100–150mg***	a) 100% primiparous	No information	a) 76	a) 65
	b) 292		b) 100% multiparous		b) 74	b) 70
Vella et al 1985	a) 161	100–150mg	a) 56% primiparous	a) Placebo	a) 72	a) 56
	b) 157		b) 61% primiparous	b) Metaclopramide 10mg	b) 74	b) 56
	c) 159		c) 63% primiparous	c) Promethazine 25mg	c) 71	c) 65
McAuley et al 1982****	a) 20	100mg	100% primiparous	a) No premedication	a) 77	a) 74
	b) 20			b) Lorazepam 2mg	b) 70	b) 52

*Post-injection numbers of participants may be lower (due to exclusion through birth or alteration in choice of analgesia)

**All studies report the mean pain scores apart from Thurlow et al (2002) who report the median pain score

***If maternal weight <70kg, 100mg given; if maternal weight >70kg, 150mg given

****Only one trial reported a statistical comparison of pre- and 60 minutes post-injection scores (McAuley et al 1982). They reported a lower pain score in the lorazepam group ($p < 0.05$) but concluded that the drug could not be used routinely because of an increase in neonatal respiratory depression

Nine trials used this method of pain assessment (Fairlie et al 1999, Jensen et al 1984, Levy 1971, Maduska and Hajghassemali 1978, Moore et al 1970, Mowat and Garrey 1970, Refstad and Lindbaek 1980, Sheikh and Tunstall 1986, Viegas et al 1993).

Twenty to 76 per cent of women reported 'no' or 'slight' pain relief 60 minutes after pethidine administration (see Figure 5.8.1).

Two trials compared different dosages of pethidine within one study (Maduska and Hajghassemali 1978, Moore et al 1970). The former found no statistically significant difference between the dosages of 50mg and 100mg with regard to pain relief. The latter, however, found that mean pain relief scores equated to just below 'moderate' relief in the 40mg group but to midway between 'moderate' and 'good' in the 80mg group ($p < 0.05$). (The Maduska and Hajghassemali trial is not included in Figure 5.8.1 as the data is not categorised matching other included trials).

3. Level of pain

This assessment compared percentages of women who reported being in various pain categories both pre-injection and at 60 minutes post-injection.

Eight groups were studied within five trials that used this method of assessment (Fairlie et al 1999, Keskin et al 2002, Moore et al 1970, Sheikh and Tunstall 1986, Wilson et al 1986). All but one trial (Keskin et al 2002) used pain categories including 'slight', 'moderate', 'severe' or 'very severe'. Keskin used the Wong Baker Faces Pain Rating Scale, a model often used to evaluate children's pain. Out of six diagrams of faces, participants chose the one that best reflected their level of pain, and this was categorised in a scale 0 (no pain) to 5 (the most intense pain). For the purposes of this review, categories 4 and 5 were translated as severe or very severe pain.

Table 5.8.3 summarises the information regarding relief of severe or very severe pain. It can be seen from Table 5.8.3 that the percentage of women categorising themselves as either in severe or very severe pain 60 minutes after pethidine administration decreased from the initial assessment in four of the eight groups. It is not easy to interpret some of the results, where at 60 minutes some women have dropped out, but the overall outcome is unlikely to be affected considering that the drop-out number was small. The most favourable outcome can be seen in the Keskin study (Keskin et al 2002) which is markedly different to the other trial outcomes. To what extent this is due to the unusual choice of evaluation tool is not clear.

Only two studies provided statistical analysis regarding the outcomes. Sheikh and Tunstall (1986) reported a statistically significant difference between the number of nulliparous women (14 per cent) versus multiparous women (0 per cent) having 'no pain' or 'mild pain' 60 minutes after pethidine administration ($p < 0.003$). Moore et al (1970) do not report a statistically significant

Figure 5.8.1 Percentages of participants with no pain relief or slight pain relief 60 minutes after pethidine injection (dosages are included).

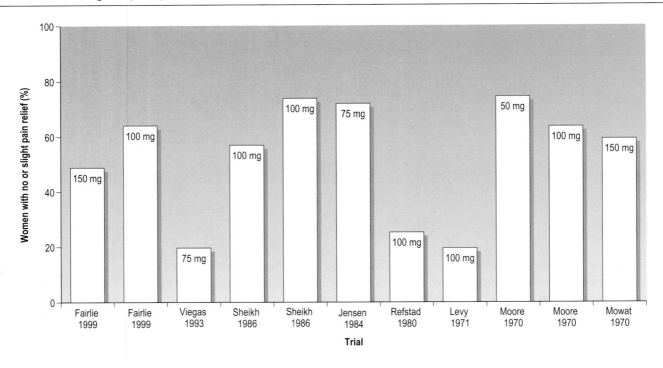

Table 5.8.3 Percentages of women grading themselves in 'severe' or 'very severe' pain pre-pethidine and 60 minutes post-pethidine administration

Author	Evaluation tool	Pethidine dose	% of women in 'severe' or 'very severe' pain pre-inj. (n*)	% of women in 'severe' or 'very severe' pain 60 mins post-inj. (n*)	Parity of women
Keskin et al 2003	Wong-Baker Faces Pain Rating Scale	100 mg	100% (n = 29)	52% (n = 25)	All primiparous
Fairlie et al 1999	Verbal pain rating 0 = No pain 1 = Mild pain 2 = Moderate pain 3 = Severe pain	150mg 100mg	100% (n = 35) 97% (n = 33)	74% (n = 35) 100% (n = 33)	All nulliparous All multiparous
Sheikh & Tunstall 1986	Verbal pain level scale: None, slight, moderate, severe	100mg 100mg	83% (n = 66) 70% (n = 33)	55% (n = 64) 75% (n = 24)	All nulliparous All multiparous
Wilson et al 1986	Verbal pain level scale: Slight, moderate, severe, very severe	100mg	68% (n = 35)	79% (no info. on numbers)	Mixed parity group (35% primiparous)
Moore et al 1970	Verbal pain level scale: Slight, moderate, severe	50mg 100mg	38% (n = 55) 40% (n = 57)	40% (n = 55) 23% (n = 57)	Mixed parity groups (76% primiparous) (49% primiparous)

n = total number of women in each group (the total number of women post-injection may be lower than pre-injection due to exclusion through birth or alteration in choice of analgesia) difference in outcomes between the 50mg and 100mg dosages.

Systematic reviews

The two identified systematic reviews (Bricker and Lavender 2002, Elbourne and Wiseman 2003) included information on intramuscular pethidine in first stage of labour (although their focus was not exclusively on pethidine but on opioids in general). In their conclusions, the reviews agreed, regarding pethidine, that:

- 'Although there are considerable doubts about its effectiveness for maternal pain relief and concerns about its potential maternal, fetal, and neonatal side effects, there is as yet no convincing research evidence to show that alternative opioids are better.'
- 'Intramuscular pethidine has the virtue of familiarity and low cost.'
- '[Pethidine] is the only opioid which can be given by midwives without prescription by a doctor.'

(NB: The Nursing and Midwifery Council has now issued advice that diamorphine and morphine also fall into this category under the Prescription Only Medicines (Human Use) Amendment Order 2004. See NMC Circular 10/2004.)

On the point of comparison of various dosages, however, the systematic reviews disagreed, as can be seen from the following quoted statements:

- 'Pain relief was similar between the doses' (Elbourne and Wiseman 2003)
  versus
- 'For . . . pethidine, the higher dose conferred greater benefit in terms of pain relief, measured as . . . pain score during labour or need for further analgesia' (Bricker and Lavender 2002).

Comparison of different dosages of pethidine

Only two trials compared different dosages within the same study (Maduska and Hajghassemali 1978, Moore et al 1970). As noted above, the systematic reviews of

Elbourne and Wiseman (2003) and Bricker and Lavender (2002) provided slightly conflicting conclusions regarding the relative effectiveness of the higher versus the lower pethidine dosages.

First, Bricker and Lavender (2002) referred to a higher pain score in labour in the lower dosage group. It appears that the Maduska and Hajghassemali (1978) trial data were used and that the pain assessments were provided by observers rather than by the labouring women themselves. The same study reports pain assessments made by the women in labour that show a statistically significantly better effect in the 80mg group than in the 40mg group ($p < 0.05$). It is unclear why Bricker and Lavender did not use this data (see Table 5.8.4).

Second, Bricker and Lavender (2002) referred to a statistically significant difference in further pethidine requirements, stating that the group receiving the lower dosage had greater need of more analgesia. Both systematic reviews combined the data from Maduska and Hajghassemali (1978) and Moore et al (1970) regarding further pethidine requirements, stating that those receiving the lower dosages were statistically significantly more likely to use further analgesia.

In the interests of clarifying the evidence regarding dosage effect, the original papers were examined. It appears that the text of Moore et al (1970) did not reflect the data presented in the tables (see text, first paragraph of 'Results' versus Table lV in Moore et al 1970). The text appears to suggest that none of the higher dosage group received further analgesia, while the table indicates that 25 participants actually opted for more analgesia. Combining the apparently incorrect text information from Moore et al (1970) with the Maduska and Hajghassemali (1978) data, it appeared that a significant difference existed, when apparently it did not. This issue was communicated to one of the Bricker and Lavender authors. This inconsistency may account for the apparent difference in further analgesia requirements. Both groups in both studies in fact used almost identical levels of further analgesia regardless of initial pethidine dosage received.

Table 5.8.4 summarises the findings in relation to comparison of two different dosages of pethidine within one trial.

Table 5.8.4 Summary of findings regarding relative effectiveness of lower versus higher pethidine dosages

Pain assessment category	Moore et al 1970 50mg v. 100mg pethidine	Maduska and Hajghassemali 1978 40mg v. 80mg pethidine
Pain relief reported at 60 mins post-injection	No statistically significant difference between dosages	80mg group reported statistically greater pain relief than 40mg group ($p < 0.05$)
Level of pain: % of women reporting severe/very severe pain	No statistically significant difference between dosages was reported	Not measured
Further analgesic requirements	No statistically significant difference between dosages	No statistically significant difference between dosages

Discussion

Pethidine, given by the intramuscular route, is a drug that is very well established in the modern labour ward setting. Midwives may wish to access research evidence that is directly related to their current working practice. The systematic reviews of Elbourne and Wiseman (2003) and Bricker and Lavender (2002) are of great value in terms of the range of information they provide to the practitioner. They present evidence regarding pethidine versus alternative analgesics, and also regarding short- and long-term side effects of the drug. However, in terms of application to practice, midwives would be left no further forward because the reviews' conclusions expressed doubt about pethidine's effectiveness for maternal pain relief, and underlined the fact that there is currently no clear comparable alternative to it.

In the absence of an alternative, midwives may find it difficult completely to discontinue pethidine use. It might be possible to avoid administering unnecessarily high dosages, however, if evidence of the relative effectiveness of different dosages were available. The systematic reviews, unfortunately, were not of practical benefit in this regard because their conclusions were not in agreement.

This lack of clarity led to further investigation of the original trial papers identified by this literature search. Data were extracted in relation to analgesic effectiveness of intramuscular pethidine, and specifically in relation to relative effectiveness of different dosages. The intention was to isolate evidence regarding pethidine's analgesic properties from the wealth of related data surrounding it, and to present the findings in an easily accessible format. The evidence could then be reviewed and the apparent conflict in the reviews' conclusions explored. Practising midwives would more easily be able to reflect on the findings of the exercise and decide on further personal enquiry.

Although it must be reiterated that the findings are difficult to interpret due to extensive confounding factors, the findings in relation to pain assessments may be summarised as below:

- Changes in VAS pain scores pre-pethidine and 60 minutes post-pethidine demonstrate suboptimal analgesic effect. (Connelly 2000 comments on the Fairlie et al 1999 study that 'the visual analogue score (VAS) is the "gold standard" of pain analysis in evaluating treatments.' He also states that 'the usual clinical goal for pain relief is to achieve a pain score = 30')
- Pain relief reported at 60 minutes post-pethidine – at best, one in five women had 'no' or 'slight' pain relief from pethidine; at worst, three out of four had 'no' or 'slight' relief.

- Percentages of women reporting severe or very severe pain 60 minutes post-pethidine decreased in only four out of eight groups studied.

Furthermore, there is little evidence available regarding relative effectiveness of different dosages of pethidine. Only two studies compared different dosages within one trial, and these date back to the 1970s (Maduska and Hajghassemali 1978, Moore et al 1970). Both studies reported similar rates of further analgesia, regardless of initial dosage, and only one of the two trials found better pain relief following a higher dosage (Maduska and Hajghassemali 1978).

These findings seem to confirm the concerns expressed by midwives, doctors and the women themselves. Midwives are left with the uncomfortable evidence that the most common form of intramuscular analgesia they offer may not consistently achieve its purpose. They are left to reflect on how/whether their everyday practice is to be affected by this information.

Discussion of the findings with a woman is, however, necessary to enable her to make a better informed choice regarding her labour analgesia. Other options are available, some more or less invasive than others. Epidural anaesthesia has significant advantages in terms of pain relief alone, but there is an association of increased length of first and second stages, increased incidence of fetal malposition, and increased use of oxytocin and instrumental vaginal deliveries (Howell 2003). Continuous support during labour may reduce analgesia/anaesthesia requirements and increase satisfaction (Hodnett et al 2003) without adding complication.

In reality, a combination of various strategies often occurs, and women may still wish to include pethidine as one of these options, despite the lack of convincing evidence. There is, therefore, still a need for well-designed studies to focus on this method of pain relief.

Conclusions

Although the confounding factors make direct comparison of the trials difficult, the evidence provided by women in first stage of labour suggests that pethidine provides suboptimal analgesic effect. Based on the evidence of the two trials that compared different dosages of pethidine, there is insufficient evidence that a higher dose of pethidine (80–100mg) is more effective in terms of analgesia than a lower dose (40–50mg).

Practice considerations

There is a need to:

- initiate focused and strictly controlled research into:
  a. the relative effectiveness of various dosages of pethidine

b. the influence of commonly used co-drugs on pethidine's effectiveness

c. comparison of pain relief between nulliparous and multiparous women

d. dosage related to Body Mass Index.

• enable informed choice by pregnant women by thorough discussion of the evidence regarding pethidine's effectiveness

• adopt alternative methods of labour management that have been shown to be effective without introducing further complications.

REFERENCES

Aly E E and Shilling R S (2000). Editorial. 'Are we willing to change?'. Anaesthesia, 55, 419–420.

Brice J E H, Moreland T A and Walker C H M (1979). 'Effects of pethidine and its antagonists on the newborn'. Archives of Disease in Childhood, 54, 356–361.

Bricker L and Lavender T (2002). 'Parenteral opioids for labor pain relief: a systematic review'. American Journal of Obstetrics and Gynecology, 186 (5): S94–109.

Chamberlain G, Wraith A and Steer P (1993). Pain and its Relief in Childbirth: Report of the 1990 NBT Survey, Edinburgh: Churchill Livingstone.

Connelly N R (2000). 'Commentary' (on Fairlie et al 1999). Evidence-based Obstetrics and Gynecology, 2: 89.

Downe S M (1997). 'Changing times: practice and practicalities'. British Journal of Midwifery, 5 (10): 629.

Elbourne D and Wiseman R A (2003). 'Types of intra-muscular opioids for maternal pain relief in labour (Cochrane Review)'. In: The Cochrane Library, Issue 4, Chichester, UK: John Wiley and Sons, Ltd.

Fairlie F M, Marshall L, Walker J J and Elbourne D (1999). 'Intramuscular opioids for maternal pain relief in labour: a randomised controlled trial comparing pethidine with diamorphine'. British Journal of Obstetrics and Gynaecology, 106: 1181–1187.

Heelbeck L (1999). 'Administration of pethidine in labour'. British Journal of Midwifery, 7 (6): 372–377.

Hicks C M (1996). Undertaking Midwifery Research. A Basic Guide to Design and Analysis, Edinburgh: Churchill Livingstone.

Hodgkinson R, Bhatt M, Grewal G and Marx G F (1978). 'Neonatal behaviour in the first 48 hours of life: effect of the administration of meperidine with and without naloxone in the mother'. Pediatrics, 62 (3): 294–298.

Hodnett E D, Gates S, Hofmeyr G J and Sakala C (2003). 'Continuous support for women during childbirth (Cochrane Review)'. In: The Cochrane Library, Issue 4, Chichester, UK: John Wiley and Sons, Ltd.

Howell C J (2003). 'Epidural versus non-epidural analgesia for pain relief in labour (Cochrane Review)'. In: The Cochrane Library, Issue 4, Chichester, UK: John Wiley and Sons, Ltd.

Hunt S (2002). 'Pethidine: love it or hate it?'. MIDIRS Midwifery Digest, 12 (3): 363–365.

Isenor L and Penny-MacGillivray T (1993). 'Intravenous meperidine infusion for obstetric analgesia'. Journal of Obstetric, Gynecologic, and Neonatal Nursing, 22 (4): 349–356.

Jensen F, Quist I, Brocks V, Secher N J and Westergaard L G (1984). 'Submucous paracervical blockade compared with intramuscular meperidine as analgesia during labor: a double-blind study'. Obstetrics and Gynecology, 64 (5): 724–727.

Jordan S (2002). Pharmacology for Midwives (Evidence Base for Safe Practice), Palgrave Publishers Limited.

Keskin H L, Aktepe Keskin E, Avsar A F, Tabuk M and Caglar G S (2002). 'Pethidine versus tramadol for pain relief during labor'. International Journal of Gynecology and Obstetrics, 82: 11–16.

Kingdom J and Woods S (1997). 'Correspondence: Opioids in labour'. The Lancet, 349: 726.

Kuhnert B R, Philipson E H, Kuhnert P M and Syracuse C D (1985a). 'Disposition of meperidine and normeperidine following multiple doses during labor. I Mother'. American Journal of Obstetrics and Gynecology, 151 (3): 406–409.

Kuhnert B R, Kuhnert P M, Philipson E H and Syracuse C D (1985b). 'Disposition of meperidine and normeperidine following multiple doses during labor. II Fetus and neonate'. American Journal of Obstetrics and Gynecology, 151 (3): 410–415.

Kuhnert B R, Kuhnert P M, Tu A L and Lin D C K (1979). 'Meperidine and normeperidine levels following meperidine administration during labor. II Fetus and neonate'. American Journal of Obstetrics and Gynecology, 133 (8): 909–914.

Lawrence Beech B A (1998). 'Pethidine – a little shot of something not so nice'. AIMS Journal, 10 (1): 7–8.

Leap N (2000). 'Pain in labour: towards a midwifery perspective'. MIDIRS Midwifery Digest, 10 (1): 49–53.

Levy D (1971). 'Obstetric analgesia – pentazocine and meperidine in normal primiparous labor'. Obstetrics and Gynecology, 38 (6): 907–911.

Liston W A (1997). 'Correspondence: Opioids in labour'. The Lancet, 349: 727.

Littler C, Sleep J, McCandlish R and Elbourne D (1997). 'Correspondence: Opioids in labour'. The Lancet, 349: 727.

Low J and Tordoff S (2000). 'Pethidine in labour'. Anaesthesia, 55: 936 (letter).

Maduska A L and Hajghassemali M (1978). 'A double-blind comparison of butorphanol and meperidine in labour: maternal pain relief and effect on the newborn'. Canadian Anaesthetists' Society Journal, 25 (5): 398–404.

Mander R (1997). 'Pethidine in childbirth'. MIDIRS Midwifery Digest, 7 (2): 202–204.

McAuley D M, O'Neill M P, Moore J and Dundee J W (1982). 'Lorazepam premedication for labour'. British Journal of Obstetrics and Gynaecology, 89: 149–154.

Moore J, Carson R M and Hunter R J (1970). 'A comparison of the effects of pentazocine and pethidine administered during labour'. The Journal of Obstetrics and Gynaecology of the British Commonwealth, 77: 830–836.

Morrison J C, Wiser W L, Rosser S I, Gayden J O, Bucovaz E T, Whybrew W D and Fish S A (1973). 'Metabolites of meperidine related to fetal depression'. American Journal of Obstetrics and Gynecology, 115 (8): 1132–1137.

Morrison C E, Dutton D, Howie H and Gilmour H (1987). 'Pethidine compared with meptazinol in labour'. Anaesthesia, 42: 7–14.

Mowat J and Garrey M M (1970).'Comparison of pentazocine and pethidine in labour'. British Medical Journal, 2: 757–759.

Nyberg K, Buka S L and Lipsitt K P (2000). 'Perinatal medication as a potential risk factor for adult drug abuse in a North American cohort'. Epidemiology, 11 (6): 715–716.

Oloffson C H, Ekblom A, Ekman-Ordeberg G, Hjelm A and Irestedt L (1996). 'Lack of analgesic effect of systemically administered morphine or pethidine on labour pain'. British Journal of Obstetrics and Gynaecology, 103: 968–972.

Priest J and Rosser J (1991). 'Pethidine – a shot in the dark'. MIDIRS Midwifery Digest, 1 (4): 373–375.

Refstad S O and Lindbaek E (1980). 'Ventilatory depression of the newborn of women receiving pethidine or pentazocine. A double-blind comparative trial'. British Journal of Anaesthesia, 52: 265–270.

Reynolds F and Crowhurst J A (1997). 'Commentary: Opioids in labour – no analgesic effect'. The Lancet, 349: 4–5.

Righard L and Alade M O (1990). 'Effect of delivery room routines on success of first breast-feed'. The Lancet, 336: 1105–1107.

Riordan J, Gross A, Angeron J, Krumwiede B and Melin J (2000). 'The effect of labor pain relief medication on neonatal suckling and breastfeeding duration'. Journal of Human Lactation, 16 (1): 7–12.

Rooth G, Lysikiewicz A, Huch R and Huch A (1983). 'Some effects of maternal pethidine administration on the newborn'. British Journal of Obstetrics and Gynaecology, 90: 28–33.

Sheikh A and Tunstall M E (1986). 'Comparative study of meptazinol and pethidine for the relief of pain in labour'. British Journal of Obstetrics and Gynaecology, 93: 264–269.

Thompson Micromedex Health Care Series (1974–2003): 118.

Thurlow J A, Laxton C H, Dick A, Waterhouse P, Sherman L and Goodman N W (2002). 'Remifentanil by patient-controlled analgesia compared with intramuscular meperidine for pain relief in labour'. British Journal of Anaesthesia, 88 (3): 374–378.

Twycross R (1997). 'Correspondence: Opioids in labour'. The Lancet, 349: 727.

Vella L, Francis D, Houlton P and Reynolds F (1985). 'Comparison of the antiemetics metoclopramide and promethazine in labour'. British Medical Journal, 290: 1173–1175.

Viegas O A C, Khaw B and Ratnam S S (1993). 'Tramadol in labour pain in primiparous patients. A prospective comparative clinical trial'. European Journal of Obstetrics and Gynaecology and Reproductive Biology, 49: 131–135.

Wilson C M, McClean E, Moore J and Dundee J W (1986). 'A double-blind comparison of intramuscular pethidine and nalbuphine in labour'. Anaesthesia, 41: 1207–1213.

Wood C M (2003). 'Audit of pethidine uptake in labour'. Derby Hospitals NHS Foundation Trust, Derby City General Hospital (internal audit).

The Practising Midwife 2005; 8(7): 16–25

More than a cuddle: skin-to-skin contact is key

Nils Bergman

The theme of UNICEF UK's Baby Friendly Initiative conference next month concerns increasing breastfeeding rates. Practising midwives generally accept that breastfeeding is important. But many health workers regard breastfeeding as beneficial but not essential, somewhat ill-suited to modern life, and essentially the mother's choice to make. So why should increasing breastfeeding rates be important, and should we expend energy on it?

I suggest that, in fact, there is nothing more important for midwives, obstetric services and health departments to do. I will now briefly sketch what I hope to elaborate in greater detail at the conference.

Baby comes first

For many years we have assumed that the fetus develops in the uterus according to an innate developmental programme, and according to how well it is fed, and that the brain develops in a linear fashion until the teenage years. We therefore make sure that basic biological needs of oxygen, warmth, nutrition and protection are provided properly at all times. We have become very skilled and competent at this, we have wonderful technology, and we have improved survival in amazing ways. Our whole health service is geared to provide this care to the newborn, and the mother is not essential for our work. After discharge our society has followed this mindset, and we provide the infant with all its needs, relieving the mother of this burden as much as possible.

That last sentence perhaps over-states the case, but is the end result of an assumption that is the foundation for our society: that the fetus and newborn is an individual entity developing to take his or her place in the world. During the past 10 to 20 years, neuroscience has advanced to a stage where we can conclude that this assumption is false. And the consequences are enormous.

After conception, the brain develops for 14 weeks according to instructions from the DNA. Thereafter,

development is dependent on stimulations of the neural cells. The neural cells multiply rapidly, and reach their maximum number at the age of 20 weeks. The synapses connect all the neural cells and reach their maximum at 40 weeks, or birth. Development is now a matter of pruning and eliminating neural cells that aren't used.

The keys are 'cells that fire together, wire together', and 'use it or lose it'. The brain does develop according to a timetable, but that timetable requires very specific stimulations at specific points for the brain to make the right connections and avoid or eliminate 'bad pathways'. The absence of the right stimulations (and, to a lesser extent, the presence of unpleasant stimulations) creates unhealthy pathways in the brain, which impact on the individual across the entire lifespan, both in physical and mental health.

There is only one way of providing all the right stimulations to the baby at the right time: the continuous uninterrupted presence of mother. The mother 'is a kind of invisible hothouse' (Hofer 1994) that stimulates the fetal and newborn brain to develop optimally.

The crucial period

The period immediately after birth is crucial for a newborn baby, and the period during which hospitals have been most active in ensuring basic needs are provided adequately. After an hour or two when we have made sure the baby is stable, we may return it to its mother. We now know that this first hour is the most important period of all for the baby, and when it critically needs to be with its mother. The scientific term is, in fact, 'critical period', and if denied the particular stimulations needed at that particular time irretrievable and permanent loss of functions result.

The specific stimulations the brain needs at birth are skin-to-skin contact and olfactory stimulation. These stimulations trigger a brain-based behaviour we call 'self-attachment', after Righard's work 25 years ago. This essential behaviour primes and sets the brain to breast-feed optimally. It is simultaneously the behaviour that starts the brain to develop the capacity to develop good relationships: breastfeeding and relationship building are synonymous to the brain at this stage.

Inseparable dyad

So, in contrast to what we previously assumed, the fetal brain grows all its neural cells before birth, and essen-tially completes its pathways in the first year or two of life. To develop into a healthy, self-contained individual, the baby must start as an inseparable dyad with mother. That 'inseparableness' is physical: tangible and tactile, it is skin-to-skin contact. The result is successful breastfeed-ing, but above all a brain that is set on an optimal devel-opmental trajectory.

REFERENCES

Hofer M A (1994). 'Early relationships as regulators of infant physiology and behaviour'. Acta Paediatr Suppl, 397: 9–18.

Further references are available on request and can also be accessed on: www.kangaroomothercare.com

The Practising Midwife 2005; 8(9): 44

To cut or not to cut?

Sharon Phillips

As a lecturer in midwifery, my job becomes more challenging and enjoyable when discussion takes place among the students within the learning environment. During a recent teaching session, the question 'whether or not to cut a nuchal cord' – that is, when the cord is wrapped around the baby's neck – provoked plenty of discussion.

When working on the delivery suite, the students had observed a variety of practices: while some midwives cut a nuchal cord, others leave it to deliver with the baby's body or slip the cord gently over the baby's head. Inevitably, the students asked what I would do in a similar situation.

Students often enjoy storytelling – perhaps this enables them to bridge the 'theory-practice gap'. Therefore, I recalled my own experience.

I had been a qualified midwife for about three years and had always clamped and cut a nuchal cord, until I observed one of my peers demonstrating and explaining that it was both practicable and beneficial, in terms of promoting physiological birth, not to do so. This had no detrimental effect on the baby; furthermore, it did not detract from the mother's natural and uncontrollable urge to push. Since this experience, I have found that the nuchal cord either slips over the baby's head, or delivers easily with the baby's body. I wondered why I ever clamped and cut.

Hard evidence

Anecdotal evidence is all well and good, but student midwives need evidence to support their practice. Therefore, following the teaching session I decided to investigate further. There are several aspects worthy of consideration regarding the nuchal cord: the utility of its detection during the antenatal period; neonatal outcomes with the presence of a nuchal cord; the possibility of the cord causing decelerations in the fetal heart rate during labour; management at birth; and the possible sequelae of clamping and cutting.

Schorn and Blanco (1991) suggest that the incidence of nuchal cord is 23–25 per cent of all vaginal births; and that normal fetal movements, together with a long umbilical cord, may result in the cord being wrapped around the fetal neck.

It is questionable whether women should be subjected to an ultrasound scan in order to detect a nuchal cord during the antenatal period. An observational study by Athanassiou et al (2000) found that the majority of nuchal cords, detected by ultrasound scan, resolved spontaneously. Athanassiou et al suggest that early detection has limited clinical utility, and appears to have little (if any) clinical impact on neonatal outcomes.

Neonatal outcomes

There have been several studies of the outcomes of nuchal cord on neonates (Collins 1999, Larson et al 1995, Miser 1992, Nelson and Grether 1998, Rhoades et al 1999), which suggest that nuchal cords are rarely associated with significant morbidity or mortality. Multiple nuchal cord entanglement is associated with a greater risk of meconium, an abnormal fetal heart rate pattern during advanced labour, and the need for operative vaginal delivery. However, there is no added risk of adverse neonatal outcome (Larson et al 1995).

Collins (1997) describes type A and type B nuchal cords that need to be distinguished at birth. Type B encircles the neck in a locked pattern; type A in an unlocked pattern. Collins (1999) suggests that type B nuchal cords are associated with stillbirths; however, it is important to remember that such events are extremely rare. In contrast, Carey and Rayburn (2000) question the role of single or multiple nuchal cord encirclement in stillbirths.

Variable decelerations in the fetal heart rate prior to birth could indicate the presence of a nuchal cord. Miser's study (1992) found that fetal bradycardia and variable decelerations in the fetal heart rate occurred twice as often in the nuchal cord group, and that multiple entanglement resulted in 'abnormal' fetal heart rate patterns. Such 'abnormalities' in the heart rate may result in unnecessary intervention.

Students and midwives should be aware of nuchal cord as a possible cause of variable decelerations of the fetal heart rate. With the presence of a nuchal cord, variable decelerations may be common during advanced first stage of labour; and, as a consequence, 'fetal distress' may be misdiagnosed. During the second stage of labour early decelerations of the fetal heart are normal occurrences, with or without the presence of a nuchal cord (Gibb and Arulkumaran 1997).

Some students have observed continuous monitoring of the fetal heart during the second stage of labour in uncomplicated pregnancies. I suggest that students should try to avoid continuously monitoring the fetus during second stage as it is uncomfortable for the woman and severely restricts her freedom to change her position. Reassurance regarding fetal wellbeing is provided by a return to normal fetal heart rate and normal variability between contractions, easily detected using intermittent auscultation.

However, I do understand that it may be difficult for students to remove the transducer if the midwife caring for the woman in labour prefers it to remain in situ, or if it is delivery suite policy to monitor the fetus continuously.

The management of a nuchal cord at birth may be anticipated by detection of variable decelerations in the fetal heart rate, as mentioned previously. Management often begins by the midwife or student feeling for a nuchal cord following the birth of the baby's head. However, the efficacy of this practice is questionable, particularly when the woman adopts a standing, squatting or kneeling position, or is in a waterbirth pool.

The tightness of the nuchal cord may determine subsequent management, although in the majority of cases it may be left and delivers easily with the baby's body (Phillips: personal observation).

Somersault manoeuvre

Schorn and Blanco (1991) describe the somersault manoeuvre for management of a tight nuchal cord. Anderson (1991) suggests this technique was developed in the early 1950s by an obstetrician, Dr Mast. The steps of the procedure are as follows (Schorn and Blanco 1991):

1. Once the nuchal cord is discovered, the anterior and posterior shoulders are slowly birthed under control without manipulation of the cord.

2. As the shoulders are birthed, the head is flexed so that the face of the baby is pushed towards the maternal thigh.
3. The baby's head is kept next to the perineum while the body is birthed and 'somersaults' out.
4. The umbilical cord is then unwrapped and the usual management ensues.

There are other potential problems when attempting to clamp and cut a tight nuchal cord: the procedure detracts from the woman's uncontrollable urge to push; and there is a risk of accidentally clamping or cutting the baby's skin. Once the cord is clamped and cut, any delay in the birth of the baby's shoulders may result in severe neonatal hypoxia.

Iffy and Varadi (1994) describe five cases of cerebral palsy where birth was delayed on account of shoulder dystocia for a period ranging from three to seven minutes – in all cases, the nuchal cord had been clamped and cut. Iffy and Varadi suggest that cutting compounds the problem of an unexpected arrest of the shoulders.

Bruce and Flamm (1999) describe a case of shoulder dystocia where the nuchal cord had not been cut and they were able to perform cephalic replacement followed by an emergency caesarean section. This resulted in a 4,900g infant with Apgar scores of 2, 7 and 9 at one, five and 10 minutes with minimal Erb's palsy which resolved within two weeks. This method of cephalic replacement is known as the Zavenelli manoeuvre (Sandberg 1985).

Physiological birth

Whenever a nuchal cord is clamped and cut prior to the birth of the baby's shoulders, the physiological process is abruptly terminated. Late clamping and cutting of the cord supports a physiological birth process (Mercer et al 2000). Student midwives develop their expertise through observation and practice: however, if they do not observe physiological birth, which includes not cutting a nuchal cord plus a physiological third stage, their practice will be restricted.

During teaching sessions it may be difficult for lecturers to provide a definitive answer to some clinical questions, such as the management of a nuchal cord. Students also need to be aware that every childbirth experience is unique and that midwives use their clinical judgement on an individual basis. Rather than attempting to provide all the answers, it is important for midwifery lecturers to stimulate appetites for knowledge and encourage students to debate and research different aspects of clinical practice.

REFERENCES

Anderson E E (1991). 'Management of nuchal cord in relation to vaginal delivery'. Journal of Nurse-Midwifery, 36 (6): 377–378 (letter).

Athanassiou A, Craigo S D, Chelmow D et al (2000). 'Is early antenatal diagnosis of a nuchal cord clinically useful?' American Journal of Obstetrics and Gynecology, 182 (2).

Bruce L and Flamm M D (1999). 'Tight nuchal cord and shoulder dystocia: a potentially catastrophic combination'. The American College of Obstetricians and Gynecologists, 94 (5): 853.

Carey J C and Rayburn W F (2000). 'Nuchal cord encirclement and risk of stillbirth'. International Journal of Gynaecology and Obstetrics, 69 (2): 173–174.

Collins J H (1997). 'Nuchal cord type A and type B'. American Journal of Obstetrics and Gynecology, 177 (1): 94.

Collins J H (1999). 'Tight nuchal cord morbidity and mortality'. American Journal of Obstetrics and Gynecology, 180 (1): 251.

Gibb D and Arulkumaran S (1997). Fetal Monitoring in Practice, 2nd edition, Oxford: Butterworth Heinemann.

Iffy L and Varadi V (1994). 'Cerebral palsy following cutting of the nuchal cord before delivery'. Medical Law, 13 (3–4): 323–330.

Larson J D, Rayburn W F, Crosby S and Thurnau G R (1995). 'Multiple nuchal cord entanglements and intrapartum complications'. American Journal of Obstetrics and Gynecology, 173 (4): 1228–1231.

Mercer J S, Nelson C C and Skovgaard R L (2000). 'Umbilical cord clamping: beliefs and practices of American nurse-midwives'. Journal of Midwifery and Women's Health, 45 (1): 58–66.

Miser W F (1992). 'Outcomes of infants born with nuchal cords'. Journal of Family Practice, 34 (4): 441–445.

Nelson K B and Grether J K (1998). 'Potentially asphyxiating conditions and spastic cerebral palsy in infants of normal birth weight'. American Journal of Obstetrics and Gynecology, 179 (2): 507–513.

Rhoades D A, Latza U and Mueller B A (1999). 'Risk factors and outcomes associated with nuchal cord: a population-based study'. Journal of Reproductive Medicine, 44 (1): 39–45.

Sandberg E C (1985). 'The Zavenelli manouver: a potentially revolutionary method for the resolution of shoulder dystocia'. American Journal of Obstetrics and Gynecology, 152: 479–484.

Schorn M N and Blanco J D (1991). 'Management of the nuchal cord'. Journal of Nurse-Midwifery, 36 (2): 131–132.

The Practising Midwife 2004; 7(7): 26–27

Smile for your sphincter

Ina May Gaskin

What is Sphincter Law? I coined the term, so let me explain. My invention of this phrase was born out of the need I saw for new thinking in the formulation of explanations of how women's bodies work in labour and birth. I believe that those terms that midwifery has borrowed from obstetrics often provide very little that really helps women – or those who attend their births, for that matter – understand why so many women's labours, especially those that take place in hospitals, fail to result in vaginal birth without some form of pharmaceutical, mechanical or surgical intervention.

According to conventional theory, the problem lies in some inadequacy in the woman, as described by the so-called Law of the Three Ps. According to this 'law', as explained by obstetric textbook author Derek Llewellyn-Jones as late as 1999, and by countless others, the woman's 'passage' may be too small, her 'passenger' too large, or her 'powers' (the frequency and intensity of her uterine contractions) too weak, and all these shortcomings are 'factors which can delay or prevent' the fetus' ability 'to negotiate the birth canal'. To me, this language reads more like an engineering problem than a description of a biological process. This is exactly what I believe we must overcome.

When I'm explaining labour to a midwifery student or pregnant woman, I would never mention anything related to the Law of the Three Ps. My own reluctance to refer to conventional medical theory arises because I think it explains so little in a practical sense about how birth really works. So why is the talk of sphincters relevant? My argument, of course, is based on the recognition that the cervix, like the opening of the bladder and the rectum, is a sphincter – and, thus, functions in ways similar to other sphincters.

Sphincters are circular muscles that surround the opening of those organs that are called upon to empty themselves at appropriate times. These openings ordinarily remain closed but have the ability to open as widely as needed when necessary. Their function and character are implicit in their name in the German language: Schliessmuskel, meaning 'closing muscle'. Each of the organs I have referred to is able to contract rhythmically as it fills, until it reaches the point of urgency at which the sphincter relaxes enough to allow urination, defecation or birth to take place.

About sphincters

The basics of sphincters are worth remembering:

- Sphincters open best in conditions of privacy and intimacy.
- Sphincters don't respond well to commands, such as 'Push!', 'Poop now!' or 'Get ready, get set, pee!'. They are not under our voluntary control.
- Sphincters are shy. Even in the process of opening, they may suddenly close when their owner is frightened or embarrassed. This is because high levels of adrenaline in the bloodstream do not usually favour (sometimes, they actually prevent) the opening of the sphincter.
- Sphincters do respond well to praise, if it comes from a trusted intimate companion or family member accompanying the sphincter's owner.
- Sphincters open better when their owner's mouth and jaw are relaxed and somewhat open.
- Sphincters open better when their owner is smiling or laughing.

We all have sphincters, and comprehend in a physical way how our own minds affect our bodies' ability to urinate or defecate according to someone's schedule besides our own, in a different place than we are accustomed to be. I would venture to say that none of us tried to balance our cheque books while sitting on the toilet even before we began to use computers for bookkeeping. We can all imagine how easy it would be to be required to poop in the presence of a group of strangers within a certain number of minutes. For many women, the early sensation of pushing feels much like the urge to poop the biggest one of your life. Now think of trying to move a baby outside of your body under less than sympathetic conditions!

This is the challenge women face every day when they are called upon to perform what should be the most intimate act of their lives in surroundings that afford them no privacy. People yell things at them that they would never (at least, with good intent) shout at someone who was trying to relieve herself of anything other than a baby. The problem is, of course, compounded by the requirement that the mother stay in the supine position while pushing. Because there is so little understanding of Sphincter Law by those who create the policies that determine how most maternity wards function, this very real law of human physiology is constantly violated. No wonder terms such as 'dysfunctional labour' and 'uterine inertia' had to be invented in an attempt, however inadequate, to explain why vaginal birth appears to be impossible in such a high percentage of births.

If we are going to be serious about reducing rates of unnecessary caesarean sections and ventouse extractions, it is incumbent upon us to organise maternity care policy in such a way as to make vaginal birth possible, even likely. This will mean drastic changes in many maternity units, both in their physical features and in what is said or done to (or for) labouring mothers.

Sphincter Law explains another phenomenon that has so far been left out of modern midwifery and obstetric texts. Students are taught that once the cervix begins to open in labour, it never closes until the baby is born. However, many other midwives (and obstetric nurses in the US) have told me that they have come across cases in which the once dilated cervix closes rather than opens, even in the presence of continued uterine contractions. I described such a case in *Spiritual Midwifery*, but have yet to see any modern textbook that describes this as a possible phenomenon during labour.

My case involved a first-time mother, a close friend, whose cervix rather easily reached 8cm in her first labour. But, at this point, her labour underwent a change. Her manner became much more serious, and she no longer laughed at the little jokes we had been making (which she had seemed to enjoy previously). When I asked her if I could check her dilation again, she agreed. Her cervix was only 4cm open. Then I suggested to my friend that she try to recover her sense of humour, and her efforts in this direction did in fact result in a re-dilated cervix and the birth of her baby within two hours (Gaskin 2002). This case, as you can probably imagine, had an enormous effect upon me, as it underlined so

profoundly the necessity of understanding the basics of Sphincter Law.

Years later, I was delighted to discover that reversal of cervical dilation had been noticed by physicians who wrote their texts during the period before most women in Britain and the US gave birth in hospitals. Consider, for instance, this quotation from one of the most-read American textbooks of the 19th century (Dewees 1847):

In 1792, I was called to attend a Mrs C, in consequence of her midwife being engaged. As I approached the house, I was most earnestly solicited to hasten in, as not a moment was to be lost. I was suddenly shown into Mrs C's chamber, and my appearance there was explained, by stating that her midwife was engaged. As I entered the room, Mrs C was just recovering from a pain – and it was the last she had at that time. After waiting an hour in the expectation of a return of labour, I took my leave, and was not again summoned to her for precisely two weeks. And Dr Lyall says, 'We have been informed by a respectable practitioner, of a labour that had nearly arrived at its apparent termination, suspended for more than two days, in consequence of a gentleman having been sent to the patient, against whom she had taken a prejudice.' Every accoucheur has experienced a temporary suspension of pain upon his first appearance in the sick chamber; but so long a period as two weeks is very rare.

I found similar statements in at least five other textbooks (Betschler 1880, Cazeaux 1884, Curtis 1846, Newman Dorland 1901, Ramsbotham 1861). I find it completely illogical to be asked to believe that labours no longer come to a halt because of impossible expectations placed upon women in labour or that cervices no longer close once dilated because levels of hormones in the adrenaline family become too high in labouring women.

Given the likelihood that women are still subject to reversed cervical dilation (a completely normal phenomenon when women are expected to give birth in atmospheres that make for high levels of hormones in the adrenaline family in their blood during labour), we need to stop labelling this behaviour as abnormal or dysfunctional and instead devise ways to improve the design of environments in which women give birth and educate the people who attend their births about how to facilitate, not interfere with, the natural process.

Crude and wrong-headed

I have one more argument to make about the choice of the term, Sphincter Law. Most women have no idea that a good deal of the care they receive in hospitals is based upon assumptions as crude and wrong-headed as the Law of the Three Ps. When you replace this inadequate formulation with something like Sphincter Law and describe the basic characteristics of sphincter behaviour, you have introduced language that can give the pregnant woman and those who may be with her in labour a better idea of what might help or hinder her during the course of labour. We midwives who see the value of preserving women's right to give birth spontaneously and physio-logically will need to have plenty of allies among the women who want to maintain these rights for themselves and for the coming generations.

A version of this article appeared in BJM, 2004, 12 (9); 540–542.

REFERENCES

Betschler (1880). Quoted in G Engelmann (1882), Labor Among Primitive Peoples, St Louis: J H Chambers. Reprinted, New York: AMS Press.

Cazeaux P (1884). Obstetrics: the Theory and Practice (7th US edition), Philadelphia: P Blakiston Son & Co.

Curtis A (1846). Lectures on Midwifery, Cincinatti: C Nagle.

Dewees W P (1847). Compendious System of Midwifery (4th ed), Philadelphia: Carey & Lea.

Gaskin, I M (2002). Spiritual Midwifery (4th Edition), Summertown, Tennessee: Book Publishing Company.

Llewellyn-Jones, D (1999). Fundamentals of Obstetrics and Gynaecology (Seventh Edition), Mosby.

Newman Dorland W A (1901). Modern Obstetrics, Philadelphia: WB Saunders & Company.

Ramsbotham F (1861). The Principles and Practice of Obstetric Medicine and Surgery, Philadelphia: Lea & Blanchard.

The Practising Midwife 2004; 7(10): 4–5

Topics for further reflection

It is interesting to me that several of the articles in this section are challenging practice, either by revisiting what we *think* we know about labour and birth – a good example being Ina May Gaskin's example on Sphincter Law – or raising questions around the difference between what we know and what happens in practice.

- Does Ina May Gaskin's 'Sphincter Law' make sense to you as an explanation of why some women may have difficult labours and/or births? Can you think of any other things to add to her list of things that help sphincters to open? Perhaps more importantly in relation to practice, can you think of ways of creating the kind of environment that women need in order to allow their cervix to open for birth?
- In the first of her articles on vaginal birth after caesarean, Rosemary Mander suggests that the concept (and nature) of a 'trial of labour' may be counterproductive. Is this concept in use in the area where you work and, if so, would you agree with the points made on the basis of your experience? If you do agree, what do you feel would need to be changed in practice in order for women choosing vaginal birth after caesarean to have more chance of a normal, vaginal birth?
- In her article on the use of pools, Ethel Burns discusses the significant advantages of the use of water pools for women in labour (which includes maternal satisfaction) yet also highlights the fact that, in many areas, excuses are given to deny women choice in this area. She also discusses the political nature of this issue, and the way in which midwives themselves may feel disempowered. Where do you stand on these issues, what are the issues in your area of practice and what (if anything) do you feel needs to happen in order for the situation to change, both locally and on a wider level?
- Virginia Howes and Kay Hardie express some deep concerns about the way in which one woman's care was affected by what she was told about local induction policies and discuss the dubious nature of some of the evidence on which current guidelines around induction of labour are based. Having read the points they make, what do you think about this issue?

Although several of the articles in this section have criticised elements of current practice – generally for not being woman-centred and based on good evidence – Pamela Hunt's article shows how we can learn so much from the simple art of telling stories and reflecting upon our experiences of attending women during labour and birth.

- If you were asked to choose three births from your own experience as a midwife from which you had learned the most, which births would you pick, and why?

Focus on . . .
Holistic Health

SECTION CONTENTS

Ice massage for the reduction of labor pain

Bette L. Waters, Jeanne Raisler

The current study investigated the use of ice massage of the acupressure energy meridian point large intestine 4 (LI4) to reduce labor pain during contractions. LI4 is located on the medial midpoint of the first metacarpal, within 3 to 4 mm of the web of skin between the thumb and forefinger. A one-group, pretest, post-test design was chosen, which used 100-mm Visual Analog Scales (VAS) and the McGill Pain Questionnaire (MPQ) ranked numerically and verbally to measure pain levels; the pretest served as the control. Study participants were Hispanic and white Medicaid recipients who received prenatal care at a women's clinic staffed by certified nurse-midwives and obstetricians. Participants noted a pain reduction mean on the VAS of 28.22 mm on the left hand and 11.93 mm on the right hand. The postdelivery ranked MPQ dropped from number 3 (distressing) to number 2 (discomforting). The study results suggest that ice massage is a safe, noninvasive, nonpharmacological method of reducing labor pain.

Keywords: labor, first stage, pain relief, acupressure, ice massage

A woman's experience of labor pain is influenced by many elements including her past experiences of pain, her coping abilities, the birth environment, and psychosocial factors. The definition of pain as an unpleasant and emotional experience resulting from actual or potential tissue damage has powered the scientific study and management of pain in recent decades. Labor pain differs from other forms of pain in that no actual trauma or tissue damage occurs. Chapman[1] describes labor pain as stimuli of receptive neurons arising from contractions of the uterine muscles, which is referred to as the visceral, pelvic, and lumbar-sacral areas. To date, labor pain management studies have focused on use of drugs that affect sensory awareness of pain, which may have the additional effect of impeding women's active participation in giving birth.

McCaffery's definition, 'Pain is whatever the experiencing person says it is, and happens whenever the experiencing person says it does,'[2] reflects the midwifery approach to labor management. This philosophy supports management options that include diverse methods for decreasing pain while not eliminating the source.

Even though there has been enormous growth in complementary alternative medicine (CAM) research in the past decade, few well-designed studies on the use of CAM in pregnancy or childbirth have been conducted. Some of the most interesting of the studies are those based in traditional Chinese medicine, which is a complex ancient system of healing that includes the use of acupuncture, acupressure (acupuncture without needles), moxibustion (stimulation of acupuncture points with heat from a burning herb), massage, diet, herbs, and exercise to promote health and treat disease. Within the framework of traditional Chinese medicine, the stimulation of acupuncture points by these treatments is a way of initiating, controlling, or accelerating body functions by stimulating energy channels (meridians) beneath the skin's surface and rebalancing the body's energy (Qi) to restore health.[3] Shiatsu – a Japanese healing modality based on acupuncture – uses massage to stimulate the energy pathways.

Despite the exponential growth of research on traditional Chinese medicine in the past decade, the mechanisms of action of acupuncture, acupressure, and moxibustion are still largely unexplained in the Western scientific model. Western research on the use of traditional Chinese medicine in obstetrics has focused on the effect of acupuncture/acupressure on nausea and vomiting during pregnancy[4,5] and on the use of moxibustion for breech version.[6] In the 1970s and 1980s, studies on the use of acupuncture for labor induction and labor analgesia were carried out, but there were problems with the study methods, including small sample sizes, the variety of methods for assessing pain, and in some studies, the lack of a control group. However, many effective CAM therapies, including massage, therapeutic touch, hydrotherapy, music, heat, and cold, are used by midwives to reduce labor pain.[7]

The purpose of this study was to evaluate the effectiveness of the use of ice massage of the energy meridian point, large intestine 4 (LI4), during contractions to reduce the woman's perception of labor pain. The energy meridian pathway is bilateral. The LI4 point is located on both the right and the left hands. Ice massage was performed on both hands, and any differences in pain sensation were measured and compared.

Background

Cooling temperatures to reduce pain

Ice or cooling applied to an injured body part is used as standard treatment of trauma, bleeding, swelling, and soft tissue injuries.[8] Ice is commonly used to reduce pain of perineal lacerations or episiotomy in the postpartum period.

The early work of Denny-Brown et al.[9] showed that cold temperature effectively blocks nerve conduction in sensory fibers. Grant[10] advocated massage with ice for the treatment of musculoskeletal pain and named his technique cryokinetics. Marshall[11] published a study using ice cube massage for the relief of chronic pain of herpes of the eye.

Melzack et al.[12,13] found that intense sensory input produced by ice massage of the web between the thumb and forefinger resulted in a 50% reduction in acute dental pain. The researchers hypothesized that the efficacy of ice massage was due to engaging the gate control pain system rather than eliminating the source of the pain.[14] They hypothesized that the positive and negative effects of the different impulses counteracted each other at the 'gate' level in the spine. When impulses reaching the spine pathway to the brain are stimulated by techniques such as vibration, scratching, or ice massage, the gate closes, resulting in a decrease in the sensation of pain. In addition, Melzack and his colleagues connected their work to acupuncture relying on the correlation between trigger points used in Western medicine that corresponded to acupuncture points used in traditional Chinese medicine.[15]

Large intestine energy meridian

The large intestine energy meridian point that Melzack used in his study on ice massage for dental pain reduction is referred to as LI4 or Hoku. The energy meridian pathway is bilateral and begins 'in the surface of the skin at the root of the index fingernail. It courses on the external part of the arm. The outward end of the shoulder blade is crossed. Then the meridian leaves the skin surface to connect with the lower part of the lung and transverse colon. It then returns to the skin surface at a point under the chin. From that point, the meridian is again buried deep within the area referred to as the double chin. It follows the lower row of dental roots, passing then to the upper line of teeth roots, crossing the front of the mouth to emerge on the skin surface and the facial point next to the nostrils'[16] (Figure 6.1.1).

Shiatsu practitioners[17] describe LI4 (also referred to as Hoku) as being located on the inner lateral midpoint of the first metacarpal. The area between the thumb and forefinger is within 3 to 4 mm of the location of an LI4 (Figure 6.1.2).

A pilot study was developed on the basis of Dr. Melzack's use of ice massage of LI4 to reduce dental pain after discovering that Aleda Erskine[18] linked dental pain, childbirth pain, and myocardial infarction under the category of 'acute clinical pain.' Acupuncture or acupressure points used for the relief of a particular pain syndrome often lie within or near the pain area, but many are located at a distance. The large intestine pathway moves from the tip of the forefinger up to the face and circles the teeth; it bifurcates at the shoulder to move downward wrapping

Figure 6.1.1 Large intestine energy meridian pathway.

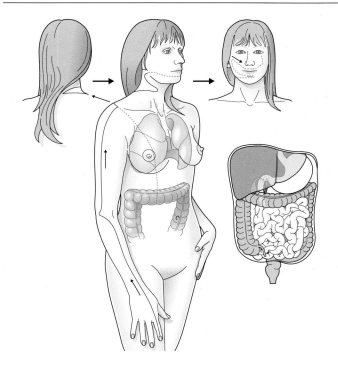

Figure 6.1.2 Large intestine energy point four, also known as LI4 and Hoku. With permission from Waters B L 1995 *Massage During Pregnancy.*

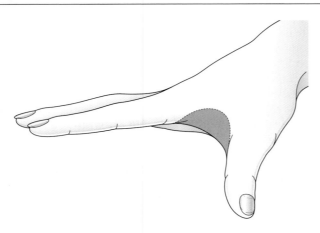

around the entire colon. At term pregnancy, the colon practically encircles the upper portion of the uterus. The location of LI4 is a point where the energy flow of the meridian is closest to the skin and can be easily stimulated with pressure, needles, or extreme cold and pressure.

The pilot study using ice massage for reducing labor pain was carried out by a researcher in 1992.[19] Twenty women were recruited to participate in this study on their admission to the labor and delivery unit at Humana Hospital, Dade City, FL. Ice massage of the energy meridian LI4 was performed during each contraction and was carried out over a 30-minute period. Data from the Visual Analog Scale (VAS) showed a mean reduction in pain of 25.15. The reduction of pain was statistically significant despite the small number of participants. The statistical standard was matched pairs *t* test. The current study expands on this previous work using a larger sample and tested efficacy of right-hand ice massage versus left-hand.

Methods

A one-group, pretest, posttest design was chosen.[20] The pretest was a 100-mm VAS. The VAS has been extensively used and validated in pain research and is considered to be a valid measure, especially in a one-time intervention study.[21,22] The pretest was used to measure labor pain intensity before ice massage and served as the control. Posttest 1 was a 100-mm VAS for both the right hand and the left hand. It was used to measure pain intensity during ice massage intervention and to compare pain intensity on the right hand versus the left hand. Pretest and posttest 1 scores were compared by using standard analysis of variance, Statistical Analysis System, Version 8.00.

Pain response differences were multiples that consisted of three elements: pain before massage, pain during massage of the left hand, and pain during massage of the right hand. These differences were identified by using Duncan's New Multiple Range test.[23]

Posttest 2 was the McGill Pain Questionnaire (MPQ) Verbal Rating Scale. The MPQ is the most widely used instrument in pain research and practice.[24,25] It consists of verbal pain descriptors designed to capture the intensity continuum of pain ranging from mild to excruciating, and ranked numerically from 1 to 5. The participant scored two questions using the MPQ: (1) What was your pain before you started the ice massage? (2) What was your pain while using the ice massage? The MPQ was analyzed by using a standard analysis of variance equivalent to a paired *t* test.[26] If data collected in posttest 2 follows the pattern of posttest 1, it is regarded as a valuable corroboration of the data.

To reduce threats to the validity, posttest 1 was administered immediately after the intervention, 40 minutes or less after scoring the pretest. This small window of time between the pre- and posttest helped to eliminate intervening events that could alter the posttest scoring. Posttest 1 was presented to the study participants on a separate sheet of paper so they could not see where they had marked on the pretest VAS. VAS tool copies were made from a master copy on the same copy machine. Posttest 2 was administered within 24 hours after the delivery. Postponing the scoring of this test until after the woman, especially the primigravida, had experienced the process of the labor and birth with full knowledge of all its intensity strengthens any corroborative data.

Study participants were a convenience sample of English-speaking Hispanic and white Medicaid recipients who received prenatal and delivery care from a clinic team of certified nurse-midwives and obstetricians at a 250-bed hospital in New Mexico. They were recruited for the study on the basis of the availability of the investigator after being evaluated and admitted to the hospital in labor by their midwife or physician. The gestational age of the participants was determined to be between 37 and 41 weeks by an early sonogram. All participants had a reactive fetal heart rate monitoring strip and were having contractions at least every 10 minutes with some cervical changes, either effacement or dilation. Women diagnosed with pre-eclampsia or chorioamnionitis were excluded from the study. Women whose labor was induced, those who had narcotics in the past 8 hours, and women with an underlying disease that precluded attendance by a nurse-midwife were excluded from the study. In addition, women dilated more than 8 cm were excluded. It was believed that the intensity of the labor contractions during this transition could decrease participants cognitive abilities and thus compromise the data obtained.

Previous research reported[27] that women found the VAS difficult to use when experiencing severe labor pain. The use of women in the early stages of labor eliminated the ethical issue of withholding pain medications they might want to use as labor progressed.

The sample size was not predetermined. The goal was to recruit as many subjects as possible within a 12-month period. Unlike many other studies[28] of non-pharmacological methods of pain relief, these participants had no prior commitment to giving birth without pain medication, and most expected to receive either narcotic or epidural analgesia at some point in the labor.

The clinical investigation protocol and consent form were approved and monitored by Memorial Medical Center's Institutional Review Board. After obtaining verbal and written informed consent, the investigator presented the pretest and explained to the subject how to mark her pain intensity at the present moment on the VAS. Ice massage was started at the initiation of the next contraction. Approximately one-third cup of crushed ice was placed in the center of a soft, thin terry wash cloth, and the four corners of the washcloth were lifted to the center and twisted to make a small ice bag. The ice bag fit snugly between the thumb and forefinger. To ensure that cold was applied only to the skin of the palm, the ice bag was placed on the medial (palm side) aspect of the hand (Figure 6.1.3).

The lateral aspect of the participant's hand was supported by the hand of the person performing the massage. The massage was stopped when the contraction ended and restarted when the next contraction began. The ice bag was rocked back and forth over the area of the web of skin between the thumb and the forefinger. The pressure of the ice bag was comparable to light scratching and was intended to mildly irritate the neuron endings in the skin.

It should be noted that the exact point of LI4 is located on the medial aspect of the first metacarpal. The skin or epidermis located directly over this point is part of the outer part of the hand and is thin. Ice massage over this area can cause breakdown of skin integrity due to cold temperatures and friction. However, the web of skin between the thumb and forefinger shown in Figure 6.1.2 is part of the thick, hard, and horny texture of the palm and can withstand the intermittent friction and cold temperatures used in this technique.[29]

The massage was carried out on one hand for 20 minutes or throughout three or four contractions, whichever occurred first. It was then repeated in the same manner on the other hand. The selection of right hand or left hand first was based on what activity the study participant was engaged in at the time the ice massage began. If she was in bed, the choice was determined by which side of the bed the fetal monitor was located. If she was walking in the halls or soaking in the Jacuzzi, the investigator accepted the participant's choice.

At the end of the massage period (40 minutes or less), the subject was given VAS posttest 1 on a separate sheet of paper. She marked on the VAS the amount of pain she experienced while using the ice massage on the right hand and the left hand. At the end of the intervention, the investigator taught a family member how to continue the ice massage if the study participant desired.

Posttest 2, the ranked MPQ designed to measure memory of pain, was completed by the participant within 24 hours after delivery.

Figure 6.1.3 Ice bag use at large intestine energy point 4 (LI4). Correct positioning of small ice bag for massage stimulation of LI4.

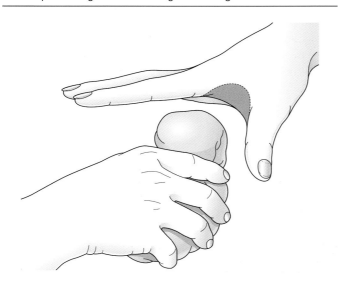

Results

Fifty-three participants were solicited for the study. Two women were excluded because they had difficulty understanding the concept of the measurement tool, one dropped out after reading the consent form, and one withdrew at her own request, leaving 49 women who completed the study. Twenty-nine were Hispanic and 20 were white. Their ages ranged from 16 to 38 years. Fifteen were multigravidas and 34 were primigravidas. Forty-one were dilated 3 or more centimeters; eight were completely effaced and 1 to 3 cm dilated at the start of the intervention. None had received any type of pain medication prior to entering the study.

The range of pain intensity on the VAS pretest was 10.0 to 86.0 mm, and the mean value of initial pain intensity was 61.53 mm. After ice massage, the right-hand mean value was lower (49.60 mm), and left-hand mean value was even lower than the right-hand (33.31 mm) (Table 6.1.1).

Table 6.1.1 Pre- and posttest 1

	Pretest	Posttest 1 right hand	Posttest 1 left hand
Mean pain response on VAS	61.53	49.60	33.31

Table 6.1.2 Memory of pain intensity scale

Mild	Discomforting	Distressing	Horrible	Excruciating
1	2	3	4	5
	2.33	3.27		
	After ice massage	Before ice massage		

Scores for posttest 2 for memory of pain intensity.

In a post hoc test of these multiples using Duncan's New Multiple Range test, it was concluded that the three means were detectably different. Although ice massage on either hand provided pain reduction, 46 participants felt less pain with left hand massage, and six felt less pain with the right.

The principal question addressed on posttest 2 was whether the memory of pain intensity, before and during ice massage, was different. Standard analysis was equivalent to a paired t test. The analysis of variance indicated a detectable difference in pain scores before and during ice massage. The mean pain unpleasantness before ice massage was 3.27, and mean pain unpleasantness after ice massage was 2.33. The verbal description of pain dropped from 'distressing' to 'discomforting' (Table 6.1.2).

Discussion

The study intervention ended on the completion of posttest 1. No attempt was made to monitor the participants' continued use of the ice massage or to change their minds about using medication. None of the participants viewed the technique as a tool to replace the use of narcotic or epidural pain relief. Three of the participants had cesarean birth, and several had labor augmentation with intravenous (IV) oxytocin following the ice massage. One participant had IV analgesia and continued to use ice massage administered by family members for 12 more hours until she was completely dilated. All of the study participants had good outcomes with normal Apgar scores.

Whatever intervention one uses, labor pains grow closer together and more intense. It should be noted that the ice massage was performed in the early hours of labor, and the effects may not be generalized to pain control later in labor. The convenience sample also restricts the study's generalizability. Other limitations are that the study was not randomized and the protocol precluded interobserver comparisons. Finally, interventions from another healing tradition (e.g., Shiatsu-based ice massage) can seem culturally foreign to Americans who may be uncomfortable using them. In this study, the application of ice massage to the Shiatsu energy meridian point, LI4, was a noninvasive, effective tool to help reduce the intensity and unpleasantness of pain from early labor contractions. It was more effective on the left hand for most of the women.

Over the years, the search for answers to controlling labor pain has focused on drugs that alter mental and sensory awareness of pain with noxious side effects of the partial paralysis of epidurals, the confusion of opiates, and the total absence of memory in the use of scopolamine. Midwife deliveries take place in homes, birthing centers, and in hospital settings where women may choose from multiple pain control methods. Dr. Reynolds[30] most astutely notes that most women in the world in remote and rural areas and Third World countries do not have access to medical procedures and drugs. Therefore, any technique that provides safe, effective pain reduction without serious side effects and that can be given by any health care professional is a definite advance. The results of this preliminary study suggest that ice massage of the LI4 may be in this category and can safely be added to the many other tools used by midwives, nurses, and physicians. Further research about this technique is warranted.

REFERENCES

1. Lowe NK. The nature of labor pain. Am J Obstet Gynecol 2002;186: S16–24.
2. Pasero C, McCaffery M. The patient's report of pain: Believing vs. accepting. There's a big difference. Am J Nurs 2001;101:73–74.
3. Budd S. Acupuncture. In: Tiran D, Mack S. Complementary Therapies for Pregnancy and Childbirth, 2nd Edition. London: Baillière Tindall, 2000.
4. Carlsson CPO, Axemo P, Bodin A. Manual acupuncture reduces hyperemesis gravidarum: A placebo-controlled, randomized, single-blind, crossover study. J Pain Symptom Manage 2000;20: 273–279.
5. O'Brien B, Relyea J, Tarerum T. Efficacy of P6 acupressure in the treatment of nausea and vomiting of pregnancy: A randomized blinded study. Obstet Gynecol 1996;174:708–715.
6. Cardini F, Weixin H. Moxibustion for correction of breech presentation: A randomized controlled trial. J Am Med Assoc 1998; 280(18):1540–1544.
7. Allaire AD. Complementary and alternative medicine in the labor and delivery suite. Clin Obstet Gynecol 2001;44:681–691.
8. Pasero C, McCaffery M. Using superficial cooling for pain relief. Am J Nurs 1999;99:24.

9. Denny-Brown D, Adams RD, Brenner C. The pathology of injury to nerve induced by cold. J Neuropath Exp Neurol 1945;4:305–323.

10. Grant AE. Massage with ice (cryokinetics) in the treatment of painful conditions of musculoskeletal system. Arch Phys Med 1964;45:233–238.

11. Marshall CM. The use of ice cube massage for the relief of chronic pain following herpes ophthalmicus. Physiotherapy 1971;57:374.

12. Melzack R. Relief of dental pain by ice massage of the hand. Can Med Assoc 1980;122:189–91.

13. Melzack R. Relief of dental pain by ice massage of either hand or the contralateral arm. Can Dental Assoc 1983;49:257–60.

14. Melzack R, Wall P. Pain mechanisms: A new theory. Science 1965;150(3699):971–978.

15. Melzack R, Stillwell DM, Fox EJ. Trigger points and acupuncture points for pain: Correlations and implications. Pain 1977;3:3–23.

16. deLangre J. Second Book of Do-In Art of Rejuvenation Through Self-Massage. Maglia (CA): Happiness Press Books, 1974.

17. Cowmeadow O. Shiatsu: A Practical Introduction. Boston (MA): Element Inc., 1998.

18. Erskine A, Morley S, Pearce S. Memory for pain: A review. Pain 1990;41:255–265.

19. Waters B. Ice Massage for the Reduction of Labor Pain. Monograph: Professional Papers, Australia/America Nurses Exchange, 1. St. Louis (MO): Barnes College Press, 1992.

20. Burns N, Grove SK. The Practice of Nursing Research: Conduct, Critique and Utilization. Philadelphia: Saunders, 2001.

21. Bodian CA, Freedman G, Hossain S. The visual analog scale for pain: Clinical significance in postoperative patients. Anesthesiology 2001;95(6):1356–1361.

22. Dexter F, Chestnut DH. Analysis of statistical tests to compare visual analog scale measurements among groups. Anesthesiology 1995;82(4):896–902.

23. Steel RGD, Torrie JH, Dickey DA. Principles and Procedures of Statistics: A Biometrical Approach, 3rd Edition. New York: McGraw-Hill Companies, Inc., 1997:201.

24. Melzack R. The McGill Pain Questionnaire: Major properties and scoring methods. Pain 1975;1:277–299.

25. Towery S, Fernandez E. Reclassification and rescaling of McGill Pain Questionnaire verbal descriptors of pain sensation: A replication. Clin J Pain 1996;12(4):270–276.

26. Steel RGD, Torrie JH, Dickey DA. Principles and Procedures of Statistics: A Biometrical Approach, 3rd Edition. New York: McGraw-Hill Companies, Inc., 1997:194.

27. Niven C, Murphy-Black T. Memory for labor pain: A review of the literature. Birth 2000;27(4):244–253.

28. Albers L. Midwifery management of pain. J Nurse Midwifery 1998;43:77–82.

29. Gray H. Gray's Anatomy, 29th Edition. Philadelphia: Lea & Febiger, 1973:1099–1100.

30. Reynold JL. Sterile water injections relieve back pain of labor birth. 2000;27(1):58–60.

Journal of Midwifery & Women's Health 2003; 48(5): 317–321

(Reprinted with permission from Journal of Midwifery & Women's Health)

Float like a butterfly . . . yoga and birth

Nerissa Fields

Yoga is a way of working with the mind and the body with the breath as the link. When you take your arm up you breathe in; when you take your arm down you breathe out. Another of the beauties of yoga is that it is non-competitive – it adapts to the needs of the individual. Yoga is often portrayed in the media as something that is not accessible to the majority: people standing on one leg with the other behind their neck; individuals in all sorts of positions that are only really appropriate if you are very supple; people jumping in and out of postures or sitting around meditating. That is yoga, but only one small aspect of it. You do not have to be young, fit, slim, healthy and supple to be able to practise yoga. You just need to find a good teacher who can adapt to your individual needs.

Yoga is mental, physical, emotional, spiritual. It does keep you fit, but as a whole person. It is not a religion; it is appropriate to those with religious beliefs and to those with none. It is a way of working with the whole person, and to some it becomes an approach to life. Yoga is practical, basic and down-to-earth, and can thus fit into our everyday life.

I teach a wide variety of groups, specialising both in pregnancy and in learning disabilities. In the latter area I work with students who have PMLD (profound and multiple learning disabilities) using yoga and aromatherapy. So if yoga can work in this area, it can work in any.

Ideal for pregnancy and labour

I run three Yoga for Pregnancy classes a week through the WEA in Leicester in term time. My classes are always full, with a waiting list, so when one woman gives birth another quickly steps in to take her place. The nature of the class is that we work on yoga movements that are beneficial while pregnant, and also on yoga movements and birth positions that might be useful in labour (explained below).

We also take time out to talk: discussion in pregnancy is so important. It is good for pregnant women to be with each other and also to be in touch with other mothers after the baby is born. We talk about whatever comes up, from fears and anxieties about the birth to various aches and pains and down-to-earth practicalities. I find this part of the session is just as important as when we are practising yoga.

I also show videos of a variety of births, as well as on breastfeeding, and postnatal depression if women are interested. Every term, women from the previous term come in with their babies and give us a blow-by-blow account of their birth. I usually ask women who have had very different births to come in so that we can hear a range of experiences. The dynamics of the group vary. Some groups continue to meet up afterwards – often for years.

I also run Saturday sessions with women and their birthing partners, focusing on how the woman and her partner can work together in pregnancy to prepare for the birth and the practical role that a birthing partner can play in labour.

Holistic approach

Yoga for pregnant women is a holistic approach, respecting the whole woman mentally, physically and emotionally.

Yoga uses the mind, body and breath to prepare us for birth – and for dealing with any eventuality.

Practising yoga while pregnant does not guarantee a perfect birth. Events can happen in labour that are out of our control, whether it is the cervix failing to dilate or not dilating enough, or a hand on the baby's head or the baby being distressed, and so forth. We therefore need to be very well prepared so as to be able to deal with whatever happens. We wouldn't climb Everest or run a marathon without preparation. That is what we are doing when practising yoga in pregnancy – preparing ourselves to handle any eventuality.

From a mental point of view, we are working on concentration, on being focused, as well as on having an open mind. We need to be clear about what type of birth we want and to go on to prepare for that birth, but always keeping an open mind.

In labour we need to work on the approach of 'letting go', 'opening up': this, combined with the breath, is a mental, physical and emotional approach. It is our birth, our baby, our labour – every birth is a one-off creative experience.

From about 34/35 weeks it is a good idea to be able to take ourselves inside, like a tortoise going inside her shell, and prepare for the birth from an internal perspective. Giving birth is not just a physical experience but a total experience, and thus it is essential to be well prepared from every point of view. Once in labour, it is important to be able to focus on the baby and on the birth in a positive, constructive and creative way.

Balancing act

Emotionally, we are working with balance while pregnant and taking that into labour so that we can be balanced and in control. Our hormones have a great deal to answer for, from the onset of menstruation to the other side of the menopause – pregnancy is no exception. Our hormones can be totally out of balance in pregnancy, and that is one of the many aspects yoga helps to deal with – bringing about that sense of balance.

However, physically (and we must be careful not to separate the physical, the mental and the emotional – these three go together) yoga helps us to stretch, strengthen and tone the whole body. Even if a woman is going to have an elective caesarean, practising yoga is still beneficial. We use yoga movements that are useful in pregnancy, and work with a variety of symptoms with which women present, from backache, sciatica, cramp and varicose veins to oedema, insomnia and heartburn. The yoga movements are adapted to the needs of the individual, taking every woman's specific requirements into account and adapting them as appropriate.

The movements

There are a whole variety of yoga movements that I find really useful in pregnancy. The muscles we use in labour are the quadriceps, the abdominals, the lower back and the whole of the pelvic area. So, although we are working with the whole body, many of the movements that we use focus on keeping this part of the body well stretched, strengthened, toned and thus able to be mobile. This includes movements such as the cat, the butterfly, pelvic tilts and pelvic floor exercises. I also have a Seven Way Stretch, both seated and standing, which I have devised for pregnant women. This includes stretching the spine upwards, a gentle sidebend, a gentle twist and a gentle backward and forward bend.

We look, too, at movements that may be useful in labour – and I say 'may' because we do not know what will be useful until the day comes. We practise many movements that include rocking and rotating the hips while in an all-fours position, kneeling, standing with or without the wall or using a chair or working with a partner for support. We also practise a whole variety of birthing positions; again, we do not know what we will want to use in that second stage of labour until the time comes. However, experimenting with a variety of postures means that we are familiar with lots of possibilities.

What is important is that women should have the choice in labour to move their body in whatever way feels comfortable and right at the time, working ideally in a way that is upright, forward and allows them to be mobile. It is important, too, to find postures to rest in that keep to the concept of being upright, forward and mobile – for example, resting against the bed or chair in the kneeling position (a partner can be sitting on the chair or on the bed and even be massaging the neck and shoulders), sitting astride a chair leaning forwards or just resting forwards over a beanbag or birthing ball. I say to women that if they lie down they might find that they never get up again!

Learning to breathe

What is really key in pregnancy and labour is the breath. This is fundamental in yoga. What we want in labour is for the breath to be comfortable, to be free-flowing, in unison with the body – mind, body, breath and contraction working together. We need to be able to breathe through the contractions and to have control over the breath. The breath is what will see us through any eventuality, whether we have a wonderful active birth, or need a ventouse, forceps or emergency caesarean – or even lose control. If we lose control we can regain it. Working with and having control over the breath is the key to staying in control.

Generally, when we teach and practise yoga, we are breathing in through the nose and out through the nose. In labour we will probably find that we want to breathe in through the nose but sigh our breath out through the mouth. It is therefore important in pregnancy to work on a whole variety of breathing exercises that give us control over our breath. Many women come to yoga when pregnant with no prior experience at all and have to learn how to breathe. All the breathing exercises practised while pregnant are the foundation for breathing in labour.

Relax!

We are all superwomen. We do everything – run the home, do a demanding job, look after children, etc, etc . . . What is rest? In yoga we work on relaxation techniques that let go of the whole of the body. It is thus important not only to get the right amount of appropriate exercise but also the right amount of rest. I can't emphasise enough how important this is.

Relaxation is fundamental while pregnant. I believe that women are still having as many 'prem' babies as ever, and one of the reasons is that they do not take enough rest and work right to the end of their pregnancy. They give up work at 35/36 weeks, thinking they have a few weeks left before the birth – and then go into labour! Last term, one woman went into labour while still at work at 35 weeks.

A spiritual experience

Finally – and this is one of the most important aspects both of yoga and of pregnancy – there is the spiritual aspect of being pregnant, of carrying this very important life. A pregnant woman needs to be in touch with her baby, to be aware of this being inside her, to be able to reach inside offering security, warmth, love. That has to be the underlying element of both pregnancy and birth. This is just the beginning of a new life for both mother and child – a new and very special path.

The role of the midwife in this new and special path is absolutely fundamental. She can be reassuring in pregnancy or even make a pregnant mother anxious. Being a midwife is one of the most powerful jobs in the hospital and in the community. It is a great pity, both for midwives and for pregnant women, that a pregnant woman does not have the same midwife or same team (though the latter does happen in some areas) in pregnancy, in labour and afterwards.

What the midwife says to a pregnant mum can have far-reaching effects: comments such as 'too small for dates,' 'too large for dates,' 'you have put on too much weight,' 'you have not put on enough weight,' 'it is important to sleep on the left side' can all cause anxiety. All these points are important but, as comedians know, 'it's the way you tell 'em'. There are some wonderful midwives from heaven who take into account how even the strongest and most dynamic of women can become very vulnerable and emotional while pregnant. This carries through to labour; women need to forget about dignity and to get in touch with their inner self, their primal self and feel free and confident to be however they want. They need the support of their midwife, and if labour doesn't go to plan they need that continued support and medical aid as well.

A personal choice

Giving birth is a one-off, creative experience, and women need to have as much control as they want. Some choose not to have an active birth, some want or need to have a caesarean, some choose an active birth and it may or may not go to plan. Whichever choice she makes it is her choice with the support of those around her. As I say to pregnant women over and over again: 'It is your birth, your baby, your labour.'

It is a privilege and a joy to work with pregnant women. As a yoga teacher it is also very important to me to join with other professionals in this area, complementing and supporting each other's work. It is a wonderful way to earn a living!

RESOURCES

Nerissa's video, 'Yoga for pregnancy and childbirth', costs £15.99 (+ £2 p&p) and is available from: Yoga with Nerissa, 30 Cambridge Street, Leicester LE3 0JP.

You can also order the video online: *www.yogawithnerissa.co.uk*

The Practising Midwife 2005; 8(1): 22–25

Giving birth on the beach: hypnosis and psychology

Sue Spencer

Imagine a distressed, labouring woman turning to you and saying, 'Just keep reminding me of my special beach, and I'll be fine.' It sounds ridiculous. Nevertheless, the image of that beach, real or imaginary, will do two things. It will give her a boost of positive energy, and focus her mind on dealing with her bodily sensations. She will continue to give birth to her baby with renewed strength and confidence. This woman will have learnt how to use hypnosis during labour.

Hypnosis is rapidly becoming a popular and effective way to prepare for childbirth, and there is a growing recognition of the importance of the psychological side of childbearing. Perinatal mental health is becoming a prominent area of concern for health professionals (Currid 2004).

For decades, the emphasis has been on the physical aspects of improving women's experience of birth, challenging the use of enemas and shaving, facilitating the most comfortable positions for birth and making delivery suites less clinical. Yet, recent research suggests that many women are still expressing a fear of childbirth, both before and after they have experienced it. Kitzinger (2001) likens the after-effects of a bad birth experience to post-traumatic stress disorder (PTSD), a term more commonly used to describe war-traumatised soldiers.

Why the fear?

What is going on? Childbirth has never been safer in the Western world. Women are bombarded with advice about the physical ways to prepare their bodies, such as good diet, moderate exercise and care of their pelvic floor. They can also gain in-depth knowledge of the physiological birth process through the copious amount of information available, from health providers, books, magazines and the internet. In addition, pain relief options have never been so comprehensive, ranging from good old gas and air to self-administered mobile epidurals.

While women need to know what to expect physically, all of my studies and experiences have produced a strong belief in the importance of a woman's psychological approach, or attitude, towards childbirth. It has an enormous influence on the way she will perceive it at the time, and come to terms with it afterwards. This holds true whether it is a home birth with candles or a high-tech one with all the extra 'e's, such as electronic fetal monitoring, epidurals and episiotomies, or an unexpected or planned caesarean section.

Using a combination of hypnosis and psychological techniques, I developed the consultancy Birthpsyche to help women confront and minimise their fears surrounding childbirth. So, what exactly is hypnosis and how can it help? In today's climate of evidence-based care and informed choice, are there any research results showing benefits?

What is hypnosis all about?

Some people think of hypnosis as a 'mind over matter' state, and this has been illustrated not just by tales of fire-walking yogis but also more recently in research on the self-regulation of blood pressure (Yen et al 1996). In 1840, the surgeon James Esdaile operated on his patients using 'mesmeric sleep' (hypnosis) for anaesthesia. However, it took until 1955 for support to come from the British Medical Association for the teaching of the therapeutic use of hypnosis in medicine.

The key elements of hypnosis are:

- Achievement of physical and mental relaxation
- Focusing the mind
- Accessing deep inner resources of strength and confidence
- Tapping into a belief in your abilities
- Suspension of conscious thoughts/beliefs.

When used for giving birth, it is the ability to reduce the fear, tension and pain cycle that is the most important aspect of hypnosis. Under the guidance of a therapist, a woman can safely learn coping skills for childbirth while in a deeply relaxed state. Gradually, and with the use of positive images and mental rehearsals, the woman can begin to accept the reality of birth and feel ready to cope with whatever happens. She can rehearse her personal coping skills and imagery to deal with contractions. Techniques for self-hypnosis can be learnt from a CD or tape, or from personal sessions with her therapist. Either way, the woman will increase her confidence in her birthing abilities.

Are there any contraindications?

The National Register of Hypnotherapists and Psychotherapists (NRHP) (2004) says:

A properly qualified practitioner will take a client's full medical, emotional and social history before deciding on a treatment strategy. There are some instances where the use of hypnosis is not recommended, or where it should be used only with care. These include epilepsy, recent electro-convulsive therapy, drug or alcohol intoxication and heart or breathing problems.

Research findings

A small study involving teenage mothers using hypnotherapy as part of their birth preparations found:

- Less need for anaesthesia or post-partum medication
- A shorter hospital stay
- Fewer babies admitted to special care.

Dr Paul G Schauble and colleagues note:

None of the patients in the hypnosis group needed surgical intervention, compared with 60 per cent of those in the non-hypnosis group. In addition, fewer patients in the hypnosis group experienced complications such as high blood pressure or vacuum-assisted delivery, opted for medical anaesthesia or oxytocin, or required medication after delivery. (Martin et al 2001)

In a Cochrane review, it was reported:

Women receiving hypnosis were more satisfied with their pain management in labour. (Smith et al 2004)

More astonishingly, a small study conducted by the University of Vermont College of Medicine, USA, evaluated the efficacy of hypnotherapy to turn a breech presentation to a vertex one. An impressive 81 per cent of the intervention group using hypnotherapy converted to a vertex presentation, compared with only 48 per cent in the control group (Mehl 1994, cited in Waites). It is suggested that the deep relaxation, facilitated by hypnosis,

played a major role in gaining the uterine space for the baby to turn.

A sense of control

One important benefit of hypnotherapy is the internal sense of control it gives the woman, once she knows how to relax herself and use positive suggestions. Feeling in control plays an important role in psychological well-being during childbirth. A woman's caregivers can also help her feel in control of her external environment by helping her into comfortable positions and understanding her preferred style of dealing with pain (Green and Baston 2003).

For some women, writing a birth plan gives them a sense of control over what will happen to them. Birth plans are loved by some and loathed by others. Choices about induction procedures, monitoring, examinations, pain relief and third stage management are ticked off as if ordering a meal or finalising the details of a longed for holiday, but they are rarely fully adhered to – for a variety of reasons. When the birth doesn't go as planned, women may either blame themselves or their caregivers. Emotions run high, and this can give a distorted view of actual events.

The bottom line

Midwifery knowledge and skills have increased rapidly over the last few decades, but large numbers of women are still experiencing a poor psychological outcome of childbirth. No matter how much 'planning' goes on, women can't physically rehearse giving birth. Hypnotherapy and other psychological techniques, such as mental rehearsal and positive imagery, can help reduce birthing anxieties and build women's confidence in their ability to cope with labour.

The research so far suggests that there will be an increased likelihood of more normal, straightforward births (Mehl-Madrona 2004). As more women become aware of the benefits of using hypnosis, or some form of psychological preparation for birth, then their caregivers will benefit, too.

Maybe you can join the women on their imaginary beach while they labour calmly and confidently! There will be less stress and more positive, triumphant births. This will lead to 'being with women' in the full sense of the phrase: as a facilitator, a guide and a trusted companion. Women will have every chance to feel positive about their labour – in both body and mind.

REFERENCES

Currid T (2004). 'Improving perinatal mental health care'. Nursing Standard, 19 (3): 40–43.

Green J and Baston H (2003). 'Feeling in control during labor: concepts, correlates and consequences'. Birth, 30 (4): 235–247.

Kitzinger S (2001). 'When a bad birth haunts you'. http://www.sheilakitzinger.com/BadBirth Haunts.htm

Martin A, Scauble P, Rai S et al (2001). 'The effects of hypnosis on the labor processes and birth outcomes of pregnant adolescents'. The Journal of Family Practice, 50 (5): 441–443.

Mehl L (1994). 'Hypnosis and conversion of the breech to the vertex presentation'. In: B Waites (2003), Breech Birth, London: Free Association Books.

Mehl-Madrona L (2004). 'Hypnosis to facilitate uncomplicated birth'. http://www.gentlebirth. org/archives/hypnbrch.html

National Register of Hypnotherapists and Psychotherapists (2004). 'Contraindications for hypnotherapy'. http://www.nrhp.co.uk/

Smith C A, Collins C T, Cyna A M et al (2004). 'Complementary and alternative therapies for pain management in labour' (Cochrane Review). In: The Cochrane Library, Issue 4.

Yen L, Patrick, W and Chie W (1996). 'Comparison of relaxation techniques, routine blood pressure measurements, and self-learning packages in hypertension control'. Preventive Medicine, 25 (3): 339–345. http://www.ingentaconnect.com

The Practising Midwife 2005; 8(1): 27–29

A time to bloom

Ishvar Sheran

Flower remedies are subtle, vibrational essences made from the flowers of plants selected for their natural healing properties. In modern times, the use of flower essences began after Dr Edward Bach discovered the well-known Bach Flower Remedies in the 1930s. Today, there are many thousands of flower essences available from companies such as The Australian Bush Flower Essences (ABFE), Flower Essence Society (FES), Original Bach Remedies, Healing Herbs and Crystal Herbs.

Flower remedies are prepared by sun infusion. Flowers are infused in water, where their energy is released by the action of the sun. This mixture is preserved in alcohol and taken orally. The dosage is generally four to seven drops taken four times a day sublingually, or four to seven drops in water sipped throughout the day. The duration of treatment can range from one day to several weeks. Generally, the longer a problem has been discernible, the longer treatment may be required to restore the positive state of health.

The essences work by flooding the body with the vibrational frequency needed to restore balance, harmony and health. In 1934 Dr Bach wrote that:

The action of these remedies is to raise our vibrations and open up our channels for the reception of the Spiritual Self, to flood our natures with the particular virtue we need, and wash out from us the fault that is causing the harm. (Scheffer 1986: 13)

White (1993) gives an account of how this process occurs. Once ingested, the essence is assimilated into the bloodstream, later entering the meridians (lines of energy that cover the body as described in acupuncture). From the meridians the essence reaches the chakras before re-entering the physical body. In this way, the entire energy field is bathed in the 'frequency' of the essence.

Most flower remedies treat disharmony in an individual's emotional and mental condition. Many physiological problems have their origins in mental distress and emotional upset, and flower remedies are used to treat the 'cause' rather than the external physical symptoms. However, some flower essences can generally be applied to certain physical states.

Flower remedies are considered by those who are expert in their use to be extremely safe (Greene 2002, Kaminski and Katz 1994). However, it may be useful to consider what this means in the current age of risk-based thinking. Flower remedies have not been 'proven' safe through scientific trials. Perhaps inevitably, there is little interest in, or funding for, such trials from the Western scientific establishment (Kaminski and Katz 1994). Equally, in the world of midwifery, there are widely used medical interventions that have also not yet been proven safe by scientific studies!

Where midwives are asked by women whether flower remedies are 'safe' during pregnancy, it may be helpful to discuss these issues and perhaps gently remind women that it is extraordinarily difficult to prove that anything is completely 'safe' at any time, and that all of their choices need to be based on careful consideration about what is right for them.

There are significant differences between flower essences and the more physical remedies, which can cause side effects. The active constituent of the flower remedy is the 'life force' or vibrational signature of the flower. Conversely, in herbal preparations the physical and chemical constituents of the plant are used. This difference may best be described as using the 'etheric' or emotional body of the flower as opposed to the physical body of the plant. Kaminski and Katz (1994) liken the effect of flower essences to our response to music or surveying a beautiful country scene. With this in mind, we can see that it is not easy to measure and judge the actions of flower remedies by scientific methods. We need new and creative approaches to evaluating the effects of vibrational therapies – which are as diverse as the effects of disease experienced by individuals.

Several flower essences can help women cope better with emotional and physical issues in pregnancy. Some of the remedies that benefit common experiences in pregnancy follow. The source of all the remedies is given to make it easy to locate them, and a list of suppliers is given at the end of this article.

Coping with pregnancy

With the enormous physical and emotional transformations that occur during pregnancy, walnut (Bach) is one of the most broadly applicable essences, as it helps an individual cope better with major change. For women who feel vulnerable, walnut or yarrow (FES) will act as an effective barrier to unwanted or unconsciously absorbed influences of other people or environments. These essences can offer protection to the pregnant woman in her increased state of sensitivity.

Both elm (Bach) and bottlebrush (ABFE) are helpful for women who are overwhelmed by responsibilities and feel unable to cope. Pregnancy, particularly first time, brings many new challenges, and it is easy for even the most capable woman to feel she cannot manage. Elm or bottlebrush will provide strength in those moments of weakness, and help restore composure.

Fatigue

Olive (Bach) and macrocarpa (ABFE) can help when a person feels totally drained and exhausted. For some women, there may be times during their pregnancy when they feel they have come to the end of their tether and are so exhausted that they cannot take any more. It can seem as if all energies are spent – physically, mentally and emotionally – and there may be a need to sleep continually. In such cases, these essences will bring a restoration of vital energies, and strengthen body, mind and spirit.

Facing difficult choices

Women are exposed to a plethora of advice and opinions about their pregnancy, birth and life in general. When there are important decisions to be made, and many options exist, it is easy to become confused. Cerato (Bach) is the ideal remedy to help resolve these situations. Cerato promotes inner knowing, and precipitates trust in one's own wisdom and decisions rather than relying on the advice of others.

Dealing with fear

Pregnancy can bring with it many fears about the future – the birth, finances and motherhood. As long as the source of the anxiety can be identified, it can be treated with mimmulus (Bach). Women needing mimmulus are often very sensitive and may fall ill as a means of withdrawing from situations they find stressful. Taking mimmulus will bring courage, and allow the woman to see things in perspective. For those whose fears are more acute and bordering on terror, rock rose (Bach) may be beneficial.

Chamomile (FES) can also bring balance and relax the nervous system at times of worry or stress (Kaminski and Katz 1994). Where women become over-anxious about others, red chestnut (Bach) can help.

Trauma

Rescue remedy (Bach) can be used in any situation that causes feelings of stress, anxiety, shock or worry. It is the most well-known flower remedy, and many women nowadays will have this around the house and may ask if it would be a good remedy for a particular situation. Rescue remedy is a composite of five essences that work as a whole to address any acute situation. While it is not a substitute for midwifery or medical care (if warranted), this remedy will quickly calm and stabilise a woman by harmonising and restoring the energetic systems of the body which become disrupted during trauma (Scheffer 1986).

I know of pregnant women who take rescue remedy when they go for hospital appointments, particularly where they are concerned that they may be kept waiting and become stressed. It is a good remedy for any kind of shock, whether this is the kind that happens to us at times throughout everyday life, or the kind that is sometimes brought on by women's encounters with the maternity services, such as during stressful screening procedures.

Physical discomfort

Morning sickness is one of the most common discomforts of pregnancy, and chamomile can help by releasing tension held in the stomach and solar plexus (Kaminski and Katz 1994). Wild potato bush (ABFE) addresses physical restrictions and feeling weighed down. It may be useful for women who feel restricted by their size, and women who are in discomfort because of frequent urination. Wild potato bush addresses the frustration of feeling encumbered by the body, and promotes renewed vitality and well-being (White 1993).

Bonding and relationships

Mariposa lily (FES) invokes the maternal instinct and promotes the feminine nurturing energy. Normally this will be naturally present in pregnancy, but it can be useful for women who feel unable to connect to or bond with their forthcoming baby. Bottlebrush can promote bonding between mother and child (White 1993).

Both women and their partners can take watermelon (FES), and this will help to create a bond between the couple. Watermelon also helps to create a positive attitude to parenthood before and after conception, and this essence is effective in reducing emotional stress during pregnancy (Keel 2002).

Conclusion

Bach intended flower essences to be a safe and simple method of home care accessible to all (Bach 1952, Kaminski and Katz 1994), and these remedies can be incorporated into women's lives and midwifery practice. At a time when natural healing modalities are increasingly popular (Larsen 1999, Tiran 2003), nature's gift of flower remedies is a simple tool that can help create holistic health.

REFERENCES

Bach E (1952). The Twelve Healers and Other Remedies, Saffron Walden: C W Daniel Company Ltd.

Greene A (2002). 'Bach remedies in palliative care'. Palliative Profile South Africa, 21 (March 2002): 6.

Kaminski P and Katz R (1994). Flower Essence Repertory, Nevada City, CA: The Flower Essence Society.

Keel M (2002). 'Flower essences and pregnancy'. Vibration Magazine, The Journal of Vibrational and Flower Essences, Nov: 7.

Larsen H (1999). 'Alternative medicine: why so popular?' International Health News, 93 (September): 1.

Scheffer M (1986). Bach Flower Therapy Theory and Practice, Wellingborough: Thorsons Publishers Ltd.

Tiran D (2003). 'Complementary and alternative medicine in maternity care'. In: Fraser D and Cooper M (2003). Myles Textbook for Midwives, 49: 919–933, 14th edition, Edinburgh: Churchill Livingstone.

White I (1993). Australian Bush Flower Essences, Findhorn: Findhorn Press.

RESOURCES

International Flower Essence Repertoire, The Working Tree, Milland, Nr Liphook Hants GU30 7JS, UK
Tel: 01428 741 5752
flower@atlas.co.uk
www.ifer.co.uk
The company stocks a huge range of flower essences from all over the world, including all those mentioned in this article.

Healing Herbs Ltd, PO Box 65, Hereford HR2 0UW, UK
Tel: 01873 890218
sales@healing-herbs.co.uk
www.healing-herbs.co.uk
Healinh Herbs are stockists of Bach Remedies made according to the original instructions of Edward Bach.

Crystal Herbs (Bach Flower Essences & Gem-Crystal Essences), 1D Gilray Road, Diss, Norfolk IP22 4EU, UK
Tel: 01379 642374
Info@crystalherbs.com
www.crystalherbs.com

Flower Essence Services, PO Box 1769, Nevada City, CA 95959, USA
Tel: 001 800-548-0075
info@fesflowers.com
www.fesflowers.com

The Dr Edward Bach Centre, Mount Vernon, Bakers Lane, Sotwell, Oxon OX10 0PZ, UK
Tel: 01491 834678
www.bachcentre.com

Australian Bush Flower Essences, 45 Booralie Road, Terrey Hills, NSW 2084, Australia
Tel: 0061 2 9450 1388 info@ausflowers.com.au
www.ausflowers.com.au

Flower remedy education

Midwives who wish to study flower remedies in depth will find further information on some of the websites listed above; a number of different types of courses are available.

The Practising Midwife 2004; 7(6): 26–29

Ginger: an essential oil for shortening labour?

Irene Calvert

In 1994 I read a research article about care during labour (Sakala 1988) and became interested that lay midwives in Canada were adding ginger to the bath water of labouring women. The author suggested that the use of the ginger appeared to relax the women and shorten their labours. I introduced this concept into my own practice and observed that it appeared to shorten labour by accelerating contractions and reducing the pain perceived by the women. In 1996 I decided to evaluate this area of my independent practice as the research for my Masters degree in Midwifery. A library search found only anecdotal evidence on the subject. This article describes the process of the study that I undertook.

The aim of the study was to determine the effects of the essential oil of ginger when placed in the bath water of a group of labouring multiparous women. The progress and the outcome for this group have been compared with the control group of women who were given the essential oil of lemongrass in their bath water.

In order to achieve this aim, the following hypotheses were developed and investigated in this study:

1. The treatment group will have a greater rate of contractions in a specific two-hour time period than the control group.
2. The treatment group will have a greater rate of cervical dilation in a specific two-hour timeframe than the control group.
3. The treatment group will have a shorter first stage of labour than the control group.
4. The treatment group will have a shorter second stage of labour than the control group.
5. The treatment group will report reduced pain intensity during labour when compared with the control group.
6. The quality of pain reported by the experimental group on postpartum recall will be different to that of the control group.

A further research objective was to investigate the possible side effects of the essential oil of ginger on the woman and her fetus/neonate.

The significance of this study was to have provided scientific evidence on the safety and efficacy of labouring in a ginger bath.

The pharmacological actions of ginger are diaphonic, antispasmodic, rubefacient and carminative (Lawless 1992). Ginger is known to inhibit the action of prostaglandins (Conroy 1992) and has been observed as having an anti-clotting action (Mills 1991). It also acts on the limbic system, which creates a feeling of wellbeing.

According to Tiran (1996), the actions of lemongrass are considered to be antibacterial, antifungal and anticarcinogenic. She also suggests that it may relieve heartburn, assist in the establishing of lactation and eliminate lactic acid during stressful times such as labour.

This research was undertaken in 1996; therefore, the references provided were current at the time of investigation.

Methodology

The focus of the study was to ascertain a cause and effect relationship between the variables; a quantitative methodology with an experimental design was chosen. In order to eliminate bias on the part of the midwife as well as the woman, a randomised controlled double-blind clinical trial was developed.

A power analysis was performed to determine the sample size for a full trial (58 women per group). The standard value of 0.05 for the significance level was set. Ethical approval for the study was obtained. The setting was a level two hospital in the North Island of New Zealand.

The researcher and other independent midwives recruited participants for this research. Women who met the selection criteria were asked to participate in the study during the antenatal period, the rationale being that a woman could make a more informed decision in this period rather then have her thought process disturbed during labour.

A general information sheet was given to the women either by their midwife or the researcher. Women could request further information from the researcher if required. Consent to participate in the research was obtained by the researcher.

Inclusion criteria

Control was maintained by strict selection criteria:

- A multiparous woman with a previous vaginal birth
- A singleton pregnancy
- Receiving continuity of midwifery care
- The cervix must be at least 3cm dilated prior to the woman entering the bath.

Exclusion criteria

- Previous vaginal surgery
- Major medical problems
- History of hypotension (soaking in the bath is known to reduce the mean arterial blood pressure)
- History of skin allergies (skin irritation is a side effect of ginger and lemongrass).

Randomisation occurred in the delivery suite, prior to the women entering the bath.

The bottles of herbal substances were prepared by a chemist using a random sampling method to obtain the numbers for the bottles.

Manipulation occurred by the experimental group receiving the essential oil of ginger and the control group the essential oil of lemongrass.

The treatment period

The treatment phase started on admission to delivery suite when the woman was in labour. The attending midwife would check that a consent form had been signed, that the woman still met the inclusion criteria and still wished to participate in the study. A vaginal examination was performed to ensure that the woman's cervix was at least 3cm dilated. The midwife then took from the locked cupboard in the delivery suite the next bottle of herbal substance. The number on the bottle was placed on all three data collection instruments as well as in the woman's case notes.

A standard bath was used which contained 228 litres of water. The bottles contained four drops of ginger and one drop of base oil or one drop of lemongrass and four drops of base oil. The chemist's rationale for these dilutions was not only to reduce the smell of the lemongrass but to ensure the substance was rendered ineffective once diluted in the bath water. When compared for smell by a group of health professionals, the different oils were not detected.

Once the woman was in the bath the content of the bottle was emptied into the bath water. The woman then mixed the substance throughout the bath water.

The women were asked to remain in the bath for at least one hour. The fetal heart rate was recorded every 15 minutes, and the maternal temperature and pulse every 30 minutes. The bath temperature was recorded prior to entering the bath and every time fresh water was added. All women agreed to undergo a vaginal examination prior to entering the bath and another two hours later.

The women all received continuity of midwifery care: this was to ensure that a midwife was in attendance should the woman decide to leave the bath, the fetal ejection reflex (Odent 1987) be instigated and the woman give birth. Women were not allowed to birth in the water due to the ability of ginger to inhibit blood clotting (Mills 1991) which could lead to a slight risk of bleeding if swallowed by the neonate.

Data collection instruments

1. Data collection sheet

This was completed by the midwife following the birth. The sheet contained demographic data as well as the information pertaining to the safety factors.

2. A visual analogue scale (VAS)

This instrument was chosen to measure the intensity of the woman's pain during the treatment period. The recordings took place prior to the woman entering the bath and every 15 minutes while in the bath. The final recording was 15 minutes after the woman left the bath.

3. A McGill pain questionnaire (MPQ)

This was used approximately 24 hours postpartum to assess the quality of the woman's labour pain.

All of the data collection instruments were returned to the researcher following the completion of the MPQ.

Statistical methods

The data was analysed using the SAS PROC NPARIWAY programme specifying the 'Wilcoxon' option. The Wilcoxon-Mann-Whitley (W-M-W) test was used to compare the contractions, cervical dilation, maternal and fetal heart rate, the first and second stages of labour, the Apgar scores and pain as indicated on the visual analogue scale and the McGill pain questionnaire, between the experimental and the control groups.

A chi test was used to test for an association between the treatment and the number of births that occurred before the second vaginal examination.

Results

The number of women who agreed to participate in the study was 47 (N = 47). The number who were randomised and finally participated in the study was 22 (N = 22). Due to the small sample size, the power to detect a difference between the two groups is greatly reduced.

Sample description

Factors that were considered in relation to their effect on the dependent variables are listed in Table 6.5.1.

Only four of the women out of the 22 research subjects had experienced a normal birth prior to participating in this study (see Table 6.5.1). The 10 women allocated to the control group resulted in nine normal births and one Neville Barnes forceps delivery (see Table 6.5.2). The latter woman had previously experienced a Neville

Barnes forceps delivery. One woman who was gravida three para two with a history of two Neville Barnes forceps deliveries had a normal birth.

The labours of the 12 women allocated to the experimental group resulted in 10 normal births, one Neville Barnes forceps delivery and one lower segment caesarean section for fetal distress. The latter woman had experienced a normal birth as a primipara. The woman who had the Neville Barnes forceps delivery had experienced a Kielland's rotation with her previous child.

The results as they relate to the hypotheses are presented below.

There was no significant statistical difference between the two groups in relation to the frequency of the contraction ($p = 0.6774$) (see Table 6.5.3), cervical dilation ($p = 0.3767$) (see Tables 6.5.4 and 6.5.5) or the length of the first

Table 6.5.1 Sample description

	Experimental group	Control
	N = 12	N = 10
Ethnicity		
European	11	8
Maori	0	2
Sri Lankan	1	0
Gravida and parity excluding present birth		
G.1.P.1	1	0
G.2.P.2	5	5
G.3.P.2	3	3
G.3.P.3	1	1
G.4.P.3	1	0
G.5.P.5	1	0
Previous birth		
Normal vaginal birth	3	1
Assisted breech	0	1
Neville Barnes forceps	2	5
Kielland's forceps	6	2
Wrigley's forceps	1	0
Unknown	0	1

Table 6.5.2 Type of birth occurring during the study

	Experimental group	Control
	N = 12	N = 10
Normal birth	10	9
Neville Barnes forceps	1	1
Caesarean section	1	0

Table 6.5.3 Frequency of contractions before and after bath

Contractions	Experimental	Control
Median per 10 mins before bath	2	2.5
Range per 10 mins before bath	1–5	1.4–6
Median per 10 mins after bath	3	3.7
Range per 10 mins after bath	2 – birthed	1.4 – birthed

Table 6.5.4 Cervical dilation of subjects before and after bath

	Experimental	Control	Both groups
Cervical dilation before bath			
Median	3.25cm	3.25cm	3.25cm
Ranges	3.0–8.0cm	1.5–6cm	1.5–8cm
Cervical dilation after bath			
Median	7.4cm	6.25cm	6.5cm
Range	3.5–10cm	3.5–10cm	3.5–10cm

Table 6.5.5 Increase between first and second measures of cervical dilation

Cervical dilation	Experimental	Control
Median increase over two hours	4.4cm	3.0cm
Minimum	0.5cm	1.0cm
Maximum	8.5cm	7.0cm

Table 6.5.6 Average length of first and second stages of labour

Stages	Experimental	Control
First stage		
Range	2–18 hours	2–18 hours
Median	5 hours 42 mins	7 hours 54 mins
Second stage		
Range	4–40 mins	6 mins–1 hour 17 mins
Median	12 mins	42 mins

Table 6.5.7 Number of sensory, affective and evaluative descriptors marked on the PRI (Pain Rating Index)

	Experimental N = 12	Control N = 11	P.value
Sensory descriptors median	15.5	19.0	p = 1.0
Affective descriptors median	3.0	3.0	p = 0.894
Evaluative descriptors median	4.0	4.0	p = 0.629
Miscellaneous descriptors median	3.0	4.5	p = 0.895

stage of labour (p = 0.5222). However, the length of the second stage of labour was considerably shorter (p = 0.0142) for the women in the experimental group (see Table 6.5.6). This result supports the hypotheses: however, due to the reduced sample size, the probability of committing a type-II error exists.

There was no statistical difference between the two groups on the visual analogue scale either before (p = 0.255), during (p = 0.964) or after the bath (p = 0.518) or on the MPQ questionnaire (p = 0.7663) (see Table 6.5.7).

Safety was seen as paramount for both the mother and the fetus/neonate. The maternal pulse rate, temperature and fetal heart rate were monitored to ensure maternal and fetal wellbeing, but no significant difference was found.

The Apgar scores for the experimental group and the control group were 9 and 9 at one minute (p = 0.1193) and 9 and 10 at five minutes (p = 0.3737), demonstrating no significant statistical difference between the groups. All of the neonates were transferred home or to the postnatal ward with their mothers. No reports of infection were recorded. No woman reported any reaction to the herbal substances.

Discussion

This study begins to address the lack of research regarding the use of essential oils by evaluating the effects of the oil of ginger when placed in the bath water of labour-ing women. The women in this study were similar in age and ethnicity. The three women who were not of European origin all spoke, and had a good comprehension of, English. The method used was a randomised controlled double-blind clinical trial.

There was no significant difference between the experimental and the control group on the frequency of uterine contraction. A difference was expected due to the increased frequency reported by Sakala (1988). Sakala's study was, however, not a randomised controlled trial, and therefore a cause and effect conclusion cannot be drawn.

Cervical dilation was classed as the primary measurement of the progress in labour. One of the requirements to participate in the study was that the woman's cervix was at least 3cm dilated. This level of dilation was set to ensure that the woman was in active labour and that the pains were not due to 'contractures'. This is a term used by Nathaniels (1992) to describe episodes of mild contractions that occur throughout the pregnancy but become stronger in the days leading up to the birth. The Bishop's score was rarely reported yet was part of the scientific protocol. The parameters measured by this tool can affect the rate of cervical dilation and the length of time spent in labour (Silverton 1993).

Women were not excluded from the study because their membranes were ruptured, as the risk of infection to the woman or the fetus does not appear to be increased when using a bath in labour (Eriksson 1996). No vaginal examination was performed on any woman with ruptured membranes until they appeared to be in active labour. In addition, both the oils used in the study have an antiseptic and anti-infective action due to the presence of the chemical aldehyde citral (Tiran 1996). Ruptured membranes can, however, accelerate labour (O'Driscoll and Meagher 1982), and could therefore influence the research findings.

There was no significant difference between the two groups for the length of the first stage of labour. In a review of studies related to the use of water in labour and birth, McCandlish and Renfrew (1993) found some studies suggested no statistical difference in the length of the first stage of labour, whereas others suggested it could be longer, and some studies felt that augmentation might be necessary.

There was no statistical difference between the experimental and the control group on the pain intensity as measured on the visual analogue scale. None of the women in the study requested any form of analgesia during the time they were soaking in the bath. On leaving the bath, a number did request pain relief: the most popular form was Entonox. The time at which the analgesia was administered was not recorded: therefore, how the effects of the analgesia related to the last assessment could not be determined. According to Gordon (1991), water acts as a form of pain relief: therefore, it is not surprising that some women required pain relief upon leaving the bath.

The sensory, affective, evaluative and miscellaneous descriptors used in the pain rating scale index of the McGill pain questionnaire were tested to determine whether there was a significant difference between the control and experimental groups. No statistical difference was found; therefore, the sixth hypothesis is rejected.

The descriptors recorded on the MPQ were almost identical to those reported in previous studies (Melzack et al 1981; Niven 1994), indicating that the quality of labour pain, for many women, is rated as severe.

Pain in labour is often difficult to assess; the degree of pain cannot always be determined by the woman's behaviour. Some women are very vocal and some become withdrawn when experiencing pain. This may be linked to the ethnic or cultural group to which the woman belongs (Bonica and Loeser 1990). Other influencing factors are the expectations of the caregivers, partner or support person as well as the expectations of the woman herself. Niven (1994) found that women who had experienced severe pain in the past coped better with labour. This was attributed to previous learnt coping mechanisms, which reduced the amount of pain perceived.

Hypotheses one, two, three, five and six were rejected. Hypothesis four was supported by the research results. The length of second stage of labour was decreased for the women in the experimental group (see Table 6.5.2). Due to the small sample size, a type-II error could have occurred and therefore no conclusions can be drawn from these results.

The research objective measured factors that related to safety such as the maternal temperature, temperature of the bath water and Apgar scores. An elevation of the maternal temperature during immersion can lead to fetal hyperthermia with its subsequent vasodilatation and hypoxia (Johnson 1996). To ensure this problem did not arise, the maternal temperature was recorded while the woman remained in the bath. To assist in the prevention of maternal pyrexia, the temperature of the bath water was also recorded.

There are many variables that can influence the type of birth experienced by a woman. In this study, only five of the 22 participants had experienced a normal vaginal birth prior to entering the study (see Table 6.5.1). This was surprising due to the parity of the women. Following this study, 19 out of the 22 women experienced a vaginal birth (see Table 6.5.2). What factors could contribute to this change? Was it continuity of midwifery care, the water, the ginger oil or a combination of all three?

For the women involved in this study, not only has it given them experience of the midwifery model and its use of alternative therapies, but consenting to the study has offered them a choice. It has empowered them to control part of their birth experience.

Limitations

A major limitation to the study was the reduced number of women who were recruited or agreed to participate in the study. This occurred as a result of the ethics committee taking six months to approve the project, coupled with the time constraints of a Masters degree. Some midwives felt they could not subject women to two vaginal examinations. Other midwives were reluctant to support the study due to the preference for using an alternative oil. It was unfortunate that the hospital midwives did not provide continuity of midwifery care, for this prevented them from participating in this project.

The study design presented as a problem for some women who had experienced a ginger bath in a previous labour. They refused to participate in the study as the researcher could not guarantee that they would be placed in the experimental group.

Due to the small sample size, the ability to generalise from the sample is severely limited. The probability of committing a type-II error exists. Given a larger sample size, the results of the study would have been more robust. This present study could serve as a pilot for further research.

Consideration should also be given to the values and beliefs of women and midwives in relation to the use of herbal substances and procedures such as vaginal examinations. However, a greater understanding of the research process by midwives would provide them with an insight into the necessity to alter one's normal practice in an attempt to provide evidence-based practice.

Implications for future research

Midwives use and recommend various kinds of oils to women for use during their childbirth experience, yet few of these practices have been evaluated – either for their anticipated effect on the woman or fetus or for their safety and cost-effectiveness.

No women or neonate suffered any adverse effects from the study. However, there is insufficient evidence to indicate that the use of oil of ginger in the bath water of labouring women is harmless. A further study with the recommended sample is required after amendments to the scientific protocol from issues discussed in this research.

REFERENCES

Bonica J and Loeser J (1990). 'Evaluation of the patient with pain'. In: J Bonica, J Loeser, C Chapman et al, The Management of Pain, volume 11, Pennslyvania: Lea & Febiger.

Conroy E (1992). 'The three faces of boran'. Soil & Health, July/August, 26–27.

Eriksson M (1996). 'Warm tub bath during labour. A comparative study of 1385 women with pre-labour rupture of the membranes after 34 weeks' gestation'. Proceeding of the International Confederation of Midwives, 24th Triennial Congress, Norway: 457–459.

Gordon Y (1991). 'Water birth: a personal view'. Maternal and Child Health, 16 (8): 431–34.

Johnson P (1996). 'Birth underwater – to breathe or not to breathe'. British Journal of Obstetrics and Gynaecology, 103: 202–208.

Lawless J (1992). The Encylopaedia of Essential Oils, Great Britian: Element Books.

McCandlish R and Renfrew M (1993). 'Immersion in water during labour and birth: the need for evaluation'. Birth, 20 (2): 79–85.

Melzack R, Taenzer P, Feldman P et al (1981). 'Labour is still painful after prepared childbirth training'. CMA Journal, 125 (4): 357–63.

Mills S (1991). Out of the Earth. The Essential Book of Herbal Medicines, England: Viking Arkana.

Nathaniels P (1992). Life before Birth and a Time to be Born, New York: Promethan Press.

Niven C (1994). 'Coping with labour pain: the midwife's role'. In: S Robinson and A Thomson, Midwives, Research and Childbirth, London: Churchill Hall.

Odent M (1987). 'The fetal ejection reflex'. Birth, 14 (2): 104–108.

O'Driscoll K and Meagher D (1982). Active Management of Labour, London: Saunders.

Sakala C (1988). 'Content of care by independent midwives: assistance with pain in labour and birth'. Social Science and Medicine, 26 (11): 1141–1158.

Silverton L (1993). The Art and Science of Midwifery, London: Apprentice Hall.

Tiran D (1996). Aromatherapy in Midwifery Practice, London: Bailliere Tindall.

The Practising Midwife 2005; 8(1): 30–34

Rebirthing birth

Anna Hewitt

The birth that has had the most profound impact upon my work as a midwife and upon my life in general is my own – when I was born. I discovered my memories of my birth, and how connected it is to my life, through 'rebirthing'.

Rebirthing

Rebirthing is an approach to personal development that uses specific breathing techniques to activate and enable the breather to access memories held in the body that relate to current issues. Rebirthing uses conscious breathing to open a connection between our conscious and our unconscious. The fact that we can breathe consciously or unconsciously allows the breath to connect the conscious and subconscious aspects of our being. Birth is an experience that most of us hold in our unconscious that can be re-experienced through breathing consciously during rebirthing.

Being born

I have re-experienced being born on several occasions during rebirthing sessions, and learnt how my birth has and is continuing to influence my life. I have re-lived my journey through the birth canal feeling extreme physical sensations and a complex array of intense emotions that seemed to be osmotically mixed with my mother's sensations, hopes and fears. I have been shocked by the harshness of my first touch, the brightness of the lights and the intensity of the sounds around me. I have also re-experienced perceiving with clarity what everyone present in the room was thinking and feeling. I have felt that my experience of birth led me to take on beliefs based on the way things seemed to be during my birth and my first moments in the world. These beliefs were made at a preverbal level and do not easily transpose into words, but I feel them in my relationships and experiences, and my expectations.

Rebirthing and midwifery

Rebirthing taught me on a personal, experiential level how acutely sensitive and perceptive newborn babies are, and how every subtlety of their first experience affects them. It showed me how much the way we touch, feel and think about a newborn baby influences their future. What I learnt through rebirthing led me to train to be a midwife. It is fascinating, and a privilege to experience and observe birth from these two perspectives. The knowledge and points of view of rebirthing and midwifery are mutually supportive and illuminating. In this commentary I want to share my insights into the importance of birth. I hope that through writing this article I can convey a sense of awareness, sensitivity and sensibility that will touch midwifery practice.

The knowledge that the physiological process of birth physically prepares a newborn for extra-uterine life is the main reason why most midwives encourage women to give birth naturally, rather than by elective caesarean section. Complications or interventions at any stage of the natural process can have far reaching physical consequences. Neonates and adults alike are, however, more than just physical bodies. In addition to priming our organs for activation and survival, the birth process instructs and can strengthen or traumatise our psyche, and enable our spirit to fully or only partially come into form. Psychological, emotional and spiritual effects are more difficult to quantify and qualify than more obvious physical trauma; there is less acknowledgement of consequences on these levels, although there is increasing acceptance of our holistic nature and substantial recent research which highlights psychosociospiritual imprinting of birth.

Historically, western psychology has presumed that the neurological immaturity of neonates limits the psychological influence of early life events. Freud (1959), did fleetingly consider that birth, representing an individual's first experience of anxiety, could be the source and prototype of later anxiety, but found this idea incompatible with his belief about the immaturity of the brain at birth. Rank, a contemporary of Freud, developed this idea, and came to the conclusion that not only anxiety, but the entire psychology of an individual relates to their birth experience (Rank 1952). Since, several psychologists and experiential psychotherapies, have presented theories that assert that the birth process has a fundamental and lasting influence on personality development, attitudes and behaviour. A variety of therapies, including rebirthing, have developed which recognise and seek to resolve prenatal/perinatal trauma. They report that it is possible to re-experience being born, and that doing so can have valuable results (Khamsi 1987). They offer comprehensive explanations of the influence of natal and prenatal events, but detailed systematic longitudinal research into the correlation between actual birth experience, personality development and birth re-experience claims is currently limited.

Studies into early intelligence, memory and perception reinforce that natal experiences are vitally important (Chamberlain 1998). Research documents that birth and prenatal memories are generally reliable (Mandler and McDonough 1995, Meltzoff 1995). Further empirical research is necessary for these findings to be incorporated into mainstream healthcare. Research based evidence is undoubtedly important, but I believe that examining the impact of birth from the experiential perspective gained through rebirthing could help us really feel the effects of interventions on the physiological journey of being born.

Birth beliefs

Most of us in western society have an underlying belief that birth is dangerous. Most of us were born in an obstetric environment, where birth has in a sense become quite safe, but where fear abounds. The focus was on delivering an alert and responsive infant and avoiding pathology and crises. The physical aspect of deliverance from semi-darkness to brilliant lights, from muffled sounds to loud noise, from warmth to relative coolness, was shocking. The transition was equally disturbing on an emotional level. Most of us were not calmly and gently welcomed. Our first moments were probably uncomfortable, panicky and confusing. Our first touch was deliberately stimulating and abrupt, not nurturing and sensitive.

How many of us live with feelings of fear, alienation and mistrust, with beliefs that life is a struggle, we need to protect ourselves, and if we show our vulnerability we will get hurt? These feelings and beliefs were instilled at birth, and then reinforced by mass thinking and societal conditioning. How many of us feel truly safe in our bodies, open in our relationships and at home in the world?

Rebirthing beliefs

Rebirthing is based on the idea that we can feel safe and happy in our bodies, relationships and in the world. It aims to release past trauma so that we can be free to live more fully. Rebirthing uses conscious deep breathing to enable us to feel how interpretations of our past experiences shape our attitudes to life, and how these attitudes are at the core of our current problems; fears, prejudices, obsessions etc. The awareness created through rebirthing can offer opportunities to reinterpret our experiences, change our attitudes and thereby change our lives. Conscious breathing can help us understand why we habitually react in certain ways, and give us the choice to respond differently.

Breathing is absolutely fundamental to life. The way we breathe has an obvious effect on our well-being. Next time you are feeling anxious take a few deep breaths and see how it helps you relax, or try breathing shallowly now and see how you start to feel a sense of panic in your stomach. When we breathe automaticaly or unconsciously our breathing pattern supports automatic or conditioned reactions. Through breathing consciously, our breath can support awareness and help us to generate our life from the choices we make in the present, rather than through conditioning or reactvity.

Generally when we are faced with overwhelming or painful events we withdraw physically, emotionally and energetically. To do this we constrict our breathing and contract away from the source of suffering. When we suppress our breathing to avoid suffering, we may evade and even forget the present time problem, but it is suppressed rather than resolved, internalised and held down by constricted breathing patterns. Many of us instinctively develop shallow breathing. When we are reminded of unresolved hurt, we habitually contract, breathe less and add to the contracted emotional scar tissue. Rebirthing uses the breath to help heal this emotional scarring.

Memory is retained in both brain cells and body cells. Experiences are stored in many ways in the body such as muscular tightness, body pains and inhibited breathing. A simple example of this is the way many people experience neck pain when they are stressed. These body memories, despite being mostly outside our awareness, influence our thinking, emotions and behaviour, and can be the cause of mental neurosis, emotional dysfunction and behavioural problems. For example a memory of being abused as a child may be stored as physical tension, and be triggered in later relationships.

Breathing deeply in the right way can activate cellular memories, releasing body pain and underlying emotions and memories. If you lie down and breathe as you would when you are running or briskly walking the energy created, which would usually go into moving your body forward, can be used to shift emotions and feelings stored in the body. When working consciously with the breath, energies held in the body start to be mobilised. A whole range of feelings, thoughts and memories will come up and the role of the rebirther is to support the process and the continuation of conscious breathing, and encourage the 'breather' to observe and move through the memories that surface, and not get further stuck in trauma or neuroses. The primary objective of rebirthing is to be free to live in a more wholesome, conscious and less reactive way, not dwell in the intricacies of trauma. This process of release through deep breathing is energising and revitalising. It actually takes up energy to hold memories down and live unconsciously and in denial. Freeing suppressed memories, feelings and thoughts can help us to feel more fully alive.

Birth: the most intense and consequential experience of our lives

Birth is probably the most intense, overwhelming experience of our life. We are thrust from a warm, watery, cushioned environment where all our needs are automatically met – out, generally into a cold, harsh, alien world about which we have everything to learn. Under the best circumstances being born is an enormous challenge, probably the biggest test of our lives. It tests us on every level of our being. The answers and conclusions we reach during this epochal event are indelibly engraved and form the foundations of who we become and how we live the rest of our lives.

At birth we are hyper-sensitive to the physical sensations and emotions, thoughts and beliefs that we encounter. Before we develop ways to screen out the incessant input that life exposes us to, we are hyper-conscious – having a greater conscious awareness of the world than we are ever likely to have again. To begin we are wide open, totally receptive and impressionable. Our first impressions are deeply imprinted, stored at an innate cellular level, and they condition our responses and reactions throughout life.

I have observed how specific birth events connect to certain life decisions, patterns and experiences. There are subtle and more obvious connections. Invasive interventions during birth have deep repercussions. From the baby's point of view, forceps and caesarean delivery are particularly shocking. I have noticed that those having been born in such extreme circumstances often create extreme and shocking life experiences.

At a concrete level forceps-born often have a tendency to migraines and headaches when under stress. At an emotional level those born by forceps frequently carry deep mistrust and suppressed anger. They may crave help whilst condemning themselves for needing it, and repelling any offers. They fear that they are unable to make it on their own, but fervently resent anyone trying to help them. They live out push/pull patterns – 'help me but go away'; having made decisions such as 'I need help, but help hurts'.

Those born by caesarean often come into their element in emergency situations or crises. They are often at ease with fast and extreme transitions, but have difficulty in processes that are gradual in nature and in completing projects step by step. They may struggle to do things on their own, and expect or feel they need others to save them. They may have a sense that they have missed out on something in life, and crave or be repulsed by physical touch having missed the tactile experience of passing through the birth canal.

People who were delivered by obstetric interventions tend to be either excessively independent, determined to do things on their own; or excessively dependant on help from others. The marker that these tendencies are trauma related is the excess. People born in a certain way seem to have made an extraordinary commitment to a specific tendency. People can, however, have similar births but make different decisions. One person may decide 'the world is a safe place' and someone else may decide 'everyone is out to hurt me'. The decisions are based on what they make their experience mean, rather than the experience per se. The connections between our birth experience and our attitudes and beliefs are, in reality, complex and variable but I have witnessed interesting generalisations relating to birth experience and life tendencies.

For example:

- Babies who were unwanted may tend as adults either to set up relationships in which they are rejected, or to make themselves indispensable so they will not be rejected again.
- People whose births were very fast often feel they need everything quickly, or they live with an underlying panic, feeling rushed and nervous.
- Those who experienced a very long labour may have a pattern of engaging in long, drawn out projects and power struggles; they may create their lives to be a struggle.
- People born prematurely may believe they are weak and helpless, or be extremely determined not to show their vulnerability. They may do things way ahead of time, or delay doing things feeling they are not ready. They may have problems with time commitments,

needing to be very early or unable to bear to be kept waiting.

- People who spent their first days in an incubator may tend to isolate themselves and have difficulties with intimacy, conveying to others that they can look but not touch. They often create a physical shield expressed as weight gain to keep them separate from the world, and dislike spending time on their own.
- People whose births were induced often have difficulty getting out of bed, in beginning projects and generally getting started. They can create circumstances where others do things for them, or push them or coerce them into doing things, which they later resent.
- Babies who maintained a transverse lie may grow into adults who are confused about their life direction and have an underlying sense that they are going in the wrong direction. They may live with a sense of misalignment between what they want to do and their survival instincts.
- People who experienced breech births have tendency to feel different, special or wrong. They may feel easily muddled, and that they do things the wrong way round. They often feel disorientated and have a bad sense of geographical direction.
- Babies exposed to drugs in labour are liable to develop drug or alcohol habits. The use of opiate-based pain relief can be linked to later heroin addiction, and inhalation anaesthesia with later substance abuse. They often struggle to live consciously, wanting to forget and remain unconscious about painful experiences. They may also feel a sense of emotional abandonment, seeking attention from others that they were initially denied.

Scientific research studies support some of the more quantifiable conclusions. For example Jacobson et al (1990) connected obstetric interventions and later self-destructive behaviour. Clearly, these generalisations are simplistic and far from exhaustive or conclusive, but I have observed that they often ring true. In my experience realising the source of certain tendencies has helped people come to terms with aspects of themselves they were previously unable to understand or accept.

Rebirthing birth choices

Rebirthing can help people comprehend why they attract certain life experiences, and why they react in specific ways. The aim of rebirthing is not regression, but through rebirthing it is possible to recall past events, including birth. Usually the experience initially is intensely physical and emotional. After physiological release, details, memories and pictures tend to become clearer. After

reliving their birth, many people have had their recall of details verified by witnesses to their birth. The most important thing is that what surfaces during a rebirthing session can lead to a deeper understanding of the subject's original responses and offer the subject the opportunity of reinterpreting the experiences.

What we learn from rebirthing can help us understand how we are creating the patterns in our life, how we have created our own limitations, and how we carry the responsibility for the choices we have made and are making. This is not about blame, guilt or recriminations. It is about accepting that we have attracted the events in our lives and that we can choose to stop letting our past traumas define our future. Rebirthing enables us to see the connection between past and current events and how we are the source of our experiences. Freedom comes when we take responsibility and are thus able to respond differently. The current societal concept of responsibility, particularly within health care, is linked more with blame, guilt and negligence and can lead to defensive and fear-based actions.

The role of the breath, the role of the rebirther and the role of the midwife

Have you ever noticed what happens to your breathing when you are anxious or frightened? How different it is to when you feel calm and relaxed? Have you ever noticed how people are breathing whilst waiting for a baby to be born? Are they all waiting with baited breath to see if the baby will make it, or channelling their anxiety into activity? Being present at a birth can activate birth trauma. Many people who are involved with birth develop unconscious defence mechanisms in order to maintain emotional control when their birth trauma gets activated. If we pay attention to how we are breathing we can become aware of all that we are feeling. Maintaining awareness of our breath makes us conscious in the present moment. This helps us act directly in response to what is actually happening, rather than through conditioned responses. When supporting a rebirth the rebirther must stay conscious of their own breath, as well as supporting the rebirthee to breathe consciously.

An essential part of all successful births is that the baby begins to breathe. Those present in many ways, obvious and extremely subtle, can help the baby learn to breathe. If everyone in the room is holding their breath and feeling afraid, the baby may sense this and become confused about what to do next (Frye 2005). The situation surrounding their first breath forms the framework of their relationship with breathing, and their relationship with life. Physiologically the first breath can be supported by the continual flow of placental oxygen. If the umbilical cord is left intact breathing can gently establish itself as the new source of life force. If it is immediately cut, the newborn can learn to breathe in a 'do or die' situation, accompanied by panic, pain and fear of separation. Early cord clamping alone may contribute to substantial birth trauma and a lasting inhibition about breathing. The instance of our first breath is imprinted in our unconscious, held in the conglomerate intelligence of the cells of our bodies; each breath we take is related to the first time that we breathed. Pioneers of rebirthing, Orr and Ray believe that the 'breathing release' associated with re-experiencing taking the first breath is the most important aspect of rebirthing and can release all resistance in life, freeing and transforming the breath mechanism and breaking the power of birth trauma over the mind and the body (Orr and Ray 1983).

The role of rebirthers is to support people to be free of their birth trauma. The role of midwives is to minimise birth trauma through their support. The support in essence is very similar though the approaches address birth from opposite directions. My involvement with both birth and rebirthing have shown me that the effects of birth are intensely complex, individual, and profound. There is a growing literature of research that illuminates the impact of birth and discusses the physical, psychological and social consequences of perinatal events. Anecdotal, clinical and experimental data are available. Two excellent websites – www.birthpsychology.com and www.birthworks.org/primalhealth/ – contain pertinent articles.

The concepts that I share are founded on my personal experiences. It may be that, as in my case, they can only be fully accepted through personal experiential validation. Actually re-experiencing their own birth could help those involved in birth support to become more aware and sensitive of the subtleties and impact of the birth experience.

If we feel how individually, birth shapes our physical capacities, strength and stamina, perceptions, expectations and beliefs – birth can be recognised as the basis of our relationship with ourselves and our relationships with others; we can see that collectively, how we are born shapes our culture and societal development, how we treat ourselves, each other and the world. If we accept the importance of birth, we see the importance of the role of midwives and how those who welcome a newborn baby into the world can influence the future of individuals, society and the planet.

REFERENCES

Chamberlain D 1998 The mind of a newborn. North Atlantic Books, Berkeley, CA

Freud S 1959 Inhibitions, symptoms and anxiety. W. W. Norton, New York

Frye A 2005 Holistic midwifery, Vol. II. Labrys Press, USA

Khamsi S 1987 Birth: etiological, developmental, therapeutic perspectives. Aesthema USA

Jacobson B, Nyberg K, Gronbladh L et al 1990 Opiate addiction in adult offspring through possible imprinting after obstetric treatment. British Medical Journal 301:1067–1070

Mandler J M, McDonough L 1995 Long-term recall of event sequences in infancy. Journal of Experimental Child Psychology 59(3):457–474

Meltzoff A N 1995 What infant memory tells us about infantile amnesia: long-term recall and deferred imitation. Journal of Experimental Child Psychology, 59:497–515

Orr L, Ray S 1983 Rebirthing in the New Age. Celestial Arts, USA

Rank 0 1952 The trauma of birth. Robert Brunner, New York

Topics for further reflection

- Some of the issues that Irene Calvert discusses in relation to her study of ginger essential oil highlight how much more difficult it is in the current climate to research holistic therapies than pharmaceutical drugs; this is a situation that may limit the options available to women in this area. Do you feel that holistic therapies should be treated in the same way as manufactured drugs as far as the requirements for evidence of safety and efficacy are concerned?

- A number of the other articles in this section cover therapies that are very difficult to evaluate within a scientific framework and, as such, they may be more difficult for some people to accept as valid. What do you think and feel about the ideas raised in these articles? If you find it hard to accept some of these ideas, can you put your finger on why this might be? If, on the other hand, you already see these therapies as valid and useful, why do you feel this is the case? Either way, does reflecting on these issues tell you more about your personal ideology in this area?

Life After Birth

The 'golden orb' of the postnatal period

A midwife's role in the process of integrating a renewed self story in a mother following birth

Sue Lennox

A time of opportunity that needs careful support

The first weeks after birth are a golden orb with woman, family and baby inside it. The size and strength of the orb varies but it can be fostered and its special properties made more conscious and enjoyable by an understanding midwife. For many women it is a time of opportunity and growth. But the orb is also easily shattered.

A golden period

The everyday and most common story of the postnatal period during my 20 years of self-employed midwifery practice is of a woman who feels good about her self and her mothering.

On the first day she is tired and elated, often awed by the sight of the baby and amazed by her own achievement. The expressions of love which almost inevitably follow for all who have been with her are happily expressed on the phone to family and friends. There is characteristically nothing reserved or conditional on that first day. This joyfulness is normal after a spontaneous vaginal birth and common even after an instrumental, ventouse extraction or caesarean section with epidural.

If the mother is at home or leaves the hospital within the first few hours she is able to breastfeed, sleep, eat and recover cocooned in what I call the golden orb: a protected space. This golden orb is protected by her family and friends through a process of increasing understanding of her vulnerability and the exquisite nature and value of this early time after birth. This is much more difficult if she is in hospital; because despite caring staff midwives it is hard for them or the woman's family to 'hold' the new mother in the same way as they can in her own home.

I work from the premise that women's construction of their story about their birth and the days which follow have implications for their future self-story and as a result affect their attachment to their babies.

Many women are secure and integrate their births straightforwardly but I believe the midwifery profession has a responsibility to ensure that we attend to the woman's sense of self within her everyday stories.

The stories which follow illustrate the midwife developing an ability to listen and to really hear the 'story behind the story'. Mostly listening to the story the mother tells about her self following her birth entails listening for signs that the experience has enhanced rather than reduced her self confidence. This enhanced self confidence in the mother is the key to caring for herself and others. Sometimes the midwife needs to use a process of reflecting back as well as listening. Occasionally problems arise and there may be a need to refer on for professional help.

Let me tell you some vignettes about how listening with this particular sort of sensitive ear to a mother's everyday story in the days and weeks following her birth makes a difference to the mother's life.

A story of the golden orb

As Ann and Jeff take their first baby, Anton, inside their house for the first time they are excited, delighted and exhausted. Anton is seated on the table in his car seat while Jeff goes out to the car to get the bag and Ann tries to sort out new baby clothes because Anton regurgitated on the way home. The baby cries, the phone begins to ring and then there's a knock on the door. It's a normal first day home.

As the midwife I rang to ask when I should visit. I had not been to the birth so when I called round Ann first updated me about everything that had happened. It all sounded fine apart from an episiotomy which I would look at later. Ann was full of praise for her caregivers and told a few funny stories about them as well.

I watched her 'breastfeed' and realised the baby was merely chomping on the nipple for 2 minutes. She handed Anton to Jeff because her nipples hurt.

Jeff was proud of his achievements during the lead up to the birth. The labour was not what he had expected but he managed to help. He was awed by Ann's strength and good temper. They were both tired but very happy.

I asked to hold Anton who was alert and needing feeding. I watched as Ann reattached Anton – this time with his lips further over the nipple so breast rather than nipple was being compressed. Anton looked ready to detach after 5 minutes and Ann thought that would be fine. I encouraged her to reattach him after a short break. We talked and he fed for half an hour. 'Ah,' she said, 'so I need to do this for longer and whenever he wants?' Like most women Ann didn't hesitate to do whatever it took to look after her baby.

When I visited the next day Ann and Jeff were having a cup of tea, Anton was asleep and this was the first time for 4 hours they had had a break. I was certainly not going to disturb Anton unless something in the story was concerning.

Ann was very pleased to see me. She wanted me to check her nipple to see if it looked alright because feeding had been quite painful and nothing seemed to be coming out. I asked about Anton's nappies and they said they had seen no urine at all. We broke open the back of a meconium-filled disposable nappy to find very moist crystals of urine. They were intrigued when I explained how the nappies are designed in this way to absorb moisture – and relieved that Anton had clearly been passing urine.

So if Anton was getting enough fluid why was he so disturbed? We talked about what is normal newborn behaviour in the first days and they began to relax because if Anton was doing normal things then they were prepared to cope with whatever it takes. I wondered how common this unconditional behaviour is at any other time in our lives.

As I visited over the next days they were keen to see me and talked about the preceding 24 hours. In a discussion in the first 4 days Ann told me how Jeff had changed plans to go in for a few hours to work in a day or two and instead had secured 10 days off work.

They had had a particularly awkward visitor the day before. Afterwards Ann felt weepy, and then Anton cried and was inconsolable for hours so they were all tired. Some cracks were appearing in the golden orb so they were taking steps to protect it. They were now using their answer phone instead of answering every call and the phone was turned off when Ann slept. Friends were being put on hold for a week or two while they just got a handle on this hugely demanding and fascinating experience of discovering and celebrating Anton and coming to grips with their new status as parents.

Ann and Jeff opened up to me as if I had known them forever. We shared stories about birthing and parenting but also about life in general. There was a sense of expansiveness in our new relationship; they trusted me and I nurtured their increasing competence and confidence with their parenting.

This quality of relationship is short-lived but significant while it lasts. Jeff went back to work at 10 days post partum and Ann waited for his return with great enthusiasm with the nights being easier than the days because he was there.

She now talked with me about her life before she met Jeff, their falling in love and her becoming pregnant when they returned from overseas where they had worked for 3 years. The birth was a complete shock to her – its power and her inability to stay in control – but she was relieved her support person and midwife were so strong and helpful throughout because it left her with a sense of pride that she was able to give birth to Anton by herself.

We also talked about her three friends who had all had caesarean sections recently and she couldn't understand why this was the case and now they had all had problems with breastfeeding as well. Her phone calls with these friends sounded difficult and sad as she said despite their initial delight and relief soon after the birth they seem frightened by their babies now.

The colour of the orb was beginning to fade as more of her social connections were being attended to and my weekly visits just became one part of the day rather than a huge source of reassurance and information. Ann integrated Anton's birth into her own life story and her relationship with Jeff was more solid than ever. I think she needed to be well supported following her birth to allow for this unique and absorbing relationship with Anton to flourish.

When finally I said goodbye I reflected again with awe on those first few days and that golden quality of love which birth seems to evoke in all of us.

Supporting and protecting the orb

Buckley (2006) in *Midwifery Best Practice Volume 4* described the hormonal basis for an altered state of consciousness in the first hours after a normal birth. The hormones oxytocin, beta endorphins and prolactin are enhanced by breastfeeding, skin-to-skin and eye-to-eye contact. Buckley explains that oxytocin catalyses feelings of love and connectedness and also explains how beta-endorphin contributes to the euphoria of the early postnatal period with prolactin helping the new mother 'to enact her instinctive mothering' (Buckley 2006). Prolactin is also thought by Grattan (2001) to have an important role in newborn brain development.

Midwives have a professional role to play in fostering and maintaining the special feelings women have immediately and for the first days after birth. In the antenatal period the midwife can suggest that the woman prepares by organising postnatal support. Buckley (2006) outlines under the categories of food, household and rest, suggestions for what Kitzinger (1991) calls a 'blissful babymoon'. This concrete help from family or friends in providing physical support in the form of child care, cooking and cleaning during the first few weeks makes an enormous difference to women's sense of well-being long term.

If the midwife has not been part of the antenatal period I have found that it is often still possible for families to arrange this help if it is gently mentioned at the first postnatal visit. The hospital lying-in time used to provide support during the early days and many people mourn its passing. Personally I find hospital postnatal wards infantilise women and I encourage early discharge if the birth happens in hospital unless it is necessary to stay because she is recovering from surgery.

As a result of The Baby Friendly Hospital Initiative and The Ten Steps, the midwifery profession is aware of its responsibility to promote mother-infant contact in the first few hours after birth (UNICEF 1991). We are less aware of how maternal confidence can be supported and enhanced long term. By celebrating and holding a special place for the mother within a family after the birth the importance of the mother in making the maternal–infant bond is underlined. The nature and strength of that bond is affected by the quality of the care the mother receives. This may be care from family and friends but it is also about the care the midwife gives.

The midwife is the happy recipient of the effects of oxytocin; the mother at times falls 'in love' with her midwife. When one appreciates the affects of oxytocin on the mother's sense of affiliation, this sense of 'being loved' can be enjoyed as a transitory projection rather than suffering a professional inflation of one's sense of worth as a midwife. Our role in this maternal projection is to send it back by acknowledging the woman's journey and to listen as she integrates the experience of the pregnancy, the birth and the new baby. When she smiles with contentment at her feat we know she knows how superb she is and, as Kirkham says, leave her with the sense that she is a woman 'who can' (Kirkham 2000).

Stories from the orb

The everyday stories of the postnatal period can sometimes be very important. Midwives' engagement with the woman's story may have an enduring effect on the mother's relationships after birth. The change, however, happens within the woman's story about herself.

About 5 years ago Mary, an ex-client of mine, left a letter in my box telling me what had happened to her following and because of my care (Lennox 2003).

I was stunned as I read Mary's story about how I came out one night to see her as a result of a phone call about her difficulty feeding. I visited her and watched her trying to feed. Little Abby would have none of it despite the fact that Mary had successfully fed an earlier baby.

I apparently asked Mary what had happened that day and her first answer was 'nothing really'. Then she remembered that her father had rung. She hadn't seen him since the birth and he rang to tell her a story about her brother. She was furious because he hadn't acknowledged her new baby or congratulated her for a successful homebirth – about which she felt very proud.

As we sat and talked Mary's anger began to abate. She fixed Abby on and the baby fed beautifully. What Mary had not told me until I received this letter was that from then on every time she became angry or upset Abby would not feed. Finally she began to address the internal anguish that she had held inside from a time in her childhood when her sister drowned. Mary had never been able to grieve for her sister but learned to bottle up her emotions until Abby came along.

Now she was writing to thank me for coming out late at night to see her and helping make the connection between her emotional states and the reason for the baby's reactions. Up until then her emotional states had been a complete mystery. She had learned how to bottle them up so well and as a result she was unconscious of her own life story. But Abby would not let her breastfeed while she was unconscious of her emotional state.

Being present to the social and emotional within the clinical environment as a midwife is challenging, however, the gems which emerge about the story behind the story make this work sustainable.

Midwifery supports the process of integrating an enhanced self story following birth

Midwives are in a unique position to offer something of great value to the woman, her baby and family, simply by being a good listener and understanding the importance of the story being told on the day of the visit.

It may be that what you hear 'is normal' or it may be something which comes out of left field and makes you alert to a sick baby. Like the day a woman told me 20 hours after the birth that her baby had been so good he had barely fed overnight and just grunted a bit. To look at this baby's face there was little sign of a problem but under his gown his heart rate and breathing showed a very different story. He was turning blue with an overwhelming infection by the time he reached hospital half an hour later. I think his treatment and successfully recovery owe something to careful listening to a story.

The common postnatal topics of conversations may seem to an onlooker merely concerned with functions such as breastfeeding, bathing or perineal and cord care. These practical aspects are important but they are at the surface level of good postnatal care; we also have a potentially privileged place in the on going development of a woman's life story, her future parenting and the baby's sense of connection with its mother. If this seems to be over claiming let me tell you a story about Jane. It shows how the story behind the story needs to be attended to if you are as a midwife really interested in mothering.

The story behind the story

Jane had a normal birth with her second child and I only met her because I was covering a colleague's births whilst she was away. Jane was very pleasant and undemanding. She was attempting to breastfeed for the first time since she hadn't been successful last time.

I feel very competent at supporting new mothers to breastfeed so I was somewhat surprised Jane was having so much difficulty until, just as she had reported to me, I saw her breast go bright red every time she fed.

I spent a good deal of time visiting her more than once a day to try and work out what was happening. It mattered to me that Jane got the help she needed to do what she wanted to do. She followed every piece of advice and was very diligent but breastfeeding was literally a trial by fire as her breasts flared up with each feed.

Finally when the baby was 2 weeks old she looked at me and said 'this is just not working'. Then she said 'I need to tell you why I think this redness is happening'.

What unfolded was a story of an old wound from her childhood and early adolescence which she had tried to ignore but which re-emerged each time she tried to feed her babies. She had been sexually abused by a neighbour but had never told anyone except her husband.

The discussions which followed did not result in Jane successfully breastfeeding her baby but it was, I believe, as important in its capacity to impact positively on her future and that of all her children.

What followed a lot of discussion about sexual abuse was Jane's horror of the effects that keeping silent had had on her life. She started on a journey of exploring her silence and coming into an adult sense of herself; reconnecting with her family from whom she had withdrawn many years before. Jane began a process of reclaiming parts of herself which had been left behind as a teenager.

When I said goodbye at 6 weeks post partum she was already a different person. The only way I can think to express that is that she felt more solid, appeared confident and sure of herself in a new way and this was merely the start for her of a new journey.

Where does professional responsibility and autonomy begin and end?

Being with, listening to, and honouring women in the postnatal period is, I believe, a very important part of midwifery. It is also a part that is often undervalued.

I sat looking at the old oak tree out of my study window and reflected on the conversation I had in relation to following up a complaint about a colleague made by a young woman on the 'complaints resolution telephone' that our local midwifery college branch operates. The midwife's position was 'If she wanted me to visit she only had to ring and let me know. I can't be expected to chase her up'.

The story was that the midwife had called to see Jill, an 18-year-old new mother with her first baby, a few days after the birth. But Jill was not home – she had left and gone to live with her mother for a while. The midwife had not been told this was going to happen – perhaps it had not been planned at all. Of course the midwife was irritated that Jill had not let her know she was leaving and wasn't there for the visit.

What I couldn't understand was why Freda, the midwife, didn't want to know what had made Jill leave where she was staying (her boyfriend's parent's house) or try and find out how she was coping. Freda felt such issues were not hers to pursue. This seemed an odd position to me – but perhaps I was being overly nosey and Freda's response was the more reasonable one?

Was the idea of autonomy and self responsibility that was being ascribed here entirely value free? Was the idea of maternal autonomy being used as an excuse for the midwife not getting involved – maybe for not caring? How much responsibility should midwives take for postnatal care? Is my sense of responsibility old fashioned? In the 21st Century are concepts such as autonomy and self responsibility more compelling than the murky concept of being 'caring'?

I have a sense that words such as autonomy and self-responsibility are being used as screens to withdraw behind – and they are described as being signs of having good professional boundaries. Is Freda seen as 'being professional' because pursuing this woman with the intention of finding out how she is would have been deemed to be interfering. Perhaps Jill's decision was an entirely adult decision of an independent and rational human act.

Concern about 'creating dependency' and the ideas and actions that diminish a mother's self confidence

Well, I could see where my colleague was coming from but it still bothered me. What Freda had done was shown Jill that she didn't care about how she was and Jill's actions had been interpreted by Freda to say the same thing.

Although I can understand Freda's frustration I believe a midwife has a professional responsibility to follow up in such a situation. When Jill rang our complaint line she had no idea that the midwife would have been put out by her actions. At the time Jill was completely absorbed in her baby.

She was in the time of the 'golden orb' but she wasn't feeling nurtured or protected. I don't think she would have left the address without telling Jill if she had felt held and protected within her orb. I think her behaviour showed how unsupported she felt. This time is about being supported and protected – notions of self-responsibility and autonomy do not sit easily alongside holding women within a protected space. The special nature of this vulnerable and uniquely loving and connected time is diminished if women are still expected to be fully autonomous and self-responsible. Freda needed to be more aware of how all-encompassing is the mother's focus on her baby at this time.

There has been talk in New Zealand in the last 5 years about not creating dependence in the birthing population. Midwives boast their women would not ring them after dark unless absolutely necessary. They argue this means that they are therefore offering a more sustainable and more appropriate service than those midwives who can be called out at any hour. There is a growing critique about the self-employed midwife pioneers claiming that they tried 'to be everything to everyone'.

Today's midwife with very strict boundaries is held up as the ideal. All women should be self responsible

individuals – and if they are not it is not the midwife's proper area of concern. Along with this model of midwife as the thinking woman's maternity provider comes a growing acceptance that midwives must share the care of individual women with other midwives, not too many but more than one-on-one. If we are to recruit and retain midwives we need models of practice that are more sustainable without placing unbearable demands on individual midwives.

I accept the need for change but in developing new models we need to be clear that the postnatal period is an exquisitely vulnerable time. It is a time when mothers are ripe for attachment – and that attachment is crucial. Midwives must understand, respect and support women in this time. They must not create dependence but they must be aware that this time holds unique possibilities.

By listening with a particularly sensitive ear to the woman's everyday story they may hear the other story emerging. In this way midwives, whether alone or sharing care, can enhance the future lives of women and their babies.

To fully explore the value of vulnerability, midwives need to stay open to the needs women express in their words or their actions. When midwives put boundaries around their work they must take account of this vulnerability. In this way they will be honouring the potency that the postnatal time has to enhance lives long term. Losing sight of the depth of our work with a shallow understanding of autonomy, responsibility and independence diminishes the value of the postnatal experience for the mother, the baby and the midwife.

REFERENCES

Buckley S 2006 Mother and baby – a good start. In: Wickham S (ed.) Midwifery best practice 4. Elsevier Science Limited, London

Grattan DR 2001 The actions of prolactin in the brain during pregnancy and lactation. Progress in Brain Research 133:153–171

Kirkham M 2000 The midwife-mother relationship. Houndmills,: Macmillan Press, Basingstoke, Hampshire, London

Kitzinger S 1991 Homebirth and other alternatives to hospital. Doubleday, London:

Lennox S 2003 Honouring the sacred in childbirth: a midwife's stories of women's developing sense of self [Unpublished as partial fulfilment for the degree of Masters of Arts (Applied) in Midwifery, Victoria University of Wellington]. Wellington: New Zealand

UNICEF 1991 The Baby-Friendly Hospital Initiative. The Breastfeeding Initatives Exchange [cited 2007 29 January]; United Nations General Assembly mandated to protect the children's rights]. Online. Available from: http://www.unicef.org/programme/breastfeeding/baby.htm

Let's ban water torture

Kate Jackson

I work in a large regional teaching hospital with more than 4,000 bookings a year. I feel moved to write the following on behalf of babies everywhere who are bathed by midwives as a 'demonstration'. I have decided to do this because of the location of my office within the maternity unit. It is right next to the nursery, and several times a day I hear the demonstration bath. It sounds like torture! So, at the risk of upsetting every midwife in the land, I extend this invitation to you all in the hope that you will reflect on these words the next time you are bathing a baby.

Alleviating anxiety

I always say to the anxious parents waiting for this event to unfold, 'Your baby will not cry when we bath him/her,' and I say this because it is true. First, I never bath a baby who is hungry or sleepy. Wait until she is ready. I usually try to get the partner in on the act if I can.

Next, I take my time. If you are in a hurry, don't bath the baby – do the urgent thing first and wait until you have time to spare. Tricky on a busy postnatal ward, I know, but make time. What is it you are busy with if not to nurture this new family and inspire them with the confidence to be great parents?

While the baby is wrapped up warmly with mum or her partner, fill the bath with really warm water. There are two important points here. 'Fill the bath': you know how much you enjoy a lovely warm bath right up to your chin, so don't put just an inch or two in. Sometimes I have water lapping over the top and I get wet and so does the floor – but it is warm and deep and the baby loves it. The other thing concerns 'really warm water'. No matter how warm the room is, the bath will be losing heat from the moment you fill it to the moment you put the child in, and we all know how long that can take. You can always have a jug of cold water ready to adjust the temperature at the last minute, but you will almost never need it.

Babies like a warm bath just as you do – so two inches of cool water will be the very thing to make her scream. Can you blame her?

Next, I tell the parents how their baby will love being returned to the element he is most familiar with. All his life, he has lived in water. Only a short time ago he was surrounded by body-temperature water, and he will love being back in it. What he might not love, though, is having all that space around him. So the next bit is really important. In a relaxed way, hold the baby firmly under his bum and the back of his neck and gently lower him in feet first. You can coo at him a bit at this point to reassure him that he is okay. When he is in up to his chin, let go of his bum and fold his arms across his chest with your free hand. You have him securely held round the back of his neck now and he will not get distressed because he cannot flail his arms around and frighten himself.

Explain to the parents that he will very soon get the hang of having space around him, but for the first few times he might not like the feeling of openness. Why should he? He was tightly packed into a uterus just yesterday. But of all the hundreds of babies I have bathed, they don't seem to mind having their legs free.

The bath is warm and deep, the baby is confident that someone has a good hold of her, she is floating in the most delicious way, and the water in her ears won't bother her – she has had water in her ears all her life.

At this point, I usually get mum or her partner to take over if they want to. Keep your voice calm and talk to the baby – everything you do will be taken in by these parents, who will either look forward to, or dread, bath times based on what you teach them without any of you even realising it.

Practice makes perfect

I don't pretend to be better at this than you – you are an amazing midwife, too – but I have just been thinking about the number of times I have done this and it has worked every time. I hear so many babies being 'tortured' in the interests of bathing, and wonder how they feel and how the parents can build on the experience somehow to get good at it.

It takes 15 minutes tops. When have you not got 15 minutes to spend nurturing your babies and parents?

One thing, though – I have never managed to ensure that the baby won't cry as I take him out and he cools down and is deprived of his lovely familiar element. If anyone has any tips for me about how to do that then I would love to hear from you. I have a lovely warm towel ready and some food handy in whatever container he gets it from and I do it as quickly as possible – but it still usually ends in tears!

The Practising Midwife 2005; 8(2): 46

Cochrane made simple
Topical umbilical cord care at birth

Tricia Anderson

What are Cochrane reviews?

The Cochrane Library is a regularly updated collection of electronic, evidence-based medicine databases, including The Cochrane Database of Systematic Reviews. Cochrane reviews, which first appeared in 1988, are used as a resource by both practitioners and researchers. For more information go to www.update-software.com/cochrane/

Fashions in caring for the neonate's umbilical cord stump have come and gone over the years in an effort to reduce the risk of neonatal infection. Care has ranged from topical application of antiseptic or antibiotic agents, alcohol wipes, drying powder, gauze dressings, bathing in antiseptic or not bathing at all, to simply doing nothing. A recent update in May 2004 of the Cochrane Review summarises the research evidence on this small but clinically important issue.

Background

Once the umbilical cord is cut, a small cord stump remains, made up of blood vessels and connective tissue covered by a membrane. This gradually necroses, dries, separates and heals. During this time it provides a potential route for infection into the baby's blood stream. In the developing world where the umbilical cord may be cut with unsterile scissors or razors, and substances such as cow dung applied to the stump, umbilical cord infections are the cause of many neonatal deaths, with neonatal tetanus causing 200,000 deaths every year. In high-income countries it is accepted practice to cut the cord using sterile scissors, and therefore cord infections are rare.

Different cord care regimes have an effect on the time the cord takes to separate. This has practical implications – a longer separation time may increase the risk of bacterial infection in developing countries. In developed countries this may have a financial implication, as local policy may dictate that midwives visit until the cord has separated.

There is general agreement that cutting the cord with a sterile implement and clean hands, and babies 'rooming-in' with their mothers (ie, mother and baby stay together at all times with no communal nursery), reduces the incidence of neonatal infections via the umbilical cord route. There is less agreement as to how best to care for the cord stump over the following days until it separates.

Objectives

This review aims to assess the difference between various approaches (antiseptic and/or antibiotic) to topical cord care compared with no routine care in preventing neonatal morbidity and mortality from infection. It aims to look at the difference between high-income and low-income countries, and to answer the question: is any intervention better than no routine cord care, and, if yes, which care is preferable?

The primary outcomes considered are: clinical evidence of cord infection (redness, swelling, smell), clinical evidence of disseminated bacterial infection (fever, meningitis, septic foci) and neonatal death. Secondary outcomes are: time to cord separation, bacterial colonisation and maternal satisfaction with treatment.

Studies included

Twenty-one studies with 8,959 participants were included. They took place from 1979 to 2003 in Canada, Israel, Italy, Norway, Spain, Taiwan, Thailand, the UK and the US. Most of the studies were small with groups of fewer than 300 babies; two were significantly larger with more than 1,200 babies (Norway and Italy). Nineteen studies looked at term babies and two at well, premature babies.

Types of intervention

Comparisons ranged between: antiseptic and antibiotic topical agents, antiseptics with no care, antiseptics with other antiseptics, antibiotics with triple dye, antiseptic powder with astringent powder, antiseptic with hydrophobic gauze dressing, daily bathing with one initial bath only (with soap, chlorhexidine or hexachlorophane) and daily cleansing with alcohol. Antiseptics included alcohol, triple dye, silver sulfadiazine, zinc powder, acriflavine, iodine, chlorhexidine and gentian violet. Antibiotics included bacitracin, nitrofurazone and tetracycline.

Limitations of the studies

The different treatments in the studies make them difficult to compare and interpretation of the pooled results difficult. The date the studies were done is relevant as routine hospital care for mother and baby, caring for babies in nurseries or rooming-in has changed over recent years. However, partial rooming-in was only practised in six of the studies; the rest had nursery-based neonatal care. Details of the individual trial quality were not provided. The majority of trials ceased at cord separation: any subsequent infections would not have been detected. All but two were in high-income, developed countries. The small numbers in the two studies that looked at premature babies limit the usefulness of their findings.

Overall results

More than 40 combinations of different antiseptics, antibiotics, placebos and no treatment were compared and assessed. Use of antiseptics and antibiotics resulted in less bacterial colonisation but there was no overall difference in the incidence of clinical infections.

None of the trials was large enough to examine the rare outcome of serious neonatal infection. There were no neonatal deaths due to infection.

Antiseptics versus dry cord care/placebo

While the various antiseptic treatments did reduce the amount and type of bacteria present, this did not impact on the neonatal infection rates. No difference was found in cord infections whether antiseptics were used or not. No severe bacterial infections or neonatal deaths occurred.

Antibiotics versus antiseptics

Less bacteria were present with antibiotics, but no clinical neonatal infections occurred in either groups in these studies. Cord separation time was less with antiseptics compared with antibiotics.

Antiseptic versus antiseptic

Many different antiseptics and regimens were studied, and none showed a convincing benefit above another. The overall rate of neonatal infections was low.

Cord separation times

Cords in the dry cord care/placebo groups took an average of eight to nine days to separate. Cord separation times suggested a trend towards a longer separation time with alcohol (up to an average of 16.9 days when daily alcohol wipes were used), but less when using antiseptic powders (an average of 5.6–8.3 days).

Overall, across all the trials, when nothing was applied to the cord stump the mean separation time was about nine days. With antiseptic powders this was reduced to about seven days. With alcohol it was increased to about 11 days, and with antibiotics or triple dye to about 12 days.

Maternal satisfaction

Three studies looked at maternal satisfaction: two found no difference; one study found significantly increased maternal satisfaction in the dry cord care/natural drying group.

Reviewers' conclusions

Studies to date in high-income settings such as the UK, where neonatal infection is rare, have not shown that antiseptics or antibiotics have any additional advantage for healthy term babies over simply keeping the cord clean and dry. There is insufficient evidence to reach any conclusion either for premature babies in NICU, or for the developing world where neonatal infection is far more frequent and severe.

Implications for the practising midwife

For healthy, term babies at low risk of infection, there is no evidence that doing anything other than keeping the cord clean is useful. This is likely to be particularly true when babies are either born at home or fully roomed-in with their mothers, as is now common UK practice.

Citation

This review should be cited as:

Zupan J, Garner P, Omari A A A (2004). 'Topical umbilical cord care at birth (Cochrane Review)'. In: The Cochrane Library, Issue 3, 2004, Chichester, UK: John Wiley & Sons Ltd.

Date of most recent review: 18 October 2004

STUDIES INCLUDED IN THIS REVIEW

Arad I, Eyal F and Fainmesser P (1981). 'Umbilical care and cord separation'. Archives of Disease in Childhood, 56 (11): 887–888.

Bain J (1994). 'Umbilical cord care in pre-term babies'. Nursing Standard, 8 (15): 32–36.

Barrett F F, Mason E O and Fleming D (1979). 'The effect of three cord care regimens on the bacterial colonization of normal newborn infants'. Journal of Pediatrics, 94: 796–800.

Dore S, Buchan D, Coulas S et al (1998). 'Alcohol versus natural drying for newborn cord care'. Journal of Obstetric, Gynecologic and Neonatal Nursing, 27: 621–627.

Gladstone I M, Clapper L, Thorp J W et al (1988). 'Randomized study of six umbilical cord care regimens'. Clinical Pediatrics, 27 (3):127–129.

Golombek S G, Brill P E and Salice A L (2002). 'Randomized trial of alcohol versus triple dye for umbilical cord care'. Clinical Pediatrics, 41 (6): 419–423.

Hsu C F, Wang C C, Yuh Y S et al (1999). 'The effectiveness of single and multiple applications of triple dye on umbilical cord separation time'. European Journal of Pediatrics, 158 (2): 144–146.

Janssen P A, Selwood B L, Dobson S R et al (2003). 'To dye or not to dye: a randomized clinical trial of a triple dye/alcohol regime versus dry cord care'. Pediatrics 111 (1): 15–20.

Meberg A and Schoyen R (1985). 'Bacterial colonization and neonatal infections'. Acta Paediatrica Scandinavica, 74 (3): 366–371.

Meberg A and Schoyen R (1990). 'Hydrophobic material in routine umbilical cord care and prevention of infections in newborn infants'. Scandinavian Journal of Infectious Diseases, 22 (6): 729–733.

Medves J M and O'Brien B A C (1997). 'Cleaning solutions and bacterial colonization in promoting healing and early separation of the umbilical cord in healthy newborns'. Canadian Journal of Public Health, 88 (6): 380–382.

Mugford M, Somchiwong M and Waterhouse I (1986). 'Treatment of umbilical cords: a randomised trial to assess the effect of treatment methods on the work of midwives'. Midwifery, 2 (4): 177–186.

Panyavudhikrai S, Danchaivijity S, Vantanasiri C et al (2002). 'Antiseptics for preventing omphalitis'. Journal of Medical Association of Thailand, 85 (2): 229–233.

Perapoch Lopez J P, Abizanda S S, Catala A G et al (1993). 'Colonization of the umbilical cord in normal neonates: comparative assessment of four antiseptic methods applied to the umbilical stump [Colonizacion umbilical en recien nacidos normales. Estudio comparativo de cuatro metodos de antisepsia umbilical]'. Anales Espanoles de Pediatria, 39 (3): 195–198.

Pezzati M, Biagioli EC, Martelli E et al (2002). 'Umbilical cord care: the effect of eight different cord-care regimens on cord separation time and other outcomes'. Biology of the Neonate, 81 (1): 38–44.

Rosenfeld C R, Laptook A R and Jeffery J (1989). 'Limited effectiveness of triple dye (TD) in prevention of colonization with methacillin-resistant staphylococcus aureus (MRSA) in a special care nursery (SCN)'. Pediatric Research, 25: 281A.

Rosenfeld C R, Laptook A R and Jeffery J (1990). 'Limited effectiveness of triple dye in preventing colonization with methicillin-resistant staphylococcus aureus in a special care nursery'. Pediatric Infectious Disease Journal, 9 (4): 290–291.

Rush J (1986). 'Does routine newborn bathing reduce staphylococcus aureus colonization rates? A randomized controlled trial'. Birth, 13: 176–180.

Schuman A J and Oksol B A (1985). 'The effect of isopropyl alcohol and triple dye on umbilical cord separation time'. Military Medicine, 150 (1): 49–50.

Speck W T, Driscoll J M and O'Neil J et al (1980). 'Effect of antiseptic cord care on bacterial colonization in the newborn infant'. Chemotherapy, 26 (5): 372–376.

Wald E R, Snyder M J and Gutberlet R L (1977). 'Group B β-hemolytic streptococcal colonization'. American Journal of Diseases of Children, 131 (2): 178–180.

The Practising Midwife 2004; 7(10): 39–41

Don't mention the 'B' word!

Jane Wallsworth

'Don't mention the "B" word!' I was given this advice by Sharon Breward, midwife and lactation consultant, as we chatted about a breastfeeding promotion session I was due to deliver to high school pupils recently. The 'B' word in question was 'breastfeeding'.

Breastfeeding describes the activity by which a mother provides the most complete nutrition for her baby. As Sharon pointed out, any emphasis on the breast is a 'turn off' for young women in Sure Start areas such as the one in which I work – Little Hulton, Salford.

Like many Sure Start areas, Little Hulton has a lower-than-average breastfeeding rate and a deeply entrenched bottle-feeding culture. Sure Start has a target to increase breastfeeding rates in the area. As the Sure Start Midwife in Little Hulton, I am working within a team of community midwives, other health professionals, parents and projects to ensure that more mothers and babies benefit from breastfeeding. Success is more likely if we avoid the 'B' word.

Images and perceptions

What is a breastfeeding mother doing? She is nourishing and nurturing her baby, and that is where the focus should be – on the process and not on the gland.

The words we use are so important because positive words inspire pleasant images and the message is well received.

Nursing mothers are giving their babies mother's milk, words that describe the unique quality of this sustenance and the special relationship between mother and baby. These lovely words evoke images of love, warmth and nurturing.

Today, we find such words quaint and old-fashioned, and use instead terms such as 'breastfeeding' and 'breast milk' – the focus being on the breast. We did ourselves no favours by abandoning the words of previous generations.

The 'B' word and the 'U' word

If we continue to use the 'B' word and call mother's milk breast milk, we should at least use the 'U' word and refer to formula as udder milk – after the gland that produces cow's milk.

Mothers who have just given birth could be asked (still in skin-to-skin contact with their newborn, of course) if they are breastfeeding or udder milk feeding. Ah, but we couldn't possibly refer to infant formula as udder milk. It's ridiculous: mothers would get upset and, besides, it is so much more than that – it is, after all, modified udder milk.

The formula manufacturer's advertising slogans would become nonsense:

'Take good care of your baby with X modified udder milk.'
'Y modified udder milk – closer by nature.'
'Z modified udder milk – because what you feed your baby now matters forever.'

If referring to cows' milk by the udder would be advertising suicide, we can see why advertising and promoting human milk by the breast has been an uphill struggle.

The female breast is a huge boon to advertising and will sell anything from newspapers to cars, but as a symbol of sexuality, not as a symbol of mothering or nurturing – and certainly not as a symbol of nutrition.

Wise infant feeding advisers recognised this by avoiding the 'B' word in slogans for the Department of Health's Breastfeeding Awareness Week:

'Mother's milk: the start of something special' (DoH 2003); and
'There's no milk like mum's milk' (DoH 1995).

Voluntary breastfeeding supporters were aware of all this long ago (hence the Nursing Mothers' Association and La Leche League). Health professionals have been a bit slow to catch on but we can make up for it now by ensuring that our words are well chosen.

The power of language

Does any of this really matter? Will changing our choice of words really have the potential to change attitudes and perceptions? I think so.

I can recall the first time I heard the term 'mother's milk'. It was 1988, my eldest son was almost six months old and I was due to go back to work. He was breastfed, despite being born at a hospital where – and at a time when – the International Code of Marketing of Breast Milk Substitutes (WHO 1981) was ignored.

I decided to wean my baby on to bottles of formula. This was harder than I had anticipated; to my surprise, he didn't know how to suck on a teat and didn't seem to like formula.

I asked my health visitor for advice. She did not suggest that perhaps I should continue to breastfeed him, that it would provide him with important nutrition and protection against infection (when he needed it most) and that the closeness and comfort of nursing would reassure both of us and help us cope with the anxiety of separation.

In fairness to her, I did not consider any of this myself, nor did any of my midwife friends. Living and working in a bottle-feeding culture had more influence on me than I acknowledged at the time.

The health visitor did suggest that I get someone else to feed my son and gave me lots of free samples of the new follow-on milk to try. Off I went, pleased with her advice and generosity.

I was back at clinic the following week, as it hadn't worked!

This time I spoke to the clinic doctor and asked her advice on the best formula to try. She seemed exasperated and said that no formula milk was as good as mother's milk, and that if my baby could not have my milk I might as well give him ordinary cow's milk.

Off I went again, not quite so happy this time, but reflecting on her words.

I had never heard anyone use the term mother's milk or say that it was better than formula for babies over six months old. I thought about why my son couldn't continue to have it (if it was, indeed, the best) and I realised that there was no good reason why he should be weaned on to cow's milk.

I continued to feed him for another six months, and all because of the words the clinic doctor used.

Midwives' choice of words

As midwives, we should always be mindful about our choice of words and the impact they have. We should make it quite clear to the antenatal woman in our care that her milk is the best nutrition for her baby and that nursing her baby is the best way to provide that nutrition as it brings unique additional psychological and physical benefits (Riordan and Auerbach 2004).

We should also be clear that formula milk is cows' milk that has been modified to provide adequate nutrition, but that it remains inferior to mother's milk.

Midwives need not worry about saying that formula is inferior – it says so on the tin!

UK law ensures that all formula must state that breastfeeding is best for babies (UK Statutory Instruments 1995), which obviously means that formula is second best.

Actually, donor human milk is second best to mother's milk (Lang 2002) – formula is third best.

Parents' choice

All parents want the best for their baby, including parents in Sure Start areas.

The reason why some mothers don't recognise breastfeeding as the best choice for them is multifactoral. We know that age, social and educational status, marital status, the partner's views, personal and family feeding history, body image, family and social support and the prevailing infant feeding culture all influence a mother's feeding choice (Bentley et al 2003).

An important factor in the choice of feeding method in my particular Sure Start area appears to be the perception that it is important for other people, particularly the partner, to be able to feed the baby.

The perception that the partner bottle-feeding the baby is 'helpful' for the mother persists even when rarely observed after the first few days or weeks. Mothers are left with most of the feeds, especially at night. Offers to feed the baby are rarely taken as an opportunity for the mother to rest; they usually 'help' her to perform some more chores!

A second perception that feeding the baby makes partners feel involved also persists. Putting the desires of partners (to feel involved) before the needs of the newborn (to obtain the best nutrition and nurturing) has occurred, in my opinion, because of a lack of knowledge about the benefits of breastfeeding and the disadvantages to health of formula feeding.

Like most Sure Start areas, Little Hulton has high unemployment and many single parent households. Perhaps lack of confidence in fathering may lead some men to adopt the traditional maternal task of feeding to strengthen their own position in the baby's life.

Many older relatives disapprove of cuddling babies, and parents are warned to avoid making the dreaded 'rod for their own back' by continuing to hold a baby who is not feeding or being winded. Feeding may be the only pleasant physical contact that fathers or partners feel they are allowed.

Lack of awareness of the importance of the mother–baby bond, sexualisation of breasts and the almost universal belief that formula is almost as good as mother's milk all contribute to parents choosing to bottle-feed (Fletcher Williams and Tappin 2002).

What can we do?

How can midwives, particularly those working in Sure Start areas, improve breastfeeding rates?

First, we can avoid the 'B' word and use the terms 'mother's milk' and 'nursing' when discussing infant feeding. If the language of breastfeeding leads to an emphasis on breasts, many women will feel it is not the right choice for them – or, if they do feel it is right, it will be for a limited time only.

Second, we can be clear and consistent about the benefits of breastfeeding. Some argue that we can only do this by also advising women about the risks of formula feeding. In an increasingly litigious age, that becomes more likely (Finigan 2004, Minchin 1998).

Midwives worry about causing feelings of guilt in mothers who choose not to breastfeed. This would occur only if mothers felt they had made a wrong decision. If mothers make an informed choice, they make a decision that is right for them at that time and they do not feel guilty.

All health professionals recognise that the choice of feeding method is the mother's, and that we should make no judgement about her choice. The focus of our work is to develop a breastfeeding culture to replace the bottle-feeding culture that leads a mother to choose to feed her baby formula milk instead of her own.

Sure Start's role

Sure Start can help by chipping away at the bottle-feeding culture that dominates many areas. All projects should be aware of the benefits of breastfeeding and should be 'nursing mother friendly'. Projects could start by making policy statements that 'Nursing mothers are welcome to feed their babies' and not 'Breastfeeding is allowed.'

Images of bottles and bottle-feeding should not be considered to be synonymous with babies. Breastfeeding, even if not common in the area, should be regarded as the normal way to feed babies.

Peer counselling programmes help to raise the profile of breastfeeding and provide mother-to-mother support for nursing mothers (Smale et al 2004).

In Salford we have La Leche League training, and the graduates are 'breast mates'. The Little Hulton group are the latest Salford mothers to complete the training. Among other things, they run a support group and a telephone helpline.

An extremely valuable part of the breast mates' work is the informal contact with people they meet in daily life. To have peer supporters who are experienced, knowledgeable and enthusiastic about breastfeeding helps to convey the idea that nursing a baby in a Sure Start area is as desirable and 'do-able' as in any other.

Tackling perceptions about maternal and paternal roles that are likely to be unhelpful to breastfeeding can be addressed during antenatal care but would be most effective long before people become parents. Having input into primary and secondary education is an ideal opportunity. The teaching sessions that the community midwifery team and I gave at the local high school were a chance to dispel some common myths about breastfeeding.

Fathers' groups can provide positive role models for fathers and suggest that breastfeeding does not exclude men from the care of their own baby. There are many ways to be a good father without feeding the baby.

Increasing breastfeeding rates

Despite my dislike of the language used to measure breastfeeding rates, there has been considerable improvement in Little Hulton.

In 2002, 11 per cent of mothers breastfed at birth (Office for National Statistics: Population Census 2001). In the first quarter of monitoring in 2004, 37.9 per cent breastfed within three days of birth (Sure Start 2004).

These two measures may not be comparable as the first is self-reporting obtained from a local population census and the second is the figure obtained from midwifery monitoring of any nursing (just one feed counts, as we wish to convey the message that mother's milk is so beneficial that even one feed is worthy of record).

Despite the difference in statistics, the community midwifery team agree that there has been a genuine increase. This can be attributed to a number of initiatives:

- Sure Start has become established in the area and purchased the La Leche Peer Counselling Course, which both health professionals and community health workers attended.
- There are seven Little Hulton breast mates sponsored by Sure Start, providing mother-to-mother support in the community. Another five mothers have completed the La Leche Peer Counsellor training and will graduate as breast mates soon.
- Salford Royal Hospitals NHS Trust (the provider of maternity services) has renewed its Baby Friendly Initiative (BFI) Certificate of Commitment, and hopes to become Baby Friendly soon.

- Community midwives have improved antenatal information about the benefits of breastfeeding.
- Hospital policies and practice are more supportive of breastfeeding due to the hard work of many midwives including Sara Blakeway, the present Infant Feeding Advisor, and her predecessor Bev Beresford.
- Midwives and health visitors work together on all the local breastfeeding initiatives.
- The majority of community midwives working in Little Hulton have attended either La Leche Peer Counsellor training or the three-day UNICEF UK Baby Friendly Initiative training.
- Little Hulton is one of five Sure Start areas in Salford that benefit from the Salford Breastfeeding Project, which is jointly funded by Sure Start and the Primary Care Trust and works to promote, protect and support breastfeeding throughout Salford.

Early indications show that a consistent, committed and well-informed approach to improving breastfeeding rates really does work, and we anticipate that even more Little Hulton babies will receive mother's milk, leading to improvements in physical and psychological health both for them and for their mothers.

We will try not to mention the 'B' word.

Acknowledgements

To Sharon Breward and Sue Saunders for inspiration. To the midwifery team working in Little Hulton: B Burt, R Day, L Barlow, L Lythgoe, J Moffat and E Saxon.

REFERENCES

Bentley M E et al (2003). 'Breastfeeding among low income, African-American women: power, beliefs and decision-making'. J Nutrition, 133: 3055–3095.

Department of Health (1995). Breastfeeding Good Practice, Guidance to the NHS, DoH.

Department of Health (2003). Ref 31636, DoH. www.breastfeeding.nhs.uk

Finigan V (2004). 'Breastfeeding the great divide. The controversy as seen through a midwifery lens'. MIDIRS Midwifery Digest, 14 (2): 227–231.

Fletcher Williams M and Tappin D (2002). Breastfeeding Education for Scottish Schools, PEACH Paper, no 14, University of Glasgow.

Lang S (2002). Breastfeeding Special Care Babies, 2nd edition, Baillière Tindall.

Minchin M (1998). Artificial Feeding: Risky for Any Baby, Victoria: Alma Publications.

Office for National Statistics (2001). Census 2001: National Report for England and Wales, London: Office for National Statistics.

Riordan J and Auerbach K (2004). Breastfeeding and Human Lactation, 3rd edition, Jones and Bartlett.

Smale M, Newburn M and Dodds R (2004). 'Peer support for breast-feeding'. NCT News Digest, 27 (July): 14–18.

Sure Start (2004). Little Hulton local monitoring, June-September.

UK Statutory Instruments (1995). Infant Formula and Follow-on Formula Regulations, no 7.

World Health Organisation (1981). The International Code of Marketing of Breast Milk Substitutes.

BIBLIOGRAPHY

Katz Rothman B and Simmonds W (2003). 'Breastfeeding: beyond milk'. MIDIRS Midwifery Digest, 13 (2): 223–226.

The Practising Midwife 2005; 8(7): 36–40

Maternal breastfeeding positions: Have we got it right? (1)

Suzanne Colson

Although exclusive breastfeeding is associated with significant health benefits, British mothers are some of the least likely in Europe to sustain breastfeeding (Hamlyn et al 2002). Knowledgeable support may be crucial in overcoming the problems that prompt early, unintended breast weaning (Renfrew et al 2005). Current breastfeeding support approaches suggest a fixed system of routine and early breastfeeding management using verbal instruction to enable mothers to learn correct positioning and attachment skills. The following points have been recently reported as best practice. To breastfeed, mothers should:

- sit in a chair with an upright back, at right angles to their 'almost flat lap'
- use a footstool (if needed) to support their feet
- swaddle the baby (if necessary), ensuring baby's arms are lying at the sides, not across the body
- support the baby on a pillow with nose and mouth in line with mother's nipple before beginning the feed
- attach the baby correctly, holding the breast, if necessary, but keeping the breast still
- elicit a mouth gape, by moving the baby against the breast and enabling the mouth to touch the nipple
- aim the baby's bottom lip as far away as possible from the base of the nipple to enable baby's tongue to scoop in as much breast as possible (Inch et al 2003a).

The theory for this kind of instruction appears to originate from three primary sources:
1. Research examining the anatomy and physiology of infant sucking (Weber et al 1986, Woolridge 1986a, 1986b).
2. Research differentiating sore nipple types and expert clinical practice (Gunther 1945, 1973).
3. Experts' practice in English problem-solving hospital/community feeding clinics (Woolridge 1995).

Infant sucking and sore nipples

A recent systematic review highlights that poor positioning and breast attachment are associated with low milk supply, nipple trauma, breast engorgement and early weaning (Renfrew et al 2000). These risk factors were first identified through landmark research carried out by Woolridge in the 1980s. Studying the mechanisms of sucking through ultrasonic examination of the buccal cavity during breastfeeding, Woolridge (1986a, 1986b) replicated and further developed earlier cineradiographic studies made of both breast- and bottle-feeding episodes (Ardran et al 1958a, 1958b). Using video recordings of ultrasound scans to examine patterns and coordination between sucking, swallowing and breathing, Woolridge (1986a, 1986b) studied six breastfed and six bottlefed infants between the second and sixth postnatal day. Mapping the anatomy of infant sucking and examining the aetiology of sore nipples, this research has been cited widely, informing practices concerning the positioning and attachment of the baby at the breast.

Woolridge's (1986a) description of normal infant sucking patterns, culminating in the finding that milk transfer involves an almost frictionless process between neonatal tongue action and maternal nipple, made good physiological sense, since experiencing pain during breastfeeding always appeared incongruent with a biological process. Woolridge (1986a, 1986b) set the gold standard for breastfeeding education.

Clinical applications centred on recommendations for teaching midwives to teach mothers optimum attachment and positioning skills to ensure effective milk transfer, breast emptying and painless feeds (Woolridge 1986a).

Challenging theory

The aim of Woolridge's (Weber et al 1986, Woolridge 1986a) pioneering research was to clarify the organisation and physiology of feeding events that occur inside the baby's mouth during a feed. Generating theories about how an infant becomes attached to the breast, Woolridge (1986a: 169) reiterated that babies are born with two primitive reflexes, the innate rooting and sucking responses enabling them to 'obtain the nutrients essential for survival'. However, mothers appeared to lack any instinctive responses, unable innately to breastfeed. Mothers, concluded Woolridge (1986a), need to learn and develop breastfeeding skills.

This theory can be challenged because it does not appear to take into account how mothers might sit or lie instinctively. Any systematic examination of neonatal positioning and attachment in relation to spontaneous maternal postures appears to have exceeded the scope of the Woolridge research (Weber et al 1986, Woolridge, 1986a, 1986b).

In the earlier cineradiographic studies made of both breast- and bottlefeeding episodes (Ardran et al 1958a, 1958b), maternal research postures are clearly described: the breastfeeding mothers observed were asked to lean over a couch with their bodies twisted so as to allow one breast to project clear from the chest wall. A nurse then 'adjusted the baby to the mother's nipple and when active sucking was established the radiographic exposure was made' (Ardran et al 1958b: 156). Although care was taken to ensure maternal comfort, these postures – suggested purely as part of a research protocol to enable close observations of breast attachment and the neonatal buccal cavity during feeds – could hardly increase knowledge about spontaneous maternal feeding postures.

Back straight, chest out!

Traditionally, in any body of literature, mothers are often shown sitting upright unsupported or upright on nursing chairs to breastfeed. Both Mavis Gunther, an obstetrician in the UK, and Karen Pryor, an American marine biologist, fervent and respected breastfeeding authorities in the 1950s to 1970s, suggested that in sitting positions mothers should sit 'bolt upright or lean slightly forward' and 'not lean backwards' (Gunther, 1973: 49; Pryor, 1973: 167). Two such upright seated postures are still widely used and promoted as the only correct way to breastfeed. These are:

- Sitting upright and holding baby in a cradle or cross-cradle position
- Sitting upright and holding baby in the clutch, rugby ball or football position.

Mothers are also advised that they can breastfeed lying down. The lying down position is usually recommended for initiating breastfeeding, especially after a caesarean section or for night feeds. Lying down, even in the artistic literature, is commonly represented in postures where both mother and baby are on their sides facing each other.

Bad for the back?

I have carried out an extensive literature search and have been unable to find any research data supporting these suggestions. However, there are some interesting postural descriptions from osteopaths. Definitions of good or correct posture emphasise alignment of the body organs that allows them to function properly. Bad or incorrect posture is that which places undue strain and pressure on any of the organs leading to their abnormal functioning with resultant pain or general bad health. The osteopathic literature is unambiguous: an upright posture where the back is at right angles to the lap is the most uncomfortable of any position, and usually becomes painful; traditionally, it is called 'the typist's position'. The typist's position is well-known among osteopaths whose treatments for predictable effects of tense trapezius and neck muscles and the tendonitis often associated with repetitive stress injury include manipulations and massage (Kapandji 1974).

Learning to breastfeed has been compared with learning how to type (Renfrew et al 2004). The argument goes something like this: when you sit straight, in an upright posture, you are well positioned; therefore, you will look better, feel better, be less tired and more accurate. In fact, these claims are unsubstantiated. It may be that sitting upright is not the most comfortable, most accurate or least tiring position for typing or for breastfeeding.

Postures where mothers are leaning back slightly, semi-reclined or flat lying are largely resting postures, not erect. Promoting relaxation and recovery, they may have a distinct advantage in that head, neck and shoulders can be fully supported. Semi-reclined postures can be just as well-aligned and balanced as erect postures, enabling full lung expansion, preventing sagging of the internal organs and exaggeration of the lumbar curve of the spine. The aim is to be stable, supported and comfortable, avoiding hunching and slumping.

One reason that has been given for sitting upright for breastfeeding is that women's breasts will 'point downwards and outwards' if they are lying back, making it difficult to latch the baby on to the breast (RCM 2002: 44). Renfrew et al (2004) also argue that lying down postures are problematic, suggesting that semi-reclined seated postures could inhibit the milk supply or cause nipple sucking. These statements are unreferenced, suggesting that this is professional opinion; authoritative statements such as these are often illustrated by a series of pictures of mothers sitting starkly upright with both feet flat on the floor and head, neck and shoulders unsupported, illustrating how to attach babies correctly to the breast using the correct seated posture.

After that, there is often a series of mothers in semi-reclined postures that are crossed out, indicating that leaning back or lying flat to breastfeed is wrong or incorrect. Again, this is unsubstantiated. However, these constant visual displays throughout the breastfeeding literature not only reinforce the widespread belief that upright sitting postures are the only correct way to breastfeed when seated, but they also assume that mothers (or, sometimes, midwives) are supposed to attach the baby to the breast.

It may be interesting to explore why some breastfeeding experts have traditionally insisted on upright sitting postures. Speculation suggests that it might have to do with etiquette, leaning back perhaps being associated with slouching or an unkempt appearance. Upright can also mean decent, honest and of good moral conduct. Or, maybe, bolt upright postures were originally thought to strengthen bone development, preventing malalignment or nerve injury; the theory could have originated at a time when the benefits of vitamin D were unknown and rickets was prevalent. Chair design is constantly changing and evolving; maybe straight-backed chairs were the only ones available in the hospital or clinical setting. Finally, it may have been thought that if breastfeeding mothers leaned back in semi-reclined or semi-flat postures, the milk could not flow upwards and out and down into the baby's mouth. Thinking in terms of bottlefeeding, and considering the effects of gravity, logically this makes sense. Equipped, however, with the understanding of the mechanisms of maternal milk release and how the baby applies 'negative suction pressure' during sucking bursts (Woolridge 1986a: 164), we can start to look beyond any association between maternal postures and the effectiveness of milk transfer.

Creating a 'problem'

A third primary source that underpins the routine verbal instruction of breastfeeding management cited above appears to originate from the nature of knowledge and clinical expertise gained during feeding clinics. Woolridge (1995: 221) reports that hospital and community clinics offer 'women with seemingly intractable breastfeeding problems' the opportunity to be taught specific positions and attachment skills to overcome them. When there are problems, his response makes good sense – a consistent approach to reorganise is probably exactly what is needed. However, to regard the initiation of any breastfeeding as problematic is culturally loaded. For example, a breastfeeding promotional video suggests that mothers must acquire coping skills to be able to breastfeed during the first postnatal week (RCM 1996). The word 'cope' comes from middle English via the French 'coper', meaning to meet in battle or give a blow with the fist. Today, coping is still associated with successful confrontation of problems: some coping synonyms are 'managing', 'getting by', 'surviving' and 'muddling through' – hardly words conjuring up images of pleasure and satisfaction.

There is a good argument to be made that it is not the act of breastfeeding that is problematic, but rather fixed attitudes and cultural beliefs that obscure the biological choice (La Leche League 1958).

Conclusion

In today's consumer world, to promote and support breastfeeding it may be more productive to encourage natural positions and introduce the concept of nurturing and enjoyment – to 'market' breastfeeding, inspired by the positive energy coming from testimonials of mothers who take pleasure in breastfeeding. That is what biological nurturing is about.

REFERENCES

Ardran G M, Kemp F H and Lind J (1958a). 'A cineradiographic study of bottle feeding'. British Journal of Radiology, 31: 11–22.

Ardran G M, Kemp F H and Lind J (1958b). 'A cineradiographic study of breast feeding'. British Journal of Radiology, 31: 156–162.

Gunther M (1945). 'Sore nipples, causes and prevention'. Lancet ii: 590–593.

Gunther M (1973). Infant Feeding, revised edition, Harmondsworth: Penguin Books.

Hamlyn B, Brooker S, Oleinikova K and Wands S (2002). Infant Feeding, London: TSO.

Inch S, Law S and Wallace L (2003a). 'Hands off! The Breastfeeding Best Start Project (1)'. The Practising Midwife, 6 (10): 17–19.

Kapandji I A (1974). The Physiology of the Joints, Vol.3: the Trunk and the Vertebral Column, 2nd edition, Edinburgh, London, NY: Churchill Livingstone.

La Leche League (1958). The Womanly Art of Breastfeeding, La Leche League International, 9616 Franklin Park, Il 60131, USA.

Pryor K (1973). Nursing Your Baby, New York: Harper and Row.

Renfrew M J, Woolridge M W and McGill H R (2000). Enabling Women to Breastfeed, London: TSO.

Renfrew M, Fisher C and Arms S (2004). Bestfeeding: How to Breastfeed Your Baby, Berkeley, CA: Celestial Arts.

Renfrew M, Dyson L, Wallace L et al (2005). The Effectiveness of Public Health Interventions to Promote the Duration of Breastfeeding Systematic review (1st edition), London: NICE.

Royal College of Midwives (1996). Breastfeeding: Coping With The First Week (videotape), Mark-It Television, 34 Gadshill Drive, Meade Park, Stoke Gifford, Bristol BS12 6UX.

Royal College of Midwives (2002). Successful Breastfeeding, London: RCM.

Weber, Woolridge MW and Baum JD (1986). 'An ultrasonographic study of the organization of sucking and swallowing by newborn infants'. Developmental Medicine and Child Neurology, 28:19.

Woolridge MW (1986a). 'The "anatomy" of infant sucking'. Midwifery, 2: 164–171.

Woolridge MW (1986b). 'Aetiology of sore nipples'. Midwifery, 2: 172–176.

Woolridge M W (1995). 'Baby controlled breastfeeding', 217–242, in P Stuart-Macadam and K A Dettwyler (eds), Breastfeeding Biocultural Perspectives, NY: Aldine de Gruyter.

The Practising Midwife 2005; 8(10): 24–27

Maternal breastfeeding positions: Have we got it right? (2)

Suzanne Colson

Biological nurturing (BN), developed from observations of successful breastfeeding, describes the holding and cuddling that most mothers naturally want to do as soon as the baby is born. During the past 25 years, I have observed and supported thousands of mothers who appear to enjoy breastfeeding in a variety of acute and community settings (Colson 1985).

Employed as one of the research midwives on the Hawdon, DeRooy and Williams team (2002) examining patterns of metabolic adaptation for healthy, moderately preterm and term but small for gestational age infants, I used BN to support breastfeeding and formally articulated the strategy for an MSc dissertation in midwifery studies (Colson 2000). Although this was a small exploratory study where comparisons were not possible, BN increased the duration of exclusive breastfeeding for this group of 'at risk' babies (Colson et al 2003).

In 2001, in conjunction with South Bank University, BN was introduced during a midwifery practice development project funded by the Department of Health and carried out in East Kent Hospitals NHS Trust (Dykes 2004). This project resulted in a peer-reviewed nurturing booklet written for mothers (Colson 2001).

An investigation into the mechanisms of biological nurturing was the subject of PhD research (Colson 2006). The thesis was awarded the Royal College of Nursing inaurgural Akinsanya Award for originality and scholarship in doctoral research. Underpinned by a mixed methods approach, both breast- and bottle-feeding mother/baby pairs were videotaped. Unexpected findings include the description of a range of sustainable breastfeeding postures and positions that appear to increase early maternal breastfeeding enjoyment, supporting pain-free and successful milk transfer.

BN has two components: a proactive mother-centred strategy emphasising baby-holding; and the midwifery assessment of maternal-infant wellbeing and milk transfer during feeding episodes.

Freedom of maternal posture

All mothers, regardless of feeding intention, are encouraged to make themselves as comfortable as possible from birth. This can be sitting upright, semi-reclined, side lying or flat lying. For my work, the word 'posture' always refers to the mother. For the mother, biological nurturing means finding a comfortable posture and offering her baby unrestricted access to the breast. This can be in as much skin-to-skin contact as desired. However, skin-to-skin contact is not a prerequisite to biological nurturing as exploratory research has suggested many mothers are reluctant to breastfeed without clothes or to undress their babies for a variety of reasons (Colson et al 2003).

Although healthy adults usually eat in upright postures, many lean back slightly. This may be a question of etiquette and, as noted previously, there does not appear to be any research data to justify the imposition of upright maternal sitting postures when feeding babies.

A BN maternal posture is defined as one that the mother says is comfortable, where there is no neck strain, shoulders are relaxed and all body parts are supported: it is pain-free, sustainable for a long period of time and thereby conducive to effective milk transfer. There are three basic assumptions underpinning BN postures contrasting them with the traditional upright postures paradigm reported previously (Inch et al 2003a):

1. Since all mothers' bodies are different, there is not one posture that will fit all needs.
2. Mothers easily find the right posture for their own needs and comfort when routine suggestions are avoided.
3. Comfortable, sustainable postures will change and evolve throughout the breastfeeding time span. Initially, they may change from feed to feed or daily.

Plenty of positions

In my work the word 'position' always refers to the baby. Biological nurturing positions are defined as those where the entire frontal aspect of the baby's body is in close juxtaposition with a maternal body contour, developing further the concept of 'tummy to mummy'. In that way, and because the areola is round, there is a potential of 360 baby positions as there are 360 degrees in a circle. Realistically, of course, there are only approximately 200 accessible baby positions.

Positioning at the breast has recently been defined as the relationship between the baby's body and the mother's, whereas attachment is the relationship between the baby's mouth and the mother's breast (Inch et al 2003b). Preliminary analysis of BN positions builds upon and further develops these definitions, bringing additional insights for the application of Woolridge's findings (1986a; 1986b). Central to the understanding of baby positions is the concept of 'lie'. I borrow the word from midwifery and obstetric antenatal fetal assessments and have redefined it to clarify BN positions in the postnatal context. The lie of biological nurturing is the longitudinal, transverse or oblique relationship between the long part of the mother and the long part of the baby.

Understanding the concept of postnatal lie can often be useful to encourage early breastfeeding for mothers undergoing caesarean section. In the first postnatal hours, many mothers are afraid that any body contact with the baby near the recent surgical site will be painful; babies are often given bottle feeds while mothers are recovering. Expanding the circumference of the theoretical breast circle to its outermost limits, mothers in comfortable semi-reclined or flat-lying BN postures can either use an over-the-shoulder position with baby in an oblique lie or try a transverse lie with the baby's body draped across her upper torso. Trying different lies often helps a worried mother to breastfeed almost immediately, thus avoiding any direct friction with her fresh wound.

It is worthwhile examining instinctive baby postnatal lie when there are common breastfeeding problems: for example, latch refusal, characterised by the baby 'fighting' the breast. Following slight modifications from traditional breastfeeding postures/positions to full BN, newborns often instinctively assume a postnatal lie on the mother's body that mirrors the antenatal lie. After a nesting-type pause, babies often self attach.

Mothers, once comfortable, are encouraged to lie their babies prone, in the close BN frontal juxtaposition previously described, for as long, as often and in as much skin-to-skin contact as desired. Again, as with maternal postures, there are basic assumptions underpinning BN baby positions, contrasting them with the traditional paradigm reported previously (Inch et al 2003a):

These include fixed ideas about:

- **The position of the baby's face**. During BN the face will certainly be near the breasts, but there is no need to line up nipple to nose or to elicit a mouth gape or routinely aim the nipple at the bottom lip. Likewise, when mothers are in semi-reclined or flat-lying postures, many babies spontaneously lead in with the chin, exhibiting searching behaviours enabling them to self attach from any angle, even while asleep. It is often the baby who latches (not the mother).
- **Swaddling**. This appears to hinder close body apposition and many innate movements.
- **The use of pillows**. These are rarely needed to support the baby as mothers often spontaneously lie back in semi-reclined or flat-lying postures where their bodies take the full weight of the baby. In this way mothers often have their hands free while breastfeeding. Pillows, however, often support the mother's body (arms, legs, back, neck).
- **Breast holding**. Some mothers want to hold their breasts, while others do not. The need to hold can change daily, even from feed to feed. Mothers are the best people to decide this and routine instruction about holding their breasts, still or otherwise, may inhibit their instinctual behaviours.
- **Nutritional needs and the place of the baby during the first 24 hours**. Most healthy term infants are born well-fed (Colson 2002). There is a physiological argument to be made focusing attention upon increasing the time of baby holding in BN postures/positions, the priority being maternal/neonatal comfort and enjoyment rather than teaching 'correct and efficient hands-off breastfeeding techniques' during the first 24 hours.

The health professional's role

During episodes of BN, many mothers and babies appear to display instinctive reciprocal feeding behaviours; midwives and other breastfeeding supporters are educated to recognise them, to learn how and when to stimulate them and to promote an environment conducive to successful milk transfer. Specifically, the midwifery focus is how to assess BN lie, neonatal awake/sleep behavioural states and milk transfer. This assessment is underpinned by nutritional physiology and a neurobehavioural theoretical framework which has inspired the concept of hormonal complexion.

Introducing hormonal complexion

Hormonal complexion is an umbrella term I am introducing to summarise the probable behavioural and mechanical effects of oxytocin (OT) and prolactin. For example, research findings suggest an association between high maternal OT pulsatility on the second postnatal day and an increase in breastfeeding duration (Nissen et al 1996).

There is also an increasing body of scientific research, mostly from animal studies, suggesting social, sexual and maternal behavioural effects – such as nesting and grooming – associated with the release of central OT. This has prompted some researchers to qualify OT as the tending, befriending, anti-stress or love hormone (Boccia and Pedersen 2002, Herbert 1994, Pedersen 1992, 2004). Although my study did not aim to examine OT pulsatility, the preceding observations, taken together with BN research video clips, introduce a compelling visual argument for the assessment of hormonal complexion as a strategy to support breastfeeding.

Along with nutritional physiology, the concept of hormonal complexion underpins BN and offers a strong theoretical framework to build upon and further develop 'the anatomy of infant suckling' (Woolridge 1986a). Traditionally, it has been thought that teaching mothers positioning and attachment (P and A) skills was the way to apply Woolridge's (1986a; 1986b) pioneering research findings concerning the organisation and physiology of neonatal suckling (Renfrew et al 2005).

How effective is routine teaching of P and A?

The background

Although 69 per cent of mothers in the UK initiate breastfeeding, 21 per cent stop during the first two postnatal weeks (Hamlyn et al 2002). The most common reasons mothers give for this early unintended breastfeeding cessation are insufficient milk and sore nipples or breasts. These statistics largely justify the development of an early, consistent, cost-effective intervention to restore confidence in the physiology of milk production and to reduce the incidence of painful breastfeeding. Based on a recent authoritative professional consensus in England, obtained from 516 respondents, the routine teaching of P and A 'using a predominantly hands off approach' has recently been recommended as the high impact solution (Dyson et al 2005: 30). But what does the research evidence say?

The research

Until 2001, there were no randomised controlled trials (RCTs) examining the impact of routine standardised teaching of P and A upon breastfeeding rates. Since then, two trials have called this practice into question. Attempting to replicate results showing positive effect from a small observational study, Forster et al (2004) randomly allocated 981 mothers to one of three groups to examine the effects of teaching standardised P and A as one of two mid-pregnancy interventions. No significant differences were found with respect to breastfeeding initiation or duration between the experimental mothers in either group and the controls.

In the other RCT, Henderson et al (2001) hypothesised that a short (30 minutes), early (first 24 hours following birth), verbal (hands-off) postnatal intervention teaching P and A would increase breastfeeding duration rates. Designed with sufficient power to show positive but not negative effect, 159 mothers were randomised to either an experimental group receiving the intervention or a control group receiving standard postnatal breastfeeding support (ie, teaching P and A by actively attaching the baby to the breast for the mother).

Surprisingly, results indicated a downward trend in breastfeeding duration rates in the intervention group, despite fewer sore nipples reported on days two and three. Experimental mothers were less satisfied with breastfeeding on four counts expressing:

1. dissatisfaction with ease of breastfeeding
2. less confidence in their feeding ability
3. scepticism that breastfeeding calmed an upset infant, and perhaps most strikingly,
4. fewer experimental mothers thought that their baby enjoyed breastfeeding.

In discussing these disappointing results, it was noted that many mothers find taught breastfeeding skills hard to achieve; the researchers could not rule out the possibility that routine 'hands-off' teaching of P and A was responsible for the lower breastfeeding rates in the experimental group.

A major limitation to the study was the possible confounding effects resulting from the researcher both delivering and assessing the effects of the intervention (Renfrew et al 2005). However, it could be argued that this limitation made these findings all the more surprising, considering that the hypothesis to which the researcher was committed, and had every opportunity to bias, proved to be ineffective.

The BN perspective does not challenge that positioning and attachment are integral to successful breastfeeding. However, in view of low, static breastfeeding duration rates in the UK for the past 20 years, it could be argued that there are gaps in the theoretical knowledge base. Once identified, they may lead us to reconsider both the nature and the timing of breastfeeding support. For example, perhaps it would be more effective if teaching of P and A was done in response to maternal request or to observed nipple sucking, rather than on a routine basis. Righard and Alade (1992) examined the effectiveness of correcting observed nipple sucking at hospital discharge (4–6 postnatal days). At four months, mothers whose babies had a faulty, uncorrected technique at hospital discharge had significantly more breastfeeding problems and earlier breastfeeding cessation. Although this small study had some confounding factors (such as the use of dummies), it may serve to increase understanding about what can happen when health professionals fail to respond appropriately to observed problems.

Developing a professional approach

Biological nurturing builds upon and further develops a similar professional approach. Using counselling skills, midwives promote maternal/infant comfort and hormonal pulsatility; midwives are taught to assess hormonal complexion and milk transfer, discreetly, so that mothers do not feel observed; changes in maternal/neonatal postures/positions are only proposed when there are problems. In that way BN introduces new ways of thinking about breastfeeding that empower mothers to find their own ways.

Based upon observations of mothers who appear to enjoy breastfeeding, my research findings suggest that there are unexplored physiological perspectives supporting successful breastfeeding. Biological nurturing is more than nipple to nose and tummy to mummy, it is more than upright or side-lying postures and cradle, cross-cradle and clutch or rugby holds, it is more than a correct sucking technique. BN is a two-person, whole-body experience introducing research evidence proposing many baby positions in three postnatal lies and a range of effective, comfortable, sustainable, pain-free maternal postures.

During the past 20 years, the low breastfeeding continuance rates in the UK have resisted national and international public health initiatives to promote and support breastfeeding (Renfrew et al 2005). Is it time to acknowledge some theoretical gaps in breastfeeding practices?

A non-prescriptive recipe for nurturing, illustrating novel maternal postures, has been published in *The Practising Midwife* (2007). The recipe is available for purchase in A3 posters and tear-off packs. Biological Nurturing workshops have been launched in London and Kent (for information, contact Joelle Temurcin: email joelledufur@yahoo.co.uk). A Biological Nurturing module is offered yearly in the context of continuing professional development (CPD) at Canterbury Christ Church University (contact the information office at the university for a module flyer). Videotapes illustrating research evidence to support practice will be available next year.

REFERENCES

Boccia ML and Pedersen CA (2002). 'Brief vs long maternal separations in infancy: contrasting relationships with adult maternal behaviour and lactation levels of aggression and anxiety'. Psychoneuroendocrinology, 26 (7): 657–672.

Colson S (1985). 'Reflexions et propos sur les rencontres du vendredi soir'. In: Association des Usagers de la Maternite de Pithiviers (ed.) Histoires de Naissance, Paris: EPI pp. 30–33.

Colson S (2000). 'Biological suckling facilitates exclusive breastfeeding from birth a pilot study of 12 vulnerable infants'. Dissertation submitted as course requirement of MSc in Midwifery Studies, London: South Bank University, June 2000.

Colson S (2001). Mother/Baby Experiences of Nurturing. Department of Health-funded breastfeeding project available from J. Dufur 4 Corunna Close Hythe Kent CT21 5EA.

Colson S (2002). 'Womb to world – adaptation from foetus to neonate from a metabolic perspective'. Midwifery Today online: www.midwiferytoday.com/articles/womb.asp

Colson S, DeRooy L and Hawdon J (2003). 'Biological Nurturing increases duration of breastfeeding for a vulnerable cohort'. MIDIRS Midwifery Digest, 13 (1): 92–97.

Colson S (2005). 'The mechanisms of biological nurturing'. PhD thesis in progress. Canterbury Christ Church University.

De Rooy L and Hawdon JM (2002). 'Nutritional factors that affect the postnatal metabolic adaptation of full-term small and large for gestational age infants'. Pediatrics, 109 (3): www.jpediatrics.org/cgi/content/full/109/3/e42

Dykes F (2004). Infant Feeding Initiatives: A Report: Evaluations of the breastfeeding practice projects 1999–2002, Department of Health online: www.doh.gov.uk/infant feeding

Dyson L, Renfrew M, McFadden A et al (2005). 'Effective action briefing on the initiation and duration of breastfeeding'. Effective action recommendations, Mother and Infant Research Unit Department of Health Sciences, The University of York (Draft for consultation).

Forster D, McLachlan H, Lumley J et al (2004). 'Two mid-pregnancy interventions to increase the initiation and duration of breastfeeding: a randomized controlled trial'. Birth, 31 (3): 176–182.

Hamlyn B, Brooker S, Oleinikova K and Wands S (2002). Infant Feeding 2000, London: TSO.

Henderson A, Stamp G and Pincombe J (2001). 'Postpartum positioning and attachment education for increasing breastfeeding: a randomized trial'. Birth, 28 (4): 236–242.

Herbert J (1994). 'Oxytocin and sexual behaviour'. BMJ, 309: 891–892.

Inch S, Law S and Wallace L (2003a). 'Hands off! The Breastfeeding Best Start Project (1)'. The Practising Midwife, 6 (10): 17–19.

Inch S, Law S and Wallace L (2003b). 'Confusion surrounding breastfeeding terms "positioning" and "attachment"'. BJM, 11 (3): 148.

Nissen E, Uvnas-Moberg K, Svensson K et al (1996). 'Different patterns of oxytocin, prolactin but not cortisol release during breastfeeding in women delivered by Caesarean section or by the vaginal route'. Early Hum Dev, 45: 103–118.

Pedersen CA (1992). 'Preface in oxytocin in maternal, sexual and social behaviours'. Ann NY Acad Sci, 652: pp. ix–xi.

Pedersen CA (2004). 'Biological aspects of social bonding and the roots of human violence'. Ann NY Acad Sci, 1036: 106–127.

Renfrew MJ, Dyson L, Wallace L et al (2005). The Effectiveness of Public Health Interventions to Promote the Duration of Breastfeeding Systematic Review, London: National Institute for Health and Clinical Excellence (NICE).

Righard L and Alade MO (1992). 'Sucking technique and its effect on success of breastfeeding'. Birth, 19 (4): 185–189.

Woolridge MW (1986a). 'The "anatomy" of infant sucking'. Midwifery, 2: 164–171.

Woolridge MW (1986b). 'Aetiology of sore nipples', Midwifery, 2: 172–176.

The Practising Midwife 2005; 8(1): 29–32

A randomised controlled trial in the north of England examining the effects of skin-to-skin care on breast feeding

Sue Carfoot, Paula Williamson, Rumona Dickson

Summary

Objective: to examine the effect of early skin-to-skin contact between mothers and their healthy full-term babies on initiation and duration of breast feeding.

Design: a randomised controlled trial comparing skin-to-skin with routine care.

Setting: Warrington Hospital, Cheshire, UK.

Participants: 204 mother and baby pairs; 102 randomised to each group.

Outcome measures: success of first breast feed, maternal satisfaction with skin-to-skin care and preference for future post-delivery care, baby-body temperature 1 hr after birth, partial or exclusive breast feeding at 4 months.

Findings: in the skin-to-skin group, 89 out of 98 (91%) babies had a successful first feed compared with 82 out of 89 (83%) in the routine care group. The difference in the success rate was 8%, 95% confidence interval (CI) (−1.6%, 17.6%); $\chi^2 = 2.7$; df = 1; $P = 0.10$. Forty-two out of 97 (43%) babies given skin-to-skin were partially or exclusively breast feeding at 4 months compared with 40 out of 100 (40%) of babies in the routine care group. The difference in breast-feeding rate at 4 months was 3.3%, 95% CI (−10.3%, 16.7%); $\chi^2 = 0.22$; df = 1; $P = 0.64$. The mean temperature 1 hr after birth was higher with skin-to-skin than routine care. The difference in means was 0.15°C; 95% CI (0.03, 0.28); $P = 0.02$. A larger proportion of mothers (87/97 [90%]) were very satisfied with skin-to-skin care, compared with 60 out of 102 (59%) in the control group; 83 out of 97 (86%) of the mothers in the intervention group said that they would prefer to receive the same care in the future compared with 31 out of 102 (30%) mothers in the control group.

Conclusions: the difference between the groups in the success rate for the first breast feed and rates at 4 months was not statistically significant. However, mothers who had skin-to-skin contact enjoyed the experience, and most reported that they would choose to have skin-to-skin care in the future. In this, the largest trial to date, previous concerns about baby-body temperature after skin-to-skin care were dispelled.

Keywords: Skin-to-skin care; randomised controlled trial; breast feeding; maternal satisfaction; temperature

Introduction

It is undisputed that breast feeding is the most superior form of providing nutrition for babies. The World Health Organization recommends exclusive breast feeding for at least the first 6 months of life (World Health Organization, 2000). Breast-feeding rates in the UK are low compared with the rest of Europe (UNICEF, 1999). In the UK, 69% of mothers breast feed their babies at birth, 55% at 1 week and 28% at 4 months (Hamlyn et al., 2000).

The UNICEF Baby Friendly Initiative was introduced in the UK in 1991 to improve breast-feeding rates and healthcare practices that affect infant feeding. Best practice is represented by the 'Ten Steps to Successful Breast-feeding', which include a number of interventions previously shown to promote breast feeding. Currently, 43 out of 343 (12.6%) maternity units in the UK have received Baby Friendly accreditation (either the UK or

Global award). Step Four of the initiative recommends early and prolonged skin-to-skin contact in the postnatal period, which should last until the first feed or for as long as the mother wishes (WHO/UNICEF, 1998). Skin-to-skin contact is defined by the Baby Friendly Initiative (WHO/UNICEF, 1998) as holding the baby naked in a prone position against the mother's (or partner's) skin between the breasts. Skin-to-skin contact is seen as a potential mechanism for promoting early breast feeding (Widstrom et al., 1987; Widstrom et al., 1990; Righard and Alade, 1990).

The evidence for recommending skin-to-skin contact is limited. Previous reviews (Bernard-Bonnin et al., 1989; Perez-Escamilla et al., 1994; Fairbank et al., 2000; Carfoot et al., 2003) have reported insufficient evidence for the effect of skin-to-skin care on the initiation and duration of breast feeding. However, a recent Cochrane review (Anderson et al., 2003), found that skin-to-skin contact had a positive effect on longer-term breast feeding, although a number of the baby physiological and attachment outcomes demonstrated little or no clinically significant differences. These authors recommended that methodological limitations of the studies to date mean that further research is required.

We report here a randomised controlled trial comparing the effects of skin-to-skin contact with routine care on the first breast-feeding experience and duration of breast feeding.

Methods

Participants

The trial was conducted between 1 April and 28 September 2002 in Warrington Hospital in the north of England. A healthy, pregnant woman was eligible for the trial if she intended to breast feed, had 'booked' at Warrington Hospital, her healthy fetus was greater than 36 weeks' gestation and she had given informed consent. A woman was ineligible if she requested either skin-to-skin or no skin-to-skin contact after delivery, or had a multiple pregnancy.

North Cheshire Research Ethics Committee approved the study. Access to undertake the study was provided by the obstetricians and senior managers within the Trust. Pregnant women were identified through the existing computer booking system at Warrington Hospital. All women who fulfilled the inclusion criteria were contacted by the clinical co-ordinator at 36–37 weeks' gestation by telephone. The women were provided with verbal information about the trial and asked if they would be interested in participating. They were assured that all information obtained during the trial would be completely confidential and would not be used for other purposes. Women who gave verbal consent were provided with written information about the trial, a consent form to sign and return and a sticker to put on the front of their 'hand-held' case notes. At the time this study was undertaken, this approach complied with the requirements of the Data Protection Act.

Interventions

In the group receiving routine care, babies were quickly dried and wrapped in a towel before being handed to their mother or partner. Mother–baby contact was interrupted for weighing, dressing and measuring the baby, or for suturing the mother's perineum after delivery. The midwife offered assistance with breast feeding when both mother and baby were ready.

In the skin-to-skin care group, the midwife placed the baby naked in a prone position against the mother's skin between the breasts as soon as possible after birth. For the purpose of the study, skin-to-skin contact was limited to mother and baby. The midwives were encouraged by the clinical co-ordinator to weigh the baby before commencing skin-to-skin contact, as this would allow skin-to-skin contact to continue until the baby showed signs of readiness to feed or the mother chose to end the contact. However, in 19 (19.6%) women, skin-to-skin contact was interrupted. In five of these cases, it was the mother's choice to interrupt the contact but, in 14 cases, the midwife decided to interrupt the skin-to-skin contact. In eight out of 19 (42%) cases, skin-to-skin contact was interrupted before the specified minimum skin-to-skin duration of 45 mins. The midwife offered assistance with the first feed when both mother and baby were ready.

Outcome assessment

The primary outcome was the success of the first breast feed. Secondary outcomes included whether the woman self-reported she was still partially or exclusively breast feeding at 4 months, maternal satisfaction with, and preference for, the care allocated as measured by a specifically designed questionnaire, baby-body temperature measured at the axilla 1 hr after delivery, the time to, and duration of, first breast feed, and the success of a subsequent breast feed before discharge.

To assess the success of a baby's breast feed, the Infant Breast Feeding Assessment Tool (IBFAT) was adapted by the clinical co-ordinator (Matthews, 1988). The IBFAT is a short assessment of baby breast-feeding competence measuring readiness to feed, rooting and hand movements, and suckling. The IBFAT also measures maternal perception of, and satisfaction with, the feeding. The first author adapted the IBFAT to include a 'latching-on' component, as a correct latch is crucial to effective breast feeding. The authors considered the amended tool (BAT) to have face validity (Figure 7.7.1).

The range of scores for each of the four components is 0–3. A total score can thus range from 0–12. A successful breast feed was defined, a priori, as a BAT score of 8 or above. The authors agreed that the baby should be able to lose one point in each category and still be considered to have had a successful feed. For example, if the baby latches onto the breast correctly after a few attempts and begins to suckle fairly well, thus losing a point from categories 3 and 4, this is considered to be a successful breast feed.

Research assistants were present as observers from the final stages of labour until the end of the first breast feed and assessed initial breast feeds. They took part in an

initial training workshop that involved viewing and assessing videotaped breast-feeding sessions. All research assistants then observed and assessed the same five breast feeds, varying in quality and length, in the postnatal ward using the BAT tool. Acceptable differences between individual assessments by a particular research assistant and the first author were no more than one point within each category, and no more than two points in total. The third, fourth and final breast feeds showed no difference in BAT scores between any assessors. The final part of the observer training involved the research assistants and first author observing a first breast feed together in the labour ward. BAT scores were identical for all assessors.

Figure 7.7.1 Scoring system for the infant Breastfeeding Assessment Tool (BAT).

Dimension	Score
Readiness to feed	
When the mother/midwife picked baby up to feed was he/she:	
a) Rooting for the breast	3
(hand to mouth movements, vocal cues)	
b) Quiet and alert	2
c) Drowsy	1
d) Deeply asleep	0
(eyes closed, no observable movements except breathing)	
Rooting (definition: at the touch of the nipple to cheek, the mouth opens and baby attempts to fix mouth on the nipple)	
When the baby was placed at the breast, did he/she:	
a) Root effectively at once	3
b) Need some coaxing, prompting or encouragement to root	2
c) Root poorly even with coaxing	1
d) Not try to root	0
Suckling (definition: sustained latch with deep rhythmic sucking through the length of the feed, with some pauses, on either/or both breasts)	
Which of the following phrases best describes the baby's feeding pattern at this feed:	
a) Sucked well on one or both breasts	3
b) Sucked fairly well	2
(sucked on and off, but needed encouragement)	
c) Sucked poorly, weak sucking,	1
some sucking efforts for short periods	
d) Baby did not suck	0
Latching onto the breast (definition: the baby grasps the nipple and the areola with a wide gaping mouth, both lips are flanged outward)	
As baby attempted to latch-on to the breast, did he/she:	
a) Grasp the breast at once and begin to suckle	3
b) Grasp after a few attempts and begin to suckle	2
c) Make repeated attempts, hold nipple in mouth, stimulate to suck	1
d) Seem too sleepy or reluctant, no latch achieved	0

Sample size considerations

A pilot study (Carfoot et al., 2004) confirmed the initial estimate of 50% for the rate of successful first feed in the routine care group. The authors considered that skin-to-skin contact would need to increase this rate in absolute terms by 25%. The pilot study indicated that such a large difference in the success of the first breast feeding was achievable.

A sample size of 154 (77 per group) was calculated to give 90% power, at the two-sided 5% significance level, to detect an increase from 50–75% in the rate of successful first breast feeds (Machin et al., 1997). The study aimed to recruit a total of 200 women to allow for losses to follow-up.

Randomisation

The trial statistician (PRW) provided a sequence of envelopes each containing the next allocation from a computer-generated randomisation list. Women were reminded of the study in early labour, and they confirmed their intention to participate at this stage. The on-call research assistant was contacted to attend the delivery as soon as possible. A sealed envelope was opened during the second stage of labour to reveal the treatment group (skin-to-skin or routine care) for the trial participant, who was informed along with the midwife responsible for her care.

Data collection

The research assistant observed post-delivery care and assessed the first breast feed in the delivery room. The clinical co-ordinator collected demographic, labour and delivery history data (past and current pregnancies) from the records. Post-delivery data collection was carried out through contact with the mothers before they left hospital and at 4 months by telephone interview.

Data analysis

Analysis followed the intention-to-treat principle. SPSS software (version 11) was used for data analysis. Confidence intervals for the differences between proportions were calculated using Newcombe's method (Newcombe and Altman, 2000). A χ^2 test was used to compare routine and skin-to-skin care in relation to success of first and subsequent feeds, whether the woman was still breast feeding at 4 months, maternal satisfaction and preference data. A t-test was used to compare baby-body temperature and time to first feed in each group. Observation of the first feed was limited to 45 mins, thus duration of feed was compared between groups using the Log-rank test.

Findings

Three hundred and twenty-five women were approached consecutively, and 244 (75%) agreed to participate. Forty women were not randomised for a variety of reasons (Figure 7.7.2).

The remaining 204 women were randomised, with 102 women allocated to each group. Two mothers were immediately withdrawn from the skin-to-skin group (one had a stillbirth, the other decided to artifically feed), whereas one was lost from the control group (withdrew consent) before the intervention phase started. These three women were not included in the analysis. The analysis followed the 'intention-to-treat' principle, with a small number of 'problem' participants analysed as per randomised group. Two mothers randomised to the routine care group requested skin-to-skin contact immediately after delivery. One mother randomised to skin-to-skin care had an emergency caesarean section, was unwell after delivery and was unable to hold her baby in skin-to-skin contact.

Although these mothers changed groups, they were analysed as belonging to the group to which they were randomly allocated.

The baseline characteristics of the participants are described in Table 7.7.1. No clinically significant baseline imbalance was noted, although there were slightly more

Figure 7.7.2 Participant flow diagram.

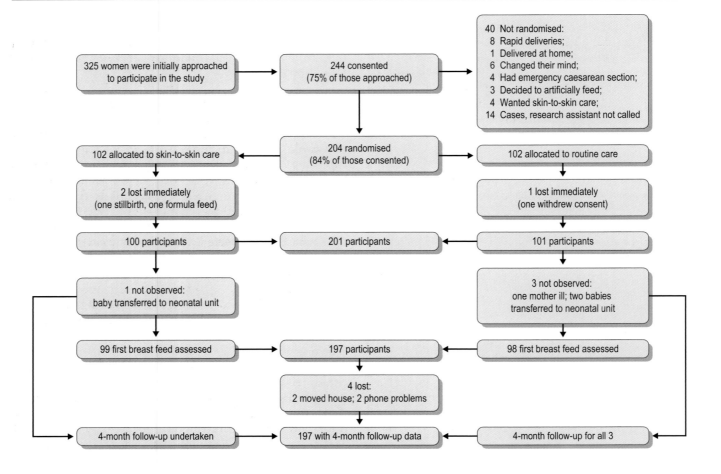

Table 7.7.1 Description of participants

Characteristics	Skin-to-skin care	Routine care
	(n = 102)	(n = 102)
Primigravidae	46 (45%)	43 (42%)
Multiparae with no previous breast-feeding experience	10 (18%)	7 (10%)
Multiparae: median duration of breast feeding (days) (minimum; maximum)	135 (14; 1080 days)	120 (3; 720 days)
Attended antenatal classes	64 (63%)	64 (63%)
Vaginal delivery	72 (72%)*	73 (72%)
Pethidine	42 (42%)*	46 (45%)
Epidural/spinal	42 (42%)*	42 (41%)
Female infant	44 (44%)	44 (43%)

*Two women had missing data because one woman decided to artificially feed and the other woman withdrew consent to participate after randomisation, thus no data were extracted from the records.

multiparous women with no previous breast-feeding experience in the skin-to-skin group; 10/102 (18%) compared with seven (10%) in the control group.

More women receiving skin-to-skin care tended to have a successful first breast feed, although there was no evidence of any effect on continuation of breast feeding at 4 months (Table 7.7.2). Eleven babies (11%) in the skin-to-skin group were cooler than normal body temperature (36.5–37.0°) during the first hour after delivery compared with 21 (21%) in the routine care group. Although the difference in temperature was statistically significant, it was not considered to be clinically important.

Time to first feed and length of first feed were comparable between both groups (Table 7.7.2). Seventy-two (37%) of 194 babies fed for longer than 45 mins from one or both breasts.

Four mothers stopped breast feeding before discharge from hospital, in two cases because the baby had difficulty latching on and in two because the baby was ill. Forty-eight (25%) subsequent breast feeds in the postnatal ward were observed by the first author, with the remaining being self-assessed by the mother. There was no evidence of any benefit from skin-to-skin contact.

Maternal satisfaction levels were high in both groups, although a greater proportion of women were very satisfied with skin-to-skin care. Eighty-seven of 97 (90%) mothers were very satisfied with skin-to-skin care, compared with 60 of 102 (59%) (P ≤0.001) in the control group. A total of 83 of 97 (86%) of the mothers in the intervention group said that they would prefer to receive the same care in the future compared with 31 of 102 (30%) (P ≤0.001) mothers in the control group.

Discussion

Although this study was successful, there were limitations. Interference from the research assistant was the most significant limitation. In some cases, the research assistant helped the mother to feed rather than the attending midwife. This tended to happen when the attending midwife was out of the room and the baby was showing signs of readiness to feed. However, this is anecdotal evidence, as this information was volunteered from some mothers at the follow-up interview before discharge from hospital or at the 4 month follow-up.

Although the rate of successful first breast feeding was not significantly different between the two groups, the findings suggest that mothers prefer skin-to-skin care, and there is no associated decrease in babies' temperatures, rather a benefit. On the basis of these findings, the authors believe there is enough evidence to offer women a choice of skin-to-skin contact in early post-delivery care.

Overall rates of successful breast feeding were higher than expected. This could be attributed to the high level of motivation of the participants, who all intended to breast feed. The success rates of the first breast feed confirmed by the findings of the pilot study were 62% in the control group. However, the observed result in the full trial for the control group was 83%. A possible explanation for this could be the presence of the research assistant in the delivery room. This may have prompted the attending midwife to ensure that she assisted the mother to breast feed.

A systematic review (Carfoot et al., 2003), conducted before the study, indicated that some skin-to-skin studies (Sosa et al., 1976; Thomson et al., 1979; Christensson et al., 1992; Christensson et al., 1995) were conducted in the context in which the control babies were separated from their mothers. In this study, there was immediate contact between mothers and babies in both groups. Under these circumstances, it is likely to be more difficult to show a large difference between the two groups.

The lack of evidence for an effect on breast feeding at 4 months was expected, as there are many factors that affect this outcome (Donnelly et al., 2000; Sikorski et al., 2001; Snowdon et al., 2001). The reasons given by mothers in this trial for stopping breast feeding included returning to work, painful breasts or nipples, too tiring, insufficient milk, difficulties with attachment and domestic reasons. These findings are similar to those of the National Infant Feeding (Hamlyn et al., 2000).

A recent Cochrane systematic review (Anderson et al., 2003) found that mothers who had skin-to-skin contact with their babies were twice as likely to be breast-feeding 1–3 months after birth. The pooled odds ratio (95% confidence interval [CI]) from a random-effects meta-analysis was 2.15 (1.10, 4.22). However, the authors

Table 7.7.2 Initial and 4-month outcomes

Outomes	Skin-to-skin care	Routine care	Difference between groups (95% CI)	Test statistic	df	P value
Success of first breast feed (BAT score 8–12)	(n = 98) 89 (91%)	(n = 99) 82 (83%)	8% (−1.6%, 17.6%)	$\chi^2 = 2.74$	1	0.10
Success of subsequent breast feed before discharge	(n = 96) 91 (95%)	(n = 101) 97 (96%)	−1.2% (−8.1%, 5.3%)		(Fisher's exact test)	
Mean temperature 1 hr after birth (°C) (sd)	(n = 97) 36.9 (sd = 0.45)	(n = 100) 36.7 (sd = 0.43)	0.15 (0.03, 0.28)	t = −2.45	195	0.02
Mean time to first feed (mins)	(n = 98) 46 (sd = 22.2)	(n = 99) 45 (sd = 22.8)	1.3 (−5.1, 7.6)	t = −0.39	195	0.70
Median (95% CI) duration of first feed (mins)	(n = 97) 40 (32, 40)	(n = 97) 35 (33, 40)	0 (−5, 5)	Z = −0.008		0.99
Maternal satisfaction with care received	(n = 97)	(n = 102)		$\chi^2 = 24.54$	1	<0.000*
Very satisfied	87 (90%)	60 (59%)				
Satisfied	10 (10%)	39 (38%)				
Fairly satisfied	0	2 (2%)				
Unsatisfied	0	1 (1%)				
Very unsatisfied	0	0 (0%)				
Preference for same post-delivery care in future	(n = 97)	(n = 102)				
Most certain	83 (86%)	31 (30%)		$\chi^2 = 61.86$	1	<0.001†
Certain	12 (12%)	35 (34%)				
Quite certain	2 (2%)	17 (17%)				
Not certain	0 (0%)	16 (16%)				
Certainly not	0 (0%)	3 (3%)				
Feeding at 4 months	(n = 97)	(n = 100)	3.3% (−10.3%; 16.7%)	$\chi^2 = 0.22$	1	0.64
Exclusive breast/partial breast	42 (43%)	40 (40%)				
Formula	55 (57%)	60 (60%)				

*P value relates to comparison of 'very satisfied' compared with the rest; †P value relates to comparison of 'most certain' compared with the rest. BAT, breast feeding assessment tool.

noted limitations in this review relating to the methodological quality of the studies, outcomes reported and variations in the implementation of the intervention. The trial reported here is larger than any of the trials included in this review, and had longer follow-up than eight out of nine studies reporting duration of breast feeding. Pooling the results from this trial with those in the review gives a combined odds ratio (95% CI) from a random effects meta-analysis of 1.89 (1.06, 3.34), a slightly smaller but more precise effect estimate, and still statistically significant.

Conclusion

The findings of this trial show a tendency for more mothers to have a successful first breast-feeding experience after a period of skin-to-skin contact with their babies than with routine care. The women also reported a higher degree of satisfaction. The study provides strong evidence that baby temperature is not adversely affected through skin-to-skin care, although there was no evidence of any effect on breast feeding at 4 months. Overall, we believe our study provides support for the implementation of skin-to-skin care.

Acknowledgements

The study was funded by a research grant from the North West Regional Health Authority. The authors would like to thank all the women who participated, as well as the midwifery staff of Warrington Hospital.

REFERENCES

Anderson, G., Moore, E., Hepworth, J., et al., 2003. Early skin-to-skin contact for mothers and their health newborn infants (Cochrane Review). Cochrane Library. John Wiley & Sons, Oxford.

Bernard-Bonnin, A., Stachtenko, S., Girard, G., et al., 1989. Hospital practices and breastfeeding duration: meta-analysis of controlled trials. Birth 16, 64–66.

Carfoot, S., Williamson, P.R., Dickson, R., 2003. A systematic review of randomised controlled trials evaluating the effect of mother/baby skin-to-skin care on successful breast feeding. Midwifery 19, 148–155.

Carfoot, S., Williamson, P.R., Dickson, R., 2004. The value of a pilot study in breast-feeding research. Midwifery 20, 188–193.

Christensson, K., Cabrera, T., Christensson, E., et al., 1995. Separation distress call in the human neonate in the absence of maternal body contact. Acta Paediatrica 84, 468–473.

Christensson, K., Siles, C., Moreno, L., et al., 1992. Temperature, metabolic adaptation and crying in healthy full-term newborns cared for skin-to-skin or in a cot. Acta Paediatrica 81, 488–493.

Donnelly, A., Snowdon, H., Renfrew, M., et al., 2000. Commercial hospital discharge packs for breastfeeding women (Cochrane Review). Cochrane Library. John Wiley & Sons Ltd, Oxford.

Fairbank, L., O'Meara, S., Renfrew, M., et al., 2000. A systematic review to evaluate the effectiveness of interventions to promote the initiation of breastfeeding. Health Technology Assessment 4.

Hamlyn, B., Brooker, S., Oleinikova, K., et al., 2000. Infant feeding 2000. The Stationary Office, London.

Machin, D., Campbell, M., Fayers, P., et al., 1997. Sample size tables for clinical studies. Blackwell Science Ltd, Oxford.

Matthews, M., 1988. Developing an instrument to assess infant breast-feeding behaviour in early neonatal period. Midwifery 4, 154–165.

Newcombe, R., Altman, D., 2000. Proportions and their differences. In: Altman, D., Machin, D., Bryant, T., Gardner, M. (Eds.), Statistics with confidence, 2nd edn. BMJ Publishing, London.

Perez-Escamilla, R., Pollitt, E., Lonnerdal, B., et al., 1994. Infant feeding policies in maternity wards and their effect on breast-feeding success: an analytical overview. American Journal of Public Health 84, 89–96.

Righard, L., Alade, M., 1990. Effect of delivery room routines on success of first breast-feed. Lancet 336, 1105–1107.

Sikorski, J., Renfrew, M., Pindoria, S., et al., 2001. Support for breastfeeding mothers. Cochrane Library. John Wiley & Sons Ltd, Oxford.

Snowdon, H., Renfrew, M., Woolridge, M., 2001. Treatments for breast engorgement during lactation (Cochrane Review). Cochrane Library. John Wiley & Sons Ltd, Oxford.

Sosa, R., Kennell, J., Klaus, M., et al., 1976. The effect of early mother-infant contact on breast feeding, infection and growth. CIBA Foundation Symposium 45, 179–193.

Thomson, M., Hartstock, T., Larson, C., 1979. The importance of immediate postnatal contact: its effect on breastfeeding. Canadian Family Physician 25, 1374–1378.

UNICEF, 1999. Towards national regional and local strategies for breast-feeding, UNICEF, London.

WHO/UNICEF, 1998. Implementing the ten steps to successful breast-feeding, UNICEF, London.

Widstrom, A., Matthiesen, A., Eneroth, P., et al., 1990. Short term effects of early suckling and touch of the nipple on maternal behaviour. Early Human Development 21, 153–163.

Widstrom, A., Ransjo-Arvidson, A., Christensson, K., et al., 1987. Gastric suction in healthy newborn infants: effects on circulation and developing feeding behaviour. Acta Paediatrica Scandinavia 76, 566–572.

World Health Organization, 2000. WHO Technical Consultant's Statement on the duration of exclusive breastfeeding. British Medical Journal 321, 958.

Midwifery 2005; 21(1): 71–79

Expression of love

Alison Baum

My first son David was born with a cleft palate and a rare syndrome called Pierre Robin which meant he couldn't breastfeed. However, by expressing, I was able to feed him exclusively on my milk until he was eight months old. (He ate solids earlier, but the only milk he drank or ate with his baby rice was mine.)

The first few months of David's life were extremely tough – we visited five different hospitals in his first five weeks. David had a very wide cleft palate, a tiny lower jaw and serious breathing problems, which meant he choked all the time. At first he was fed by a naso-gastric tube, but at 10 days old the tube came out and we graduated on to a special squeezy bottle. Without any roof to his mouth David had no suck, but he still made the action with his mouth and lips – so when he went to suck we would gently squeeze the bottle.

The biggest breakthrough came when we were taught 'side-lying', a technique whereby I fed David his bottle lying on a pillow, on his side. Any excess milk dribbled out of his mouth and was therefore less likely to overwhelm him. But his feeds were still incredibly precarious. They were like an amazing silent dialogue, with me responding to his every move, ever watchful not to squeeze too much lest he get overwhelmed and choke.

For the first 10 weeks I also tried to see if David would feed from the breast, but he became distressed and it was cruel as he couldn't get any milk out – quite simply, he had no suck. Although David couldn't breastfeed, I was determined that he should at least benefit from drinking my expressed milk. I started expressing on day one and didn't stop until David was eight months old. Above and beyond the normal benefits of breastmilk there were four main reasons that gave me the momentum to express:

1. We knew that David would have an operation to repair his cleft palate at six-and-a-half months old, and I wanted him to have all the immunity I could give him. Before David's operation, everything he drank (and ate) came out of his nose, and breast milk is known to be far less irritating than formula on the nasal passages.
2. We knew that sometimes milk went the wrong way into David's lungs, and once again breast milk is far better tolerated than formula. Indeed, David never got a chest infection, and we are sure that my milk was the reason why.
3. David, like many cleft palate babies, had severe glue ear, and breastfeeding has been shown to help the condition.
4. I hoped that if I managed to express until David had his operation to repair his cleft palate, he would be able to breastfeed afterwards.

Basically, I felt helpless with so much of what was going on with David medically, but expressing was something I could do – a difference I could make.

Exclusive expressing

If you express all your milk for your baby because he or she is unable to breastfeed it is called exclusive expressing. Exclusive expressing is tricky because the breast doesn't get the normal stimulation of the baby sucking at the breast. To keep the milk flowing you have to express as often as the baby would feed from the breast. At the beginning that was at least eight times a day and once during the night. Lots of research has shown that expressing with a double-electric pump can help (Jones et al 2001). It has been shown to increase yield and fat content, and it allows you to express more quickly.

The only trouble with double-pumping is that it is not terribly practical – put simply, you just haven't got enough hands! I sat there like a lemon holding both collecting funnels on my breasts; I couldn't even turn the machine on myself, let alone drink a glass of water!

I am sure I would have given up expressing much earlier if I hadn't tracked down the Easy Expression Halterneck bra from the United States. It kept me sane and happy, as I was able to have a life while I expressed. The Halterneck holds the funnels of the collecting sets comfortably in place, which freed me up to eat and drink, play with David and talk to my friends and family on the phone, all while I expressed. It was fantastic to be productive in more ways than one!

To keep my milk supply going I had to express in the night, even after David was sleeping through – I didn't mind, as the Halterneck freed up my hands to allow me to read my way through the first three Harry Potter books!

The old saying 'there is no point crying over spilt milk' just doesn't apply when you've spent 30 minutes making it. But with the Halterneck the collecting funnels were safe, and even though I am very clumsy I managed to avoid any mishaps. In fact, I found that my milk yield increased using the Halterneck, probably because I was so much more relaxed while I expressed. It got to the point that I was so ahead of David's demands that there was no room in the freezer for any Häagen-Dazs! I am proud to say I was even able to donate milk to my local milk bank at Queen Charlotte's Hospital in west London.

I had used the Halterneck for almost six months when I realised that no one else in the UK knew about it. I was determined to make it available to British women – it had made such a huge difference to my life that I wanted other mums to benefit, too. So I hooked up with the manufacturer in the US, and set up my own company, Express Yourself Bras. I am now the exclusive distributor of the Halterneck in the UK.

From strength to strength

David recovered well from his cleft palate repair operation and went from strength to strength. He never got the hang of breastfeeding, which wasn't surprising as many of his associations with it had been negative – such as being squirted in the eye as I frantically tried to hand-express into his mouth! But the breastfeeding didn't matter as he was doing so well, and for the first time he was happy.

David needed hearing aids for about six months, until he had a grommet operation when he was a bit over a year. The grommets were amazing – he could hear properly for the first time, and his talking just took off! Two years and two sets of grommets later, we are back with the hearing aids. He is very proud of his new moulds – embossed with the Manchester United flag!

David has a wonderful cheeky grin and a fabulous sense of humour. He started school this September and is getting on great – if it weren't for his hearing aids you wouldn't have any inkling of his terrible start in life. He is amazing – we are so proud of our first little miracle boy.

Second time round

When I became pregnant again my hopes of breastfeeding were re-ignited, but once again things didn't go to plan. Joshua was born a month early and there were problems with his feeding from day one. Everyone was telling me the latch was perfect, but I could only tell if he was feeding by looking at him – so much for 'toe-curling' stuff! Also, my husband, a paediatrician, had looked and noticed that there was a translucency to Joshua's palate, and he thought he might have spotted a bifid uvula. We were concerned that Joshua had a submucous cleft palate, but we were reassured that everything was fine and that we should just be mum and dad.

Unfortunately, any issues about Joshua's feeding soon became irrelevant: he wasn't holding his temperature and wasn't feeding well, and when he started deteriorating rapidly on day eight they did a lumbar puncture and found he had viral meningitis. He was desperately ill, and I started expressing for him in earnest. I would sit by his incubator, my hand resting on his head while I double-pumped for him. The care Joshua received was excellent; he was a real fighter and pulled through.

When we were back on the transitional care ward, my concerns about Joshua's feeding became more prominent. But I was again told to relax and believe in my abilities as a breastfeeding mother. For days my time on the pump was rationed and I was encouraged just to feed Joshua on the breast, but I felt he could only take from my breasts if they were full and that he couldn't drain them properly. We were finally discharged on a Thursday, I was told to go home, do loads of lovely skin-to-skin and discard the pump. In the end, I so wanted to believe Joshua was fine and that this would work that I did what I was told. It felt like a fantasy: not real, but wonderful, breastfeeding properly for the first time.

On the Monday, my husband and I took Joshua to Great Ormond Street. The consultant took one look in Joshua's mouth and announced that he had a classic and significant submucous cleft – the skin layer was there, but none of the musculature was behind it, and there was a 'notch' in his hard palate. It turns out that to diagnose a cleft it is not good enough just to 'look' – you also have to 'feel'.

We were, of course, devastated by the diagnosis, but I knew I would be able to long-term express, so that Joshua, like David, could at least benefit from my milk. As soon as I got home I started to express but, to my utter dismay, nothing came out – my milk had gone. The five days of no expressing and the previous week of limited expressing had done the damage – in the hospital I would pump for only three minutes as I felt I was being rationed; I'd make 180ml in this time, but in retrospect I was just taking off the fore-milk, not draining the breast to stimulate more production.

While I'd been in hospital and Joshua had been very poorly and IV fed, I had expressed more milk than he needed. On the day of Joshua's diagnosis, my extra milk was on its way to the milk bank at Queen Charlotte's, but we managed to intercept it and get it to our home freezer instead. So my challenge was to re-lactate and get a sufficient supply going before the supply of my expressed breast milk (EBM) ran out.

Family support and expert help

It was an incredibly difficult and stressful time. My family was a huge support, as was Liz Jones, the neonatal feeding advisor at North Staffordshire Hospital and now a good friend. Liz is also an academic and an international expert on exclusive expressing. I was angry with the health professionals who had not listened when I'd voiced my concerns about Joshua's suck, but more angry with myself for listening to them. If I had not known what I knew through my experience with David I would have given up, not realising that re-lactating was an option.

We are so lucky that I managed to re-lactate and avoid Joshua having formula as he turned out to be extremely dairy intolerant. His extreme and painful constipation was only resolved when I removed all dairy from my diet. So I don't want to imagine what would have happened if I'd given up on expressing and put him on formula.

Because Joshua's cleft wasn't as severe as David's had been, he could also take some milk directly from me. As he got older he got better and stronger at the breast, but unfortunately his suck was never strong enough to take all he needed directly from me or to empty my breasts – when I tried a couple of times to stop expressing and just breastfeed him, my milk supply plummeted. However, I would put him to my breast for most feeds, either before or after his bottle of expressed milk.

I used the Halterneck, of course, and became masterly at double-pumping at the same time as feeding Joshua his bottle of EBM – I often chatted on the phone at the same time as well! I also found that I could sit David on my lap and read him stories while I double-pumped. Being able to give David attention in this way helped stave off the 'little green devil'!

I have to confess that I had been taking my Halterneck and my double electric pump for granted until I accidentally left them at home when I went to my close friend Louise's for dinner when Joshua was coming up to five months old. My initial panic subsided when I realised

that I could borrow Louise's hand-pump (Louise had recently given birth to Sadie). The most frustrating 40 minutes ensued; in double the time I only managed to express a quarter of what I normally make. My hand ached and I was extremely stressed, but Louise looked surprisingly relieved.

She explained that if I – 'the queen of expressing,' as she calls me – had only managed to make such a small amount, then she didn't feel nearly so bad about how hard she had been finding hand-pumping. (That said, many mums do get on fine with a hand-pump.)

When Joshua was five months and the operation to repair his cleft palate loomed, I got on the phone (while Joshua slept and while I expressed) and spoke to some of the mums to whom I'd sold expressing bras over the previous two years. It was utterly uplifting to find out how much the Halterneck and alternative Bustier have helped so many other mothers to give their babies the very best. I've spoken to mums returning to work, mums wanting their partner to do the odd night feed, mums with sick or premature babies and mums of twins or triplets. They've each got their own remarkable story to tell.

Immediately post-operation, Joshua found breastfeeding less painful than feeding from a bottle, but I found it a nightmare – the stitches in his mouth dug straight into my nipple which was extremely painful. Fortunately, my husband had the cunning idea of getting breast shields – thank goodness for all-night chemists! I only needed to use the shields for four days, because the stitches started to dissolve and the pain eased.

Post-op was also tough because Joshua's new improved suck was better than his swallow – so, whether he was feeding on a bottle or at my breast, he was often overwhelmed by the milk and choked. But six weeks post-operation Joshua mastered the 'suck, swallow, breathe' pattern. I gradually increased his time at the breast while decreasing the expressing and top-ups of EBM. Finally, seven months after Joshua was born, I achieved my dream of being a fully breastfeeding mother.

Giving something back

Soon afterwards I started my training to be an NCT breastfeeding counsellor, and embarked on an intensive nine-week Sure Start course to become a peer support breastfeeding mum. It was then I realised that normal mums with normal, healthy babies often struggle with breastfeeding. Primarily it boils down to a lack of information, misinformation, conflicting information and a lack of support.

I then made a huge decision, to take voluntary redundancy from the BBC – where I'd been a producer/director for almost 10 years – and to launch a new website (www. expressyourselfmums.co.uk) to help bridge the gap between wanting to breastfeed and actually being able to do it.

Express Yourself Mums, which has been live since January 2005, is a central resource for breastfeeding mums and the healthcare professionals who support them. I've recently joined forces with another mother, Carly, who had a tough time breastfeeding her daughter Izzie as she was constantly being told that Izzie – though healthy, alert and with plenty of wet and poo-filled nappies – wasn't putting on 'enough' weight. Carly gave in and started to top up as directed, only to discover that the growth charts that were being used for Izzie were designed for bottle-fed babies. Together we plan to support mums and healthcare professionals to have a positive impact on breastfeeding rates in the UK.

In the information zone on our website there are in-depth articles by international experts such as Dr Jack Newman and Rebecca Glover. In our product zone we sell tried and tested specialist breastfeeding and expressing products.

Facility for midwives

I'm delighted to have received a grant from UnLtd – an organisation that gives out millennium funding to social entrepreneurs – and I'm using this money to ensure that midwives can order free, colourful A5 leaflets and posters about Express Yourself Mums from the dedicated healthcare professional page of our website.

Our product zone has a section aimed specifically at healthcare professionals, offering a range of valuable teaching resources and equipment for hospitals and clinics.

Our range is constantly growing and improving. We've started selling Suzanne Colson's excellent booklet on bio-logical nurturing. If you order free leaflets for display in your clinics we will send you a brochure that highlights the products that you might be interested in for your hospital/clinic.

Sharing experiences

Express Yourself Mums is also a place where women can share inspiring success stories and problems overcome – an online community with a positive twist. Mums are encouraged to share their experiences and ideas online, to give their feedback on products and tell their stories with the gritty honesty you'd share with your sister or best friend.

Express Yourself Mums is also the first specialist retailer that triggers a donation (of up to £2.50) to charity with every purchase: – for most products sold, the customer can choose which breastfeeding or baby charity to support from a list of 12.

Alison Blenkinsop, midwife and International Board Certified Lactation Consultant, wrote recently: 'I am very pleased to promote the Express Yourself Mums website – I often give the internet link to mothers I help. I know they'll find a lot of useful information here.'

I now spend my time addressing conferences, talking to healthcare professionals and spreading the word that help is at hand. Never in a million years could I have imagined that this is what I'd be doing. Life throws stuff at us all, and I guess I've decided to pick it up and run with it. Yes, both my miracle boys had a tough start, and the last four years have been an incredible rollercoaster ride for our family, but at least I feel other people are learning from our experiences and hopefully benefiting from this knowledge.

REFERENCE

Jones E, Dimmock PW and Spencer SA (2001). 'A randomised controlled trial to compare methods of milk expression after preterm delivery'. Archives of Disease in Childhood (fetal neonatal ed), 85 (2): F91–F95.

The Practising Midwife 2005; 8(10): 29–34

Breastfeeding peer support in Doncaster: the next stage, learning from each other

Mavis Kirkham

Peer supporters have been working to support and encourage breastfeeding mothers in Doncaster since the start of Breastfriends Doncaster in 2000 (Kirkham 2000). The training for these volunteers was based upon an enablement model developed by Mary Smale during her work as a National Childbirth Trust (NCT) breastfeeding tutor. She has since published this work as a teaching pack (Smale 2004).

The training and work of the first two sets of volunteers was evaluated (Curtis et al 2000). This evaluation demonstrates both the value of their work and the sensitivity and complexity of relationships between volunteers and midwives.

Training for peer supporters has continued, mainly within Sure Starts in various parts of Doncaster, but there are not enough training courses to produce and maintain a network of breastfeeding peer supporters across the area.

Two years ago the opportunity came for funded part-time work to consolidate and co-ordinate breastfeeding peer support. There were many applicants. Not surprisingly, the successful candidates had trained as Breast-friends. Originally there were two posts and their holders worked closely together. Financial cut-backs led to the loss of one post and the post-holder now plans to train as a midwife. The other post continued, funded, via a series of temporary contracts, through the skill and commitment of the Head of Midwifery, Vivienne Knight.

Daniella Thornton has held her twenty-two and a half hour per week job for two years now. Her job title is 'Breastfeeding Service Development Officer – Grade B'. Her work demonstrates what breastfeeding peer supporters can achieve for women and for midwives. This article was developed from a conversation with Daniella in September 2006. As this article was completed (February 2007) we heard that Daniella's continued employment had been ensured.

A friend with experience

Daniella spends three mornings each week on the post-natal wards where she meets all the breastfeeding mothers and gives them her contact details. Her point of contact with them is her own experience as well as her extensive knowledge. Daniella has breastfed her own three children.

Doncaster has a three-generation history of bottle-feeding and many new mothers have no friends or family with any experience of breastfeeding. Daniella is therefore the only woman many breastfeeding mothers know who has experience of breastfeeding and who they can turn to with queries and questions about what is normal and what they can expect. On booking, some women now state 'I'm going to breastfeed. I know Daniella'. This is a great change, in this culture of bottle-feeding, from the statement 'I'll try to breastfeed' with the implied likelihood of failure for a woman who knows no-one who has done this before.

Professionals give Daniella's phone number to mothers with problems. She deals with an average of seven phone queries from women each week and can make home visits if wanted. She has become widely known. Recently she went to a football match and the woman next to her said 'Are you that breastfeeding woman from Doncaster? My sister's best friend had a baby and she talked to you . . .'

The small number of breastfeeding peer support volunteers in the community means that Daniella spends most of her time giving direct support to mothers, rather than training or co-ordinating volunteers. Clearly there is a limit to what one woman can do.

Relationships with professionals

Relationships between midwives and peer supporters can be difficult, with some midwives feeling that peer supporters are encroaching upon their area of expertise. Some midwives and health visitors chose not to work with peer supporters when Breast Friends Doncaster was first set up and some may have seen them as a threat (Curtis et al 2000). Daniella is very conscious of how her work could be seen by midwives and stresses that 'I see myself as extra support for mums and staff'. She has worked consciously and empathetically to develop these relationships. 'I'm happier getting on with people . . . you don't tell people what to do or undermine what they do. I'd be miffed if people undermined me.'

Developing trust and positive relationships with staff has been a slow process. 'It's taken six years: four voluntary and two employed to get the right relationships with midwives.' During 2006 she feels that 'everything has slotted into place' and she has become 'an expert resource for professionals'. She averages one phone call a week from midwives, mainly those on the postnatal wards, some community midwives and some health visitors use her expertise and some do not. She now receives occasional calls from children's nurses and paediatricians, following her support for a breastfeeding paediatric nurse.

Parallels with midwifery

Enjoying the job

Listening to Daniella, I am struck by the parallels with midwifery, particularly midwifery before it was professionalised and birth became highly medicalised. She enjoys her work, 'it's not just a job'. She respects, quietly supports and empowers women.

Listening and developing relationships

Daniella thinks that 95% of her work is listening and her listening skills are well developed. She feels it is vital that she can 'take time to sit with women and let them talk and I get the problems'. 'It's not always breastfeeding, often it's what's behind it. They blame the breastfeeding because that is easier. Often it is the situation she finds herself in, plus breastfeeding difficulties.' Daniella's reputation in the community is such that women clearly find her attention and understanding to be empowering.

Reporting on her job after one year Daniella wrote:

'I found that a lot of the mums really liked the fact that they had a chance for a non-rushed, one-to-one chat with someone who is non-medical and who has breastfed their own children. This I feel helped them relax and open up about any problems they were having, their fears/expectations, what they should expect in the future, etc.'

Appearing non-rushed is a skill, not just a reflection of time available but such chats only happen if they are prioritised. Many midwives feel that such conversations embody the relationships with women from which they derive great job satisfaction and which they find pressure of work now makes it hard for them to achieve (Kirkham et al 2006). It is to the great credit of Daniella and the midwives who work with her that they have developed a service where women's needs are the priority and such support for breastfeeding is possible. Hopefully it also frees up some midwife time.

Time and resources

Daniella does not see herself as working just the hours for which she is paid, 'because I enjoy it'. She fills in a rota for the hours she works, 'but the phone is on 24/7'. Like many midwives (Kirkham et al 2006), she feels the impact of lack of resources upon her work. She tries to visit women within 24 hours of a request, but that is difficult now she is the only peer supporter in post. Losing the other peer support post, and insufficient volunteer peer supporters leaves her relatively isolated. There are volunteer peer supporters in some Sure Starts, but they only cover relatively small areas and funds for further training courses are drying up. Therefore, Daniella lacks peers to whom she can refer women or with whom she can discuss issues. Many midwives share this experience because of pressures of work upon themselves and colleagues (Kirkham & Morgan 2006, Kirkham et al 2006).

Though employed by the midwifery service, Daniella supports some women long after they have passed into the care of their Health Visitor. She finds that 'there are lots of problems after babies are six weeks old'. As a result of her experience of women in isolation with regard to breastfeeding, she likes to maintain contact with women who have had problems for two weeks after the problems are resolved. Most of this support is given in her own time.

Support

Since Breastfriends training was developed from a voluntary sector model, Daniella values and develops her own support network. She can access good telephone support through her original trainer, Mary Smale, and the NCT breastfeeding network. Through them, she has access to a great pool of expertise, which is essential in situations that individuals encounter rarely. For instance, she supported a woman who had had extensive treatment for childhood leukaemia and enabled her to successfully breastfeed; she also gained knowledge relevant to this woman's care which she fed back to midwives.

The NCT breastfeeding network also gives Daniella opportunities for facilitated reflection upon her work with her peers. Many midwives feel they lack support (Ball et al 2002, Stapleton et al 1998) and are not trained to develop and value their own professional support network. Daniella's support is excellent, but it is entirely voluntary and unfunded. In this, it parallels the emotional support of family and friends, which enables many midwives to go on practising in the face of stress and challenges at work (Kirkham et al 2006). Caring and listening seem little valued within the NHS with all its pressures towards action. This is particularly true around breastfeeding (Dykes 2006).

In terms of time and subjects of concern, Daniella's job lacks boundaries. She does not encroach upon professional areas of expertise and encourages women to raise concerns with appropriate professionals. Yet some women's worries do not fit the expertise of midwives, health visitors or doctors and when what is wanted is a listening ear, she listens. She enjoys developing her knowledge of breastfeeding and her interpersonal skills. Recently she has started working through interpreters and her work has been observed by midwives on the Return to Practice Programme. The service she gives is excellent but she works far more than her paid hours. Since she is happy in her work, this may be seen as acceptable. The aim of breastfeeding peer support is cultural change and, when most women in Doncaster have friends and family who have successfully breastfed, the need for professional peer support will wane. For the present, however, Daniella is dedicated and relatively isolated. Dedication and isolation can lead to burnout. More training for volunteers and another peer support post would alter this situation, but funds are scarce and the very existence of Daniella's job is unusual. Daniella's skills and confidence are such that I am sure she will go on to have a successful career and will probably not always work around breastfeeding. She certainly feels that her work as a peer supporter has been enabling for her.

In conversation with Daniella, I am struck by the parallels between her experience and that of many midwives (Kirkham & Morgan 2006, Kirkham et al 2006). Yet midwives are not aiming to work themselves out of a job, there are many more of them, their work is more defined and constrained, and stress, isolation and burnout are common. It does seem that cultural change is needed within maternity services if midwives and peer supporters, separately and together, are to fully achieve their potential. When I discussed this with Mary Smale, she said that midwives and peer supporters encounter similar issues around breastfeeding and suggested 'some regular joint forum in which they can see their similar situations and become more skilled not just in knowledge but in mother-centred communication'. Such a forum would also give support and recognition to those who feel isolated. Meanwhile, the mothers and midwives of Doncaster appreciate a very special service.

REFERENCES

Ball L, Curtis P, Kirkham M 2002 Why Do Midwives Leave? Royal College of Midwives, London

Curtis P, Stapleton H, Kirkham M, Smale M 2000 Evaluation of the Breastfriends Doncaster 2000 Initiative. WICH, University of Sheffield

Dykes F 2006 Breastfeeding in hospital. Routledge, Oxford

Kirkham M 2000 Breastfriends Doncaster 2000. Practising Midwife 3(7): 20–21

Kirkham M, Morgan RK 2006 Why midwives return and their subsequent experience. Department of Health, London (www.nhsemployers.org and www.rcm.org)

Kirkham M, Morgan RK, Davies C 2006 Why do midwives *stay*. Department of Health, London (www.nhsemployers.org and www.rcm.org)

Smale M 2004 Training breastfeeding peer supporters: an enabling approach. Available from The National Childbirth Trust, London

Stapleton H, Duerden J, Kirkham M 1998 Evaluation of the impact of the supervision of midwives on professional practice and the quality of midwifery care. English National Board for Nursing, Midwifery and Health Visiting, London

Topics for further reflection

Postnatal care has, as I have discussed in previous volumes of *Midwifery: Best Practice*, been relatively neglected by comparison to other areas of midwifery. It is, then, really heartening to read work such as Sue Lennox's article about the concept of 'the golden orb'. As well as providing insight into the ways in which we can help women create their self-stories, this article also raises some interesting questions about the environment of birth and postnatal care, which links with some of the articles in Section 2. It is, for instance, much easier to see how women can be within the orb while they are in their homes, and, as Sue notes, less easy to protect the women who remain in hospital.

- Do you find the concept of the golden orb a useful one for your practice? How could you apply it in the area where you work? Do you agree with Sue that part of a midwife's role is to help women create their self-stories and, if so, what are your experiences in this area? (You may also like to compare Sue's thoughts with those that Lorna Davies shared in Section 3.)

When I first read Kate Jackson's article on bathing babies, two things really struck me. The first of these was the way in which she managed to describe a practical exercise so well through the written word, and the second is the way in which, throughout the article, she consid-ered how a baby would be experiencing the bath. It made me wonder whether, if we thought more aspects of practice through in the same way, what else we might seek to change about our approach?

- Have you ever considered birth, or resuscitation, or having a vitamin K injection or PKU test from the perspective of the baby? If you were a baby experiencing one of these things, do you think you would like to have you as your midwife?! Having thought these things through from a baby's perspective, is there anything you might change about your practice?

Suzanne Colson discusses several concepts which are relatively new to the area of breastfeeding, and she and Jane Wallsworth both offer food for thought around the terminology that we use in this area.

- What are your thoughts about the language we use around breastfeeding? (The question of what mother's milk is called in other languages arises again in the next section).
- Do Suzanne's thoughts about positioning resonate with your experience? If you have breastfed your own child, what positions did you end up feeling most comfortable with? What is the experience of the women you work with? Is this something that you could explore further in practice with women?

Focus on . . .

Working/International Stories

SECTION CONTENTS

Empowering women in Nagorno-Karabakh

Susan Burvill

Nagorno-Karabakh (NK) is a beautiful, mountainous area just inside the borders of Azerbaijan, and a former Soviet occupied territory. It is inhabited by ethnic Christian Armenians, who enjoy their own dialect, culture, history and food. It is a war-torn area, which at the moment exists in the precarious position of a ceasefire. The four-year war with Azerbaijan (1991–1994) left more than 20,000 dead and 1.5 million displaced, causing major damage to the infrastructure.

It is not recognised by the world as an independent state, despite having its own government, language and national flag. NK lives in a state of uncertainty – this is an area crying out for a system of justice and a humane rational approach from the international community.

Health services have been reduced to almost nothing in many areas; economic difficulties and bad transportation have put women and children at particular risk. Infant mortality is estimated at around 28/1,000, with morbidity rates poorly reported.

Rebuilding hospitals

I worked with Family Care, an Italian organisation that focuses on mother and child healthcare. The funding for the majority of its work in Armenia and NK came from USAID (US Agency for International Development). The first task was to upgrade and sometimes rebuild bombed-out hospitals and clinics. Many labour wards had no windows – just plastic sheets – in temperatures dropping to −20°F in winter. Many had no running water, drugs or trained staff. One midwife spent the four years of the war helping women have babies in a collapsed underground car park.

I have now made several trips to NK, as well as to the main part of northern Armenia. Journeys to NK involve going via Yerevan, the capital of Armenia, as NK air space is kept strictly clear of planes due to the ceasefire. I am usually laden with medical items and my own luggage.

I am picked up and taken by Land Rover over the mountains into NK, a six-hour bumpy road to the capital Stepanakert. The awesomeness of the snow-capped mountains and Mount Ararat as we leave Armenia contrast with the desperate sights of bombed, ethnic-cleansed villages and people's homes. Farmlands heavily mined to prevent reoccupation by Islamic owners who have fled to Azerbaijan in the war stretch into the horizon. The Lachin corridor, as it is called, is the 'the no-man's land' between Armenia and NK and must be traversed to enter NK. Rail-lines and other main roads have long been destroyed or fallen into bad repair.

Like most of the ex-Soviet bloc outside the major centres of power, a visit is like travelling back in time to the 1940s. I have worked and lived in Africa and India where poverty can be seen everywhere, but in NK and Armenia it is more a poverty of the spirit, of the human psyche. I am not a political scientist, but it would appear that communism was not nourishing to the human spirit.

Recent visits have taken me to remote mountain villages to meet with village leaders, midwives and local women. The people I met and their faces will stay with me for many years. The trips to these isolated places up and down endless mud tracks left me aching from head to foot and awestruck at the loneliness of some of these communities.

Empowering women

One of the main objectives of the consultancy work was to empower local women through education about their reproductive health. With this in mind I was able to set up 11 antenatal classes in clinics, villages and hospitals. But, first, it was important to ensure that midwifery knowledge was accurate and not based on misleading custom and practice. This was a real challenge. Many midwives had years of practical skills but no theoretical basis on which to change practice.

The NK and Armenian media enjoy interviewing overseas workers. On two occasions I had my voice dubbed into Karabaghy and Russian for local TV stations. Once I was invited to give a talk in northern Armenia to student midwives: when I arrived, the room was full of more than 100 people – doctors, midwives, students, nurses and the television cameras! I swallowed hard and got on with it. I aimed to cover the basics:

- Maternal choice (non-existent; the concept was strange to them at first)
- Environment and support
- Freedom to move in labour and birth (women are in the lithotomy position for the birth, and often in communal rooms in the major units)
- Eating and drinking in labour (not allowed).

None of these topics appear in the Soviet 'procedures' for childbirth, which are taught verbatim to students. Halfway through this presentation to a very quiet, attentive audience, a midwifery lecturer stood up and said: 'Why do you come here and say women should be able to mobilise and be upright for birth? We always did it that way until the West told us to do it differently. We never had delivery beds before the Soviets came and brought Western ideas – we used birthing stools and ropes tied from ceiling beams for women to hold on to!'

This was a very pertinent point, applauded by the audience. Some of the younger midwifery students were in tears as the reality of midwifery in Armenia today is far removed from the vision I was offering, especially as many of them will be having their own babies in this system.

Human endurance

The personal stories are haunting, and often full of courage and human endurance that we in the West would find hard to imagine. I have many individual stories, too numerous to mention, of births and emergency transfers in lorries down cold, dark mud tracks. However, I would like to share one story.

I was teaching a midwife how to conduct antenatal groups in the regional unit when I was called to the labour ward. A woman in heavy labour with a baby in a breech position had been transferred by truck over the mountains from a remote village. The midwife and doctor in her village had no facilities and no experience to deal with this. They had received no information or training for many years – this is not uncommon. They had no up-to-date textbooks or journals, and lacked essential clinical skills. The staff asked me to help.

The village woman did not speak Russian, the 'educated language' of doctors and hospital staff. She was terrified. According to hospital routine her husband had

been told to leave and was waiting, frightened, out in the cold. The staff spoke over the woman as if she were an interesting case to observe, not a woman about to give birth to her baby – a most intimate and personal event, I believe.

The room filled with all types of people; the lights were turned up, and the din was unbearable. I looked around, trying to make sense of all these people in conversation with each other. The room was very cold, and midwives, doctors, cleaners – in fact, everyone – were in woollen socks and sweaters. I remember thinking, 'Rome was not built in a day', so I concentrated all my attention on the woman and worked with my interpreter (who I thought would pass out at being thrust into a birth situation!). I got the expectant mother out of lithotomy and encouraged her to do as she wanted. She was obviously frightened, looking at the others for permission to move off her back. She eventually moved on to her side with a sigh of relief when the first leg popped out.

A beautiful baby boy was born without any problems, legs first, into this very cold room. Much to the paediatric nurse's horror, I gave the mother her wailing baby to feed and cuddle. The mother was overjoyed but shocked – having your baby skin-to-skin after the birth is just not done. The midwives and doctors kept saying, 'We don't do it like that . . .'.

The placenta followed physiologically with the cord intact. Syntometrine is rarely used, but the process of placental 'delivery' can be a haphazard mixture of pulling and manual removal – and often leads to bleeding.

Despite hospital routines that would baffle the most patient among you, and obstructive corruption involving the handing over of money to the hospital staff (even though maternity care is supposed to be free), I managed to get the woman and her baby out of the door and into a taxi with her husband. She was a poor woman from the 'no-man's' area in Lachin who could not afford the bribes for food and kind treatment. As she left she said she had nothing to give except milk from her cow. I was deeply touched by her plight. I could see by her hands that she worked the land morning to night. Her husband was ground down by the life he led, and desperate, but loved his new family dearly.

Word of this birth spread into the regions, which raised my professional status no end! Being seen to 'perform' for those people was pivotal – earning respect is imperative if you want to initiate change.

Acute training need

The Armenian midwifery profession has much work and development to do, not least the establishment of its own association or college. Many so-called midwives have not received any formal training, but progressed from nursing because no one else in the village could offer maternity care. Others trained under the Soviet system more than a decade ago, and have worked in total isolation since. Many of the young trained midwives do not want to work in the villages, but remain in the towns where modernisation is occurring. The older midwives in the villages remain in isolation, and the plight of women when these skilled practitioners retire and die will constitute a serious humanitarian problem.

The midwives, obstetricians and paediatricians also need to receive a living wage. Many in the villages had not been paid for many months, and even when they are it is a pittance – encouraging the corruption ubiquitous in the larger regional centres.

Raising women's profile

My job was to raise the profile of women by concentrating on their reproductive health and empowering them to take control of their lives by questioning and changing for the better the issues that affect them and their families. I was, however, a drop in a vast ocean of need – the funding for this project has, unfortunately, ended.

People often ask if the NK and Armenian people are angry about what has happened to them under the Soviets and in the ongoing struggle with the international community. But I would say 'no'. I feel that some are just miserable and sad, and are getting on with life the best they can. Despite this, I experienced extraordinary hospitality and warmth. I am grateful for the experience of working with these people and for the wisdom born of arduous lives that they imparted to me on my visits.

Acknowledgements

I would like to thank the management of Addenbrookes NHS Trust for supporting me and giving me the time to go on the 2002 trip; and the midwives and women of Armenia – especially my interpreters, Nuneh and Anna, without whom I would have been completely lost.

The Practising Midwife 2004; 7(2): 15–18

Birth and death in Sierra Leone

Sarah Bush

For a year, British midwife Sarah Bush worked in northern Sierra Leone with the medical aid agency Médecins Sans Frontières (MSF). Sierra Leone has been devastated by a decade of civil war during which time health services collapsed. MSF runs a surgical programme in Magburaka district hospital and also supports the paediatric and obstetrics/gynaecological ward. Despite considerable improvements to healthcare in Magburaka, the majority of women admitted to the obstetrics/gynaecological ward during Sarah's stay arrived too late; their babies were already dead. It was then a question of trying to save the mothers' lives. Sarah describes case histories of some of her patients, and explains how her anger at the preventable suffering she witnessed has driven her to return to Sierra Leone to try and improve the situation for women there.

When I arrived, the country was post-war and relatively calm due to the presence of the United Nations forces, but the health infrastructure was in pieces and there was a critical lack of trained health staff. There was only one midwife in the hospital, and she was working in the antenatal care clinic. The majority of the women admitted on to the obstetrics/gynaecological ward arrived too late with no fetal heartbeat. Within one year there were 620 births, including 302 caesarean sections, 42 cases of eclampsia and 35 incidences of ruptured uterus. There were 158 stillbirths and 27 maternal deaths (some of which were gynaecology cases or due to indirect causes such as malaria and cardiac problems).

After returning home, I began to sift through my memories and I felt angry. There is a wealth of literature (WHO and Unicef 1996, Fransen 2003) highlighting maternal mortality and the huge disparity between the wealthiest nations and the poorest. Three-quarters of maternal deaths are due to abortion, obstructed labour, haemorrhage, sepsis and hypertensive diseases of pregnancy (Stekelenburg and Roosmalen 2002). Nevertheless, these women die silently in the most torturous ways imaginable, unattended by any health professional, far away from medical facilities and with no access to public transport.

I have remembered many women's stories. The bleak statistics reveal the hard facts, but I want to illustrate the human experience of millions of women's lives through four simple, true, everyday stories.

Easter's story of septic abortion

Easter was a young girl: she did not know her true age, but she looked no more than 13 or 14. She was tiny, emaciated and extremely pale. She was fortunate to have found transport, and had spent eight hours on a bad road. Easter did not speak Temne, the regional language, so it was difficult for her to give a clear history. The story she related, confusing at times, was that she had been raped. Five days previously, she had paid a local woman for an abortion and had been held down and a sharp instrument used. She blacked out. When she awoke, she was covered in blood and felt weak.

On examination, she had a high pyrexia, with tachycardia and hypotension. She had a very tender and distended abdomen with all the signs of acute peritonitis. Her uterus felt palpable of around 16 weeks. We had a very basic laboratory; she was negative for malaria but her HB was 3.0. The only donor she had with her was her sister; she was not compatible, and we had no blood in the blood bank.

Without any ultrasound or investigative tests, operations have to be performed purely on clinical judgement. During the laparotomy, her abdomen was found to be full of clots of blood. She had a perforation of the right lateral side of the uterus, which was already gangrenous and necrotic. There was pus in the right ovary and Fallopian tube. Easter had to have a hysterectomy and removal of the right Fallopian tube and ovary.

A few days later Easter's father arrived. He had been working in the fields and had walked two days to find her. He was a compatible donor and donated blood. After the operation Easter did not speak, but cried a lot – she was empty. It was difficult for the local staff to console her.

- Thirteen per cent of maternal deaths in developing countries are due to unsafe abortion (WHO 1997).
- Complications of pregnancy and childbirth are the leading cause of death among women of reproductive age (WHO and Unicef 1996).

Mabinty's story of obstructed labour

Mabinty was 18, and this was her first baby.

She had been tended by a traditional birth attendant, but it had been five days since the contractions began and the head was 'headstuck', although visible. She lived a two-day walk from the hospital, so they had tried everything. She had taken native herbs, they had tried fundal pressure to dislodge the stuck baby and attempted a form of episiotomy with a knife. She was in unbearable, endless pain. After a few days Mabinty was becoming weaker and ill with fever. The family carried her by hammock to the nearest road, which took many hours, and waited half a day for a car to pass by.

Mabinty was obviously septic when she arrived. On vaginal examination, she was fully dilated, the head felt low but had excessive caput and moulding. The scalp of the baby's head was already visibly macerated and offensive; it was obvious that no fetal heart would be heard. Mabinty was prepared for a craniotomy, and anaesthetised with ketamine.

A craniotomy, if possible, is always preferable to a caesarean section, as there is less risk of infection or ruptured uterus with subsequent pregnancies. I found it hard to be present for the craniotomy. Mabinty had tissue necrosis of the vaginal wall up to the cervix, and some debridement was done.

After the operation she had to wash her genitalia regularly in a plastic bowl with mild antiseptic, and was on IV antibiotics. By the second day, as all the dead tissue continued to slough away, she became incontinent and developed a large vesicovaginal fistula (VVF). Although she used torn-up cloth to soak up the urine, and washed obsessively, she smelt constantly of urine.

Urinary incontinence is a huge stigma. Women become ostracised. Mabinty's husband abandoned her, and she was left with a limp because the pressure from the obstructed labour had caused loss of sensation and drop foot due to permanent damage to the sacral nerves. She managed to walk again but dragged her foot behind her.

- Obstructed labour is the cause of 8 per cent of deaths in the developing world (WHO 1997).

- It is estimated that 500,000 to one million women worldwide now live with a fistula, and are incontinent of urine and often of faeces (Unicef 1996).
- More than a quarter of women living in the developing world suffer with a short-term or chronic illness due to pregnancy and childbirth (Unicef 1996).

Isata's story of eclampsia

Isata's family told me that she had not felt well for a long time. It started with unbearable headaches – she could feel something crawling in the front of her head, and she could not see well. It became so bad that she found it difficult to walk and the headache just would not go away. Her hair was shaved off to try and ease the pain, and she tried many different native herbs.

It was Isata's first baby. She arrived at the hospital in a battered car. It was the rainy season, and the road had been almost impassable. Isata was fitting continuously on the back seat of the car, foaming at the mouth and her breathing was very laboured. Her mouth was full of blood due to biting on her tongue; the family thought that she had been possessed by devils.

Isata was not in labour. The cervix was tightly closed, posterior and thick, and she palpated around 38 weeks pregnant – the fetal heart was heard. She was deeply comatosed from hypoxic brain injury caused by repeated fitting. Isata was screened for malaria, as cerebral malaria can cause fitting, but it was negative. She had a caesarean section immediately after magnesium sulphate and hydralazine had been administered. Isata never regained consciousness, and had obvious signs of severe brain damage. She eventually died of pneumonia and sepsis. Her baby just managed to survive. The family carried Isata home in a hammock, the same way in which she had arrived.

- Eclampsia is the cause of 12 per cent of maternal deaths in the developing world (WHO 1997).
- One vial of magnesium sulphate costs 33p; one vial of hydralazine costs 54p.

Hanna's story of postpartum haemorrhage

Hanna had already had six children, three of whom were still alive; this time, she wanted a girl. The traditional birth attendant who had attended her previous deliveries came as soon as her contractions started, and she had progressed quickly – the baby came out screaming, and was a very fat girl. Then Hanna started to bleed violently and fast – it would not stop. The family carried Hanna to the hospital in a blanket, which was wringing with blood. By the time she arrived she was pale and gasping and the bleeding had stopped. She was almost white, peripherally shut down and died as we tried to perform a cut-down for IV access.

Five days later the distraught father of the baby came to the ward. He told us that there was no other 'suckling mother' who could feed the baby, so they had been feeding the infant water. A tin of baby's powder milk cost more than a week's wages; with three other children to support, it was not an option. The baby was dehydrated, losing weight and crying weakly. The maternity ward was completely full, and the paediatric ward crowded with children sleeping on the floor. To admit the baby was not an option, and would not solve the situation. We bought the father one tin of milk, and the national staff explained how to boil the water and how much powder to use. We told him to go to a charity in another town that might be able to help, knowing that the baby had only a very slim chance of survival.

- Twenty-five per cent of all maternal deaths in the poorest parts of the world are due to haemorrhage (WHO 1997).
- One vial of methylergometrine costs 6p.

A human rights issue

The reality for the majority of women in the world is very different from the westernised ideal of the birth plan and the expected perfect birth experience. In Africa as a whole, the lifetime risk of dying during pregnancy and childbirth is 1 in 16; in some parts of the continent it is much higher, due to extreme poverty and war. In Sierra Leone during the war, it was estimated that the lifetime risk was 1 in 6 (WHO and Unicef 1996).

Maternal mortality in the developing world is a complex human rights issue, with many contributing factors such as a general lack of political will, poverty and gender inequality (Fransen 2003). What is so unacceptable is that less than 1 per cent of maternal mortality in developed countries is due to the above causes (CEMD 2002), highlighting the fact that when resources and services are available these deaths are avoidable (WHO and Unicef 1996). The repercussions of maternal deaths affect the whole society, and it is the children who suffer the most.

I hope not to upset or offend people reading this article – I know it's graphic, but this is the reality for millions of women. During my time with MSF I have also been privileged to see the positive side of Sierra Leone – I have stories, too, of miracles, happiness, dancing, laughter and the will to live. I have learnt much from the people of Sierra Leone. Despite the tragedies, there is hope, and there is also much room for improvement – of which I hope to be a part.

As I write, I am back in Sierra Leone, having signed up for another nine months. My job now has changed, and I am involved in training within some of the MSF-supported hospitals and clinics on obstetric emergencies and arranging workshops for the maternal and child health nurses (MCH). The MCH nurses often work in remote areas – alone, with limited resources and with no access to public transport. If we can improve their skills and their ability to detect problems early, lives can be saved. Expatriates from Médecins Sans Frontières won't stay here forever.

It is essential we leave education and knowledge behind us.

Want to get involved?

Médecins Sans Frontières is always looking for qualified midwives to work in aid projects overseas.

If you have current NMC registration and would like to make a real difference to the lives of women and babies in the developing world, please contact MSF. You can find out more or apply online at www.uk.msf.org or call the human resources department on 020 7404 6600.

REFERENCES

CEMD (Confidential Enquiry into Maternal Deaths in the United Kingdom) (2002). Why Mothers Die, 1997–1999, London. RGOG Press.

Fransen L (2003). 'The impact of inequality on the health of mothers'. Midwifery, 19: 79–81.

Stekelenburg J and Roosmalen J (2002). 'The maternal mortality review meeting: experiences from Kalabo District Hospital, Zambia'. Tropical Doctor, 32: 219–223.

Unicef (1996). The Progress of the Nations, New York: Unicef.

WHO and Unicef (1996). Revised 1990 Estimates of Maternal Mortality: A New Approach, Geneva: WHO.

WHO (1997). Maternal Health Around the World (wall chart), Geneva: WHO.

The Practising Midwife 2004; 7(2): 11–14

Caring for mama and pikinini in Papua New Guinea

Jennifer Cameron

In September 2003 I visited Goroka, in Papua New Guinea. My journey began in my hometown of Bendigo, Australia. One of my obstetric colleagues visits Goroka Base Hospital several times a year as a volunteer doctor for AusAid. He encouraged some of our local midwives to volunteer and share expertise and knowledge with the Gorokan midwives and nurses. He is very enthusiastic and persuasive, and before I knew it I was on my way!

Papua New Guinea is the largest developing country in the South Pacific region. It comprises 463,000km^2 of land area and 600 separate islands (AusAid 2002). It is divided into provinces, and most of its 5.2 million people live in rural villages, with approximately 20 per cent in urban areas such as Goroka, the capital of the Eastern Highlands Province. Although Papua New Guinea has abundant natural resources, it does have a moderate debt burden: it is estimated that 22 per cent of people live on less than US$1 per day (World Bank 2001, cited in AusAid 2002).

Approximately 650 distinct languages are spoken in Papua New Guinea: however, most professionals can speak English, and most town folk speak a mixture of local dialect and English known as 'Pidgin'.

Goroka is located in the Eastern Highlands of Papua New Guinea, about 5,000 feet above sea level. It is lush and green, and because it is temperate there is minimal risk of malaria. My first view of the highlands was from the aircraft: we flew over stunningly beautiful velvety green hills, swathed in mist and cloud. On the ground Goroka was lush and green but also wet and very muddy as it had been raining heavily. We were met at the airport by the Director of Nursing, and were ferried to our accommodation in the 4WD ambulance-cum-taxi.

Access in Papua New Guinea is dictated by its geography. Extensive, thick forests and steep mountains have made road construction difficult, and the only way to get to Goroka from the capital of Port Moresby is by air. Goroka sits on the Highlands Highway, which runs across the middle of Papua New Guinea, giving Goroka road access to the towns of Madang to the east and Mount Hagen to the west. In Goroka there is a public bus system that ferries people from the surrounding villages to the town and back via the Highlands Highway and other assorted rough dirt tracks.

Goroka Base Hospital has 300 beds and is the only referral facility for the Eastern Highlands Province (population 120,000). It has one working telephone located in the office of the CEO. Our first task was a tour of the hospital. It was bigger than I had imagined: medical, surgical and children's wards; maternity and special care baby nursery; A&E and an outpatients' department; theatre and a psychiatric ward. (The latter held three patients, all psychotic from using marijuana which grows wild around the villages.)

Pathology, blood bank, pharmacy, radiology and a sterilising department formed part of the hospital complex. There was also a medical research centre attached, its main function being to carry out research into malaria.

General health picture

There is an abundance of fresh vegetables in Papua New Guinea, and people generally eat well, although meat protein is limited in some areas. Health problems include malaria, tuberculosis, HIV and STDs. Violence and tribal fighting still occur in Goroka, and disputes are sometimes settled with spears – a patient presenting to A&E with a spear sticking out of his body is not uncommon. Domestic violence is frequent, with men and women as both instigator and victim. Polygamy occurs, and jealousy from the wives often results in injuries to the husband – particularly on the acquisition of a new wife or any suspected infidelity.

Maternity care

Goroka Base Hospital caters for 3,000 births per year. The following statistics illustrate the average workload for the unit (Hoffman and Mayall 2002):

- Booked: 2,199
- Unbooked: 433
- Referred: 333
- Total: 2,865

Another 1,000 births occur in nearby villages or in outlying health centres where the referrals originate.

Overall, the perinatal mortality rate (PNMR) is approximately 36:1,000 (see Table 8.3.1). For Papua New Guinea generally it is 58:1,000; for Australia, 6:1,000; and, for the UK, 8.3:1000. The main causes of infant death are very low birth weight, septicaemia, birth asphyxia and congenital syphilis.

Maternal mortality in PNG generally is 26:10,000 births. The main causes are malaria, eclampsia and post-partum haemorrhage. In Australia the maternal mortality rate is <1:10,000, but higher for indigenous women.

The maternity unit consists of a discrete labour ward, a postnatal area located in the children's ward, a special care baby nursery and an antenatal clinic located in the hospital grounds. Antenatal screening consists of haemoglobin estimation and a venereal diseases research laboratory for syphilis.

The labour ward comprises six birth beds, all in one room. The beds can be screened off from each other but there is no real privacy. This was probably the area that affected me most strongly: the women laboured, birthed, bled or convulsed inches from each other. Women experienced births, both live and still, in this one room.

Women usually present in early labour. Some have walked in from their villages in the surrounding hills. On arrival they are greeted by the midwife, and their history details are taken. They are then admitted to the labour ward. Here they remain, walking about, or resting, until second stage. No relative or companion is present. The birth beds are made up with a draw sheet only. Where possible the women are expected to bring their own bed linen to the hospital.

Women birth on their backs and in stirrups – episiotomy is routine. We were able to provide the midwife in charge with some best practice information relating to intrapartum care and birthing positions. A copy of the WHO (2003) publication Managing Complications in Pregnancy and Childbirth was given to the ward as a guide. (The hospital has now implemented some of the recommendations, and women are more active in labour and are encouraged to be upright for birth.)

Once she has birthed the mother gets up and showers, cleans the shower and then collects her baby and sits outside the labour ward to be handed over to the postnatal nurses. She will be discharged later that day or the next day. If she has no one to collect her and no money, she will walk back to her village carrying her baby or transporting it in a 'bilum', a knitted string bag.

At birth, and once the cord is clamped and cut, the baby is taken to a resuscitation area. Here, he or she is dried and examined. Once the baby is stable, IMI Vitamin K, prophylactic antibiotic eye drops, hepatitis B vaccine and oral Sabine vaccine are given. We noticed that neonates were routinely suctioned at birth, and so we provided some further education about current best practice in this area.

Accepted practices

Many intrapartum practices originated in the 1970s and '80s when there was a resident obstetrician in Goroka, and reflect the accepted practices for that era. The midwifery and nursing staff had continued the practices as they had no knowledge of recent relevant research. This is an important area of need in regional hospitals in Papua New Guinea.

It was important to be diplomatic and use a sensitive approach in the area of practice change. The midwives and nurses in Goroka are working in difficult and poorly equipped conditions, and do amazingly good work.

There are three to four midwives in the unit, and several nurses. Most of the nurses are general nursing students who do a maternity rotation as part of their course. There is always a midwife in charge, who performs the vacuum extractions and most of the perineal repairs. The nursing students also learn how to repair perineal wounds.

The implication of a lack of appropriately skilled staff was brought home to us during our visit. A woman had undergone an elective caesarean section that day. This was her fifth pregnancy, and she was carrying twins. The indication for the caesarean was 'pikinini sleep cranky,' Pidgin for 'baby is in a transverse or unstable lie.' In fact, both twins were in a transverse lie. A longitudinal lie would be expressed as 'pikinini sleep straight.' The mother haemorrhaged during the caesarean section, was transfused and then transferred in a stable condition to the ward for postoperative care.

Table 8.3.1 Perinatal deaths at Goroka Base Hospital, Papua New Guinea

	Stillbirths	Neonatal deaths	Total
Booked	29(1.3%)	7(0.33%)	36(1.63%)
Unbooked	23(5.31%)	11(2.54%)	34(7.8%)
Referred	20(6%)	15(4.5%)	35(10.5%)
Total	72(2.5%)	33(1.5%)	105(3.66%)

The ward was extremely busy that evening, with three women admitted in a shocked state from ruptured ectopic pregnancies. Ectopic pregnancy is common in Goroka because there is a high incidence of STDs, with resulting tubal damage. Some time during the evening, while the staff were busy stabilising the three women with ectopic pregnancies, the mother of the twins died from a further postpartum haemorrhage. There were just not enough staff to care for her.

She had four other young children at home plus the newborn twins. This was the closest I had been to maternal death, and it hit home just how fortunate we are in Australia.

Susu-mama: breast milk only

Exclusive breastfeeding is the norm in Goroka. In Pidgin, milk is 'susu' and breast milk is 'susu-mama'. In the special care baby nursery (SCBN) the sick and premature infants receive only 'susu-mama': there is no formula in the hospital. The premature infants are mostly cared for by their mothers who sit on the floor in the nursery with their baby on their lap or in a bilum. Each time the baby stirs it is offered the breast or expressed breast milk from a cup. The SCBN was fairly basic: two ancient incubators (1960s), one oximeter, a set of phototherapy lights and several standard nursery-style cots for the babies.

Conclusion

The fact that the hospital at Goroka ran at all was amazing: one working telephone; one sterile theatre gown to wear all day when operating; resterilised gloves and equipment – not to mention the occasional dog trotting through the ground floor!

The Papua New Guinea people are inherently happy and friendly, and are very appreciative of any help that comes their way. We were made incredibly welcome, housed in the hospital flats and very well looked after by the local people, including the AusAid administrator.

Goroka is relatively safe, but one night I was woken by a volley of loud bangs. I froze in my bed as it sounded like gunshots, but none of the abundant dogs in the neighbourhood barked or stirred so I assumed it was nothing out of the ordinary and went back to sleep.

It was an amazing two weeks, and I learnt so much in a short time. It made my previous 30 years in maternity care seem almost ordinary – almost!

Acknowledgement

The author would like to thank the Department of Nursing, La Trobe University, Bendigo, for supporting this visit to Goroka.

REFERENCES

AusAid (2002). 'About Papua New Guinea'. www.ausaid.gov.au/country/png/png_intro.cfm

Hoffman I and Mayall P (2002). 'Our views of Goroka'. Volunteers E-News, Issue 2, December 2002, www.abc.net.au/science/ slab/png/

World Bank (2001). World Development Indicators 2001, Washington DC. Cited in AusAid reference above.

World Health Organization (2003). Managing Complications in Pregnancy and Childbirth, Geneva: WHO.

FURTHER READING

Shorter D (n.d). 'Healthcare in PNG: a personal story'. www.abc.net.au/science/ slab/png/

ABOUT AUSAID

AusAID manages the Australian Government's official overseas aid program, helping developing countries reduce poverty and achieve sustainable development.

www.ausaid.gov.au

On mission with Médecins Sans Frontières

Karsten Bidstrup

The desire to make a difference brought Pia Thorsø Sørensen, a Danish midwife, from the clinical maternity ward in Roskilde County Hospital in safe, suburban Copenhagen to the village of Madhu in the humid jungle of northern Sri Lanka.

Background

Madhu is situated very close to the frontline that has separated the island for years. It is a holy place surrounding a Catholic church, blessed by the presence of The Lady of Madhu, a local saint who apparently performs a miracle every now and then . . .

Both the Tamils and the Sinhalese consider the area holy, so Madhu has been relatively peaceful during the civil war. Madhu has therefore been the obvious sanctuary for Tamil refugees throughout the 20-year-long, bloody conflict.

The concentration of refugees in the area attracted some large NGOs in the early 1990s, among them the medical aid agency Médecins Sans Frontières (MSF).

On call around the clock

MSF runs the small hospital in Madhu, and Pia is in charge of the maternity ward. It is a full-time job in every sense of the word, since she is often on call around the clock.

There is no doubt about what motivates her: 'It's all about doing something good,' she says. 'But you must want to do it, not feel it's an obligation.'

And it definitely takes some willpower when the Tamil nightwatchman calls her again, at 2:30am after a 14-hour working day and only a few hours of sleep. 'Pia Aka, Pia Aka, please come to the hospital,' he whispers as he knocks on the door of her tocul (round hut).

Aka means big sister; it is a loving and respectful nickname that makes one think of the difference between the relatively small Tamils and the healthy Scandinavian woman.

The transportation from MSF's compound to the hospital is by four-wheel-drive with a rotating beacon, light inside the cabin and all windows rolled down. Those regulations are upheld by The Tamil Tigers in order to avoid shooting. The Tigers must be able to see who is driving around the village at night during curfew. Sometimes the request for Pia to come to the hospital is a false alarm, but lengthy births often demand her presence.

At the hospital in Madhu and the mobile clinics in the surrounding area, the local staff work closely with the MSF team. Apart from Pia, the team includes logisticians, doctors and nurses from all over the world. They each run different parts of the hospital and offer free medical assistance to those in need.

'We are not obligated to travel the world to help people, but it is a privilege to be able to do so,' Pia says. 'I think working with MSF is fantastic. Experiencing people's gratitude is quite moving, and it is a rush to realise it all matters. One feels so appreciated. Of course, work at home is also appreciated, but in Sri Lanka things are not taken for granted because there is nowhere else to go.'

'Once you are left with nothing but your bare hands your skills are truly put to the test,' says Pia.' A stethoscope made of ash wood (the local women refer to it as a musical instrument) is Pia's sole tool during antenatal consultations, and at the hospital in Madhu there are no high-technology scanners, no Entonox and no anaesthetists offering epidurals.

'The options we have in Western Europe have created a need and why not take advantage of those options?' Pia reflects. 'However, the Tamils know there are no anaesthetics here. We can offer paracetamol as a common pain killer but it has no effect during birth. These are two different realities.'

Overcoming language barriers

Mokungo means push and was obviously the first indispensable Tamil word that Pia mastered. Usually, the daily communication is in English, but when that is not sufficient the interpreter takes over. A nun, Sister Teresa, is often present during births and antenatal consultations. Pia's predecessor surely wished that Sister Teresa had been there one day when she kept saying 'mutele, mutele' to a woman giving birth, firmly believing it meant push. It made the poor woman and everyone else in the room look around nervously for a crocodile!

A bizarre birth

Pia cannot help smiling when she recalls one of the more humorous events in a number of bizarre episodes she experienced in the small hospital in Madhu.

'A young man told his even younger brother to take his pregnant wife to the local hospital because her waters had broken and labour had set in. She was a primi, and got on to the back of the small moped and off they went along the muddy, pot-holed track through the jungle.

The ride took some time and the young man was terrified – he kept up speed in the hope of reaching the hospital in time. However, unfortunately the woman began to give birth. By the time the two arrived at the hospital it was all over, and I was able to pull out a very tiny baby from the woman's trouser leg.

The little girl had a birthweight of 1.7kg, but she was quite healthy. In fact, the whole situation seemed to affect the poor brother the most – he was in a state of shock.'

An abrupt end

Pia's assignment in Sri Lanka came to an abrupt end when she was struck down with the feared tropical disease dengue fever during one of the epidemic outbreaks that occurs at frequent intervals. The disease is potentially fatal, especially if caught twice; and, since the risk was too high if she remained on the island, MSF sent Pia home immediately.

'But of course I would do it again,' she insists. 'There's always a labouring woman who needs a midwife . . .'

Karsten Bidstrup is a Danish photographer who has travelled extensively with Médecins Sans Frontières.

MSF is always looking for qualified midwives to work in projects around the world. They are looking for midwives with:

- Training in both nursing and midwifery, with current NMC registration
- Minimum of two years' experience post-qualification
- Minimum of three months of travelling and/or work experience in a developing country
- Experience in supervising and managing others
- Ability to train and coach other health workers
- Available to work for a minimum of nine months

Please go to www.uk.msf.org or call us on +44 (0)20 7404 6600

To be as effective as possible in MSF's emergency operations in South-East Asia, MSF are sending only highly experienced volunteers who have already worked with them in other emergencies.

The Practising Midwife 2005; 8(2):17–18

Contraception education in Brazil

Barbara Hastings-Asatourian

My visit to Brazil in October 2004 came about after I launched the resource, 'Contraception: the Board Game', and began to investigate the potential of bringing the concept to an international audience. This article represents a combination of my observations on fertility, sexual health and sex education in Brazil. It includes information gathered from discussions with non-governmental organisations (NGOs) and private providers, from a commissioned UK Trade and Investment research paper and sources of statistics recommended to me by the NGOs.

Brazil has a population of 181 million and is the world's fifth largest country. More than 32 million of its inhabitants are aged 10–19. While there, I heard Brazil referred to as 'third world,' with extremes of wealth and poverty, exemplified by infamous suburban settlements or 'Favelas'. Just 10 per cent of the population own 51 per cent of Brazil's wealth, yet 18 per cent (32 million) live in poverty, many young people literally begging on the streets. The average life expectancy is 67 years for men and 72 years for women (UKTI 2004).

Fertility

Brazil's total fertility rate declined steadily from 6 per 1,000 in the 1940s to 3.3 in 1986 and to 2.44 in 1994. (Replacement level is 2.2.) Projections indicate a total fertility rate of 1.8 in 2020. In 1996 the crude birth rate was estimated at 21.16 births per 1,000 population, compared with 42.1 from 1960–65 (Country Studies 2004a).

Larger families have become less affordable than in the past, when young children worked at home, cost their parents very little, and supported their mother and father in their old age.

The Catholic laissez-faire approach, while not actively promoting family planning, did nothing to stop contraception. The resulting demographic change came about by women themselves taking control. NGOs told me that very few people give religious reasons for not using contraceptives.

One significant contributor to the population decline was that in the 1980s, as many as a third of women having caesareans were illegally sterilised because doctors could earn an attractive fee (Mirsky 1995).

In the 1980s, as a result of public opinion and the women's movement, the Ministry of Health began to include family planning services in an integrated women's health programme. The 1988 constitution included the right to family planning. The Family Planning Law took effect in 1997, regulating sterilisation, making it available in the public health network, but forbidding it during childbirth. At the same time legislation enabled other birth-control alternatives. Oral contraceptives became available 'over the counter.'

A large BEMFAM survey of 1996 found that 40 per cent of women in stable relationships had been sterilised. The average age at which women underwent this procedure was 28.9 years in 1996, compared with 31.4 years in 1986. In contrast, in 1986 only 0.8 per cent of men had had a vasectomy, compared with 2.6 per cent in 1996. This continued to contribute to a decline in Brazil's fertility rate. About 65 per cent of Brazilian women use contraceptives (Country Studies 2004b).

In the early 1990s, 1.4 million abortions were performed each year, almost all technically illegal: there was approximately one abortion for every two live births. Although abortion in Brazil is legal only in cases of rape and danger to the mother's life, the law has never been strictly enforced. Back-street abortions explain the country's position as having the fifth highest maternal mortality rate in Latin America, estimated at 141 deaths per 1,000 births. Recent statistics show that 219,834 teenagers had abortions between 1999 and April 2003 (Country Studies 2004b).

Teenage sex

Teenage fertility rates remain high:

- Births among teens aged from 10–19 climbed from 565,000 in 1993 to 698,000 in 1998, but are now showing signs of decline.
- Between 1993 and 2002, the teenage birth rate fell from 37.7 to 32.2 births per 1,000 pregnancies.
- Ministry of Health figures show that 210,946 Brazilian teenagers gave birth between 1999 and April 2003.
- One in 10 Brazilian girls aged between 15 and 19 has at least two children.
- Fifty per cent of Brazilian teenagers who become pregnant have their first child by the time they are 16.
- Only 14 per cent of sexually active teenagers between 15 and 19 say they use contraceptives.

(International Planned Parenthood Federation 2003, Singh 1997, United Nations Population Information 1995, 1996)

Sex education

In spite of having a well-developed educational system, Brazil has high levels of illiteracy. Although education is compulsory, and free from seven to 14 years, more than two million children do not go to school. At secondary level this number is estimated to be three million (UKTI 2004).

Issues relating to sexual awareness and sex education in Brazil parallel those in the UK. Television and new technologies openly deal with sexual issues. For many reasons there is still a lack of comprehensive sex education nationally in schools, in spite of evidence that prolonging the school career and providing comprehensive sex education in school has a positive impact. Young people with five or more years of education are more likely to delay sex, more inclined to use contraceptives, and less likely to have an unplanned pregnancy. Use of condoms during the first sexual experience is increasing, as is condom use during the most recent sexual encounter.

The issue of who should deliver sex education remains contentious. In one survey, 47 per cent of teachers said they felt ill prepared to teach sex education to children; and, as in the UK, many Brazilian parents find talking to their children difficult. One Brazilian survey reported that only 32 per cent of parents discussed sex with their children, and 50 per cent claimed never to have done so. However, one study found that when sex education was available at home, teenagers were much more likely to use contraception (Boender et 2004; IPPF/WHR 2001).

HIV/AIDS epidemic

Around 1.6 million people are living with HIV in Latin America. In 2003 around 84,000 people died of AIDS, and 200,000 were newly infected. In Brazil national prevalence is well below 1 per cent, but alarming infection levels above 60 per cent have been reported among injecting drug users in some cities (UNAIDS 2004). When AIDS emerged in the 1980s, the Brazilian government directed its efforts to the south. In 1987, it established a programme to respond more widely to the epidemic and to identify partnerships with NGOs, private-sector companies and international development agencies.

In 1993 and 1998, the World Bank substantially funded prevention, treatment, testing and capacity building. AIDS prevention programmes were launched throughout the country. Initially, these targeted those at highest risk but later, between 1993 and 1997, they focused on behavioural intervention, information, education and communication initiatives, as well as on providing support to AIDS patients. The project also funded research centres and groups such as sex workers and indigenous tribal councils. During this time these organisations distributed condoms and educational material to 500,000 people, provided specialised orientation to 200,000, and trained 2,000 community workers.

A decline in new AIDS cases and morbidity levels among the leading risk groups followed, probably resulting from free anti-retroviral medication and an increased number of treatment centres. UNAIDS has consequently selected this programme as a 'best practice' example. Typically, however, 80 per cent of Brazil's HIV/AIDS budget is spent on treatment and less than 10 per cent on prevention (Pan American Health Organisation 2000).

Schools programme

The National Schools Prevention Programme had two stages. The first involved 13–19 year olds; the second, 4–12 year olds. Training was delivered by distance learning via the open television channel, which has now reached 52,000 schools and around 30 million students aged from four to 19 (Chequer et al 1998).

One study of 11–19 year olds found inconsistent understanding of the facts about pregnancy and the spread of disease. Only 20 per cent of students knew that there was risk of pregnancy prior to the menarche, and only 50 per cent of boys believed pregnancy could result from first intercourse (Blanc and Way 1998, Singh et al 2000).

Yet, one international survey of 15–19 year olds found that Brazilian adolescents did demonstrate the highest knowledge of protecting themselves. An estimated 90 per cent of Brazilians understand STD/AIDS transmission fully, and the Brazilian government feels that the objective of the first phase of prevention has been achieved. Nevertheless, a third of reported AIDS cases occur in young Brazilians aged from 15–29.

In Brazil, as internationally, those living in poverty and in disadvantaged circumstances are at greatest risk of teenage pregnancy and HIV/AIDS. But with low levels of school attendance in poorer areas, school-based programmes are not reaching those most in need. An approach that does not rely on literacy or school attendance is clearly needed (Gigante et al 2004).

The wealthier areas in southern Brazil have a better social infrastructure and benefit more from the work of health agencies than northern areas. Young people in the south are more likely to use contraceptives – although consistent condom use is doubtful as the south has a higher prevalence of AIDS.

Sex trade

Sex work is often used to meet immediate economic needs, and therefore the longer-term impact of unprotected sex is not immediately considered. Abstinence-only schemes or those promoting faithfulness (eg, Uganda's ABC programme – Abstinence, Be Faithful, Use a Condom) are unlikely to have relevance for sex workers (UNICEF 2002).

Perception of relationship stability and risk has highlighted gender differences. For example, when asked if they were in a stable relationship at the time of their first sexual experience, 45 per cent of boys in one study replied yes compared with 94 per cent of girls (Magnani et al 2001). In one sample from the Alan Guttmacher Institute (1998), Brazilian young men averaged 2.6 sexual partners in the previous year. While the women reported improved attitudes to safer sex following an intervention, no significant differences were found in the men. These differences may result from social pressures, in common with stereotypes experienced in the UK – for example, the dual standards surrounding the carrying of condoms (Population Council 2003).

There is also a macho male culture in Brazil that begins very early. One NGO provided me with a selection of excellent educational materials for challenging male stereotypes and domestic violence, and suggested that sex-specific programmes might be a solution in issues such as violence, peer pressure, alcohol and drugs. The Working with Men project uses traditional music (forro) in such initiatives (Galvao et al 2002).

I was very impressed by the explicit messages of both safer sex and negotiation in the context of adolescence, and issues such as alcohol and peer pressure. The quality of materials, although very different from UK resources and much less reliant on computer technology, was also high.

Throughout my visit, it became clear that factors influencing sexual health and the challenges faced by governments, NGOs and the general public are similar internationally. Poverty and inequality feature prominently in AIDS prevalence, in teenage pregnancy, and in general health breakdown. Clearly, the most successful political initiatives are those operating neither in isolation from, nor in competition with, other main players, but those that – through a spirit of generosity – collaborate, draw from and build on each other's expertise.

Acknowledgements

Thanks to the British Consulate in Brazil, BEMFAM – Bem Estar Familiar no Brasil, Instituto Promundo, Instituto Kaplan, Instituto Papai and GTPOS – Grupo de Trabalho e Pesquisa em Orientação Sexual, for generously sharing information and resources, and sources of statistics.

REFERENCES

Alan Guttmacher Institute (1998). Into a New World: Young Women's Sexual and Reproductive Lives, http://www.agi-usa.org/pubs/new_world_engl.html

Blanc A K and Way A A (1998). 'Sexual behaviour and contraceptive knowledge and use among adolescents in developing countries'. Studies in Family Planning, 29 (2): 106–116.

Boender C, Santana D, Santillan D et al (2004). The So What Report: A Look at Whether Integrating a Gender Focus Into Programs Makes a Difference to Outcomes. An Interagency Gender Working Group Task Force Report. Population Reference Bureau. Accessed October 2004 at http://www.prb.org/pdf04/TheSoWhatReport.pdf

Chequer P, Pimenta C, Barrios J and Brito I (1998). Monitoring and Evaluation: Brazilian National STD/AIDS Program. Carolina Population Center, page 7. Accessed October 2004 at http://www.cpc.unc.edu/measure/publications/pdf/sr-01–04country_report_br.pdf

Country Studies (2004a). Brazil. U.S. Government Printing Office Online Bookstore. Accessed October 2004 at http://www.countrystudies.com/brazil/fertility.html

Country Studies (2004b). Brazil. U.S. Government Printing Office Online Bookstore. Last accessed October 2004 at http://countrystudies.us/brazil/28.htm

Galvao Adriao K, Medrado B, Lyra J and Nascimento P (2002). 'Working with men on health and sexual and reproductive rights from a gender perspective: the experience of the "Oficinas De Forro" in Brazil'. In: Cornwall, A and Welbourne A (eds). Realising Rights: Transforming Approaches to Sexual and Reproductive Well Being. London: Zed Books.

Gigante DP, Victora CG, Goncalves H et al (2004). 'Risk factors for childbearing during adolescence in a population-based birth cohort in Southern Brazil'. Rev Panam Salud Publica, 16 (1): 1–10.

International Planned Parenthood Federation (2003) Country Profiles: Brazil. Accessed October 2004 at http://ippfnet.ippf.org/pub/IPPF_Regions/IPPF_CountryProfile.asp?ISOCode=BR

IPPF/WHR (2001) Working in Schools: Sex Education in Brazil. Spotlight No 3. http://www.ippfwhr.org/publications/serial_article_e.asp?SerialIssuesID=34&ArticleID=141

Magnani RJ, Gaffikin L, Seiber EE et al (2001) 'Impact of an integrated adolescent reproductive health program in Brazil'. Studies in Family Planning, 32 (3): 230–243. Abstract accessed October 2004 at http://www.cicred.org/rdr/rdr_uni/revue104-105/18-104-105.html#18.21.A

Mirsky J (ed) (1995) Private Decisions, Public Debate: Women, Reproduction and Population, Marty Radlett Panos.

Pan American Health Organisation (2000). 'Update on HIV/AIDS surveillance in the Americas.' Epidemiological Bulletin, 21 (3). Accessed October 2004 at http://www.paho.org/english/dd/ais/EB_v21n3.pdf

Planned Parenthood Federation of America. 'Teenage pregnancy facts'. http://www.teenwire.com/views/articles/wv_20000114p023_pregnancy.asp

POPIN (1995, 1996). Population Today (monthly newsletter. Accessed October 2004 at http://www.un.org/popin/popis/journals/poptoday/

Population Council (2003). Selected DHS Data on 10–14-year-olds/Brazil. Annexe to Facts about Adolescents from the Demographic and Health Survey: Statistical Table For Program Planning. The Population Council. Accessed October 2004 at http://www.popcouncil.org/pdfs/gfdreports/annexes/annex_brazil.pdf

Singh S (1997). 'The relationship of abortion to trends in contraception and fertility in Brazil, Colombia and Mexico'. Family Planning Perspectives, 23 (1): 342–352.

Singh S, Wulf D, Samara R and Cuca Y (2000). 'Gender differences in the timing of first intercourse: data from 14 countries'. Family Planning Perspectives, 26 (1): 21–28, 43.

UKTI (2004). Overseas Marketing Information Service Report, BRA0238. Rio de Janeiro: UKTI (Commissioned by the author).

UNAIDS (2004). Report on the Global HIV/AIDS Epidemic, Geneva: UNAIDS.

UNICEF (2002).Young People and HIV/AIDS: Opportunity in Crisis, Geneva: UNICEF.

FURTHER READING AND RESOURCES

Csillag C (1999). 'Sex education is key to combating AIDS in Brazil'. Lancet, 353: 2221.

Kaiser Network. 'Teenage pregnancy statistics'. http://www.kaisernetwork.org/daily_reports/rep_hiv.cfm

USEFUL WEBSITES

Brazilian Government: www.brazil.gov.br
Brazilian Ministry of Health: www.saude.gov.br
World Bank: www.worldbank.org

The Practising Midwife 2005; 8(2): 21–24

Home thoughts from abroad

Lorna Davies

In May 2005, I became one of an apparently increasing number of 'migrant midwives' seeking a better life in New Zealand when I took up my new post as a lecturer in midwifery at a polytechnic in the South Island. I am also a very part time self-employed midwife, carrying a small but manageable caseload of women. In this article I would like to share with you some of my observations and reflections on midwifery in Aotearoa, the 'Land of the Long White Cloud'.

I had harboured the desire to work as a midwife in New Zealand for many years and arrived in the country experiencing equal measures of trepidation and anticipation. I had followed the re-establishment of the profession in New Zealand with interest and admiration. I had become increasingly disenchanted with what I perceived as apathy within the ranks of midwifery in the UK and the acceptance of what I considered to be a less than optimal maternity service. The dawning of the renaissance of midwifery in New Zealand following the Nurses Amendment Act in 1990, had been followed by the publication of *Changing Childbirth* (DoH 1993) in the UK in 1994 and with it the potential for the privilege of autonomy that had been granted to our sister midwives in New Zealand. The opportunity for women to be able to enjoy the benefits of continuity of care and carer, was within our grasp. In the eyes of the international midwifery community, the ground-breaking partnership model that was introduced in New Zealand was hailed as a flagship, and there was an expectation that other countries would follow suite. In 2004, 10 years after the publication of *Changing Childbirth* (DoH 1993), New Zealand celebrated the launch of its own Midwifery Council, whereas in the UK, the dream of *Changing Childbirth* had become a fond but distant memory and the best that the government could offer maternity services was a maternity 'module' within the Children's National Strategic Framework (DoH 2004). In spite of the development of the partnership-based model proposed by the Independent Mid-

wives Association (Francis and van der Kooy 2004) and more recently, the 'One Mother One Midwife' campaign (Abbott 2005), I remained disillusioned and felt that I needed to believe that a midwifery model of care was truly achievable. New Zealand also offered a lifestyle that we could not afford to enjoy in the UK, so my long-held dream became a reality when I left for the other side of the world with my family.

So was New Zealand going to be the 'land of milk and honey' that I was anticipating?

There is little doubt that the opportunities are available here for midwives to practice as autonomous practitioners. The organizational framework supports the recognition of the midwife as the 'guardian of normal birth' (MoH 2007). About half of the midwives working in New Zealand are self employed (Midwifery Council 2006a) and are remunerated by the Ministry of Health for providing a comprehensive package of care for women throughout their childbearing episodes under the provision stated within Section 88 of the New Zealand Public Health and Disability Act (MoH 2007). They can choose where, when and how they wish to work. They may work within a sole practice linking with other midwives for back-up purposes to enable them to take time off to attend other births, etc, or they may work within a group practice, partnering or forming other arrangements to meet the needs of the group practitioners. They may offer a range of birthing choices such as place of birth, which in theory allows women the opportunity to shop around and find a midwife who shares her philosophy. They can cut their cloth according to their needs and lifestyle at any given time by increasing or decreasing their caseload of women. For example a midwife with few family commitments may choose to take on the maximum recommended caseload of 5–6 women per month (NZCOM 1997), whereas someone with a young family may choose to take only one woman a month in order to spend more time at home with her children. (Midwifery Council of

New Zealand 2007). The flexibility available is one of the very positive aspects of this way of working.

Midwives are sometimes employed to provide a similar package to self-employed midwives by a District Health Board (DHB), as salaried employees with a little less flexibility as a result, but with the security of tenure that salaried employment has to offer. The usual option of DHB employment is to work as a 'core' midwife in a hospital setting providing rostered shift cover in a maternity facility.

Hospitals fall into three categories: tertiary, secondary and primary. Tertiary or base hospitals are large consultant units offering standard obstetric and neonatal care. They are generally based in the larger cities and women with specific obstetric and medical needs will travel sometimes extensive distances in order to receive specialist care. The secondary units are smaller less specialized hospitals that may have a visiting if not permanent obstetric and/or paediatric services. The primary hospitals are small 'cottage style' hospitals that frequently serve as maternity hospitals, similar to those that could be found in the UK up until the 1960s. They are similar to the existing birth centres in the UK.

Once she has established that she is pregnant, a woman is entitled to seek out a lead maternity carer (LMC) with whom she will enter into a contract for the duration of her pregnancy, birth and between 4–6 weeks postnatally. Primary maternity care is financed by the Department of Health (DoH) and is free of charge to women who are nationals or have permanent residency. LMCs can be midwives, obstetricians or GPs with a Diploma in obstetric care, but 78% of women opt for a midwife to provide care and support during their childbearing experience. (NZHIS 2007).

The New Zealand College of Midwives 'Partnership Model' (Guilliland & Pairman 1995) which underpins the organization of maternity care in New Zealand through Section 88 (MoH 2007) ensures that the delivery of care is a collaborative affair, with women clearly staking their claim in the process. Women generally seem to be very well informed about the services on offer and their rights. New Zealand has some of the strongest patients' rights legislation in the world, and this is reflected in maternity services (HDC 2007, Womens' Health Action 2007). All midwives are expected to work in partnership with women, providing or supporting continuity of midwifery care throughout the woman's childbirth experience. The discussions that take place on the road to decision making can be awesome, and the woman's decision is, in the eyes of the legal system, absolute.

From an admitted subjective viewpoint, the concept of risk does seem to be slowly but insidiously gaining ground here. This is quite interesting because the issue of litigation is hardly an issue here. New Zealand has a no-fault personal injury insurance cover, the Accident Compensation Claim scheme (ACC), which means that the indemnity insurance costs (a service provided via membership of the New Zealand College of Midwives for self-employed midwives) are affordable. Clearly the midwife can still be held to account professionally and can be issued with disciplinary action and in extreme cases, struck off the register. Here, it seems to be the media that the midwifery profession are wary of. New Zealand is a small country in terms of population and even the cities have a small town feel about them. Being discredited by the media seems to instil as much fear as being sued does in the UK.

From an anecdotal perspective, it would seem that the less than positive representation of midwifery within the media is having an impact on recruitment at the moment, and there is a national shortage of midwives as acute, if not worse, than that currently experienced in the UK (NZCOM 2006, RCM 2006). To compound this situation, the average age profile of midwives practising in New Zealand is now recognized to be 50+, which leaves the profession with a demographic time bomb ticking away. (Midwifery Council 2006a). In order to address this problem, midwifery is flagged up as a skills shortage profession with Immigration Services (NZIS 2006) and consequently many of the midwives currently registering with the Midwifery Council are overseas applicants.

This scarcity (particularly of LMC midwives) can mean that women's choices are sometimes curtailed. This is particularly evident in certain geographical areas. In theory, women have free rein to choose, after consultation with their midwife, where they feel would be best placed for them to give birth. In many areas, unless she has located and pinned down a midwife practically before the test result has confirmed her state of pregnancy, she may be left with very little choice of midwife, and in some cases without a midwife at all.

This shortage may also mean that midwives inadvertently end up taking on a greater caseload than they can realistically handle which may impact on the quality of care that they are able to offer or cause situations of burnout and all that that entails for the individual, their family and the midwifery profession at large (Hunter 2001). The New Zealand College of Midwives recommends a caseload of no more than 5–6 women a month (NZCOM 1997) but it is common knowledge that there are midwives who have a far greater number of women in their caseload.

It would seem that the interface between the primary service provided by the self-employed LMCs and the DHB workforce is perceived as tenuous at times by some practitioners in some areas. As we previously discussed, within the secondary and tertiary hospital facilities, core midwives may be involved in providing care for women who require secondary obstetric care and whose LMC midwife has handed their care over to the secondary service. They are also expected to support the LMC midwives during labour and birth and in the early postnatal period. Although relations between LMC midwives and core staff are generally cordial, there are clearly times when both parties may feel that there is a conflict of interest and this can lead to an adversarial sense of 'us and them'. For example, if an LMC feels that the core staff are not following her instructions in her absence, or if the core staff feel that an LMC is not visiting a woman in the postnatal period and expecting core staff to fill in in her absence, then the potential for a breakdown in relations is created. I understand that the New Zealand College of Midwives and midwifery managers are aware that there is a problem and are working at ways of bridging the differences between core staff and self-employed midwives in order to improve relations and working conditions. Some attempt to hold regular forums where hospital staff and independents come together to thrash out any problems relating to the interface are also held in some areas.

The way in which self-employed midwives are funded can also give rise to frustration. For example self-employed midwives are only given their full payment for birth when the woman has a normal vaginal birth. If the woman has an elective caesarean section, even though she may be with the woman for the surgery, she loses out financially. However, if the woman requires a caesarean section after the establishment of labour, then the midwife receives payment for the labour and birth module in its entirety. This can also lead to some confusion in terms of responsibility. Although the tertiary facility may in such a situation be taking over in terms of management, the LMC midwife has built up a relationship with the woman over a number of months and as her advocate would normally wish to remain involved in her care.

All midwifery educational programmes within New Zealand are undergraduate and 'direct entry'. It would appear that few nurses, who are given little concession from an educational entry perspective, opt to enter midwifery programmes, which means that New Zealand now has over a decade's worth of graduate midwives who have no formal 'nursing' qualification, thereby altering the profile of the profession quite extensively. The undergraduate programmes here are quite different from midwifery programmes in the UK. Although the students do access the hospital system to gain some skills and experience in the first couple of years, that clinical experience may be less than overseas registrants have grown to expect. The practice experience of the students is almost exclusively spent with self-employed midwives providing continuity of care. The number of practice placement hours is slightly less than those of students in European programmes. However, this is something that is being addressed as part of a review of midwifery education, where it is proposed that the hours in New Zealand programmes are brought

into line with current EU requirements (Midwifery Council 2006b). There has been some criticism by both practitioners, fellow health professional bodies and the media about the confidence levels of new graduates. This concern is also being attended to by the aforementioned midwifery education review and the proposal to extend the number of practice hours within programmes. Additionally, the Clinical Training Agency (CTA), which is a unit of the Ministry of Health, has recently prime-pumped a pilot mentoring scheme for newly qualified midwives for the next 2 years (NZCOM 2006). The Midwifery First year in Practice scheme (MFYP) offers newly qualified self-employed LMCs, as well as public and privately employed midwives, the opportunity to develop the specific knowledge and skills required to progress from a competent to a confident midwife with the support of a firm mentoring structure. This involves ensuring that they have a clearly identified mentor who will receive funding for supporting the new graduate midwife and for attending updates during the year of mentorship. The new graduate also receives financial support for attending study days and updates, and remuneration for income lost during time spent on mentorship issues. This is a positive move which will be closely monitored, and it will be interesting to see what the outcomes demonstrate following the introduction of the programme.

I was surprised to discover that whereas in the UK midwives have been expected to be able to provide evidence of professional updating by decree of the Midwives Act (1901) and more recently by the introduction of PREP, in New Zealand this was not the case until recently. Although there has been the availability of Masters and Doctoral Studies here for some time, the opportunity for access to continuing midwifery education has only recently started to gain momentum. As a result of the passing of the Health Practitioners Competence Assurance Act 2003, the issue of professional development has now become a mandatory component of the re-registration process for all health professionals. The Midwifery Council have responded by making aspects of the professional competency requirements mandatory and the midwives are required to attend a triennial Technical Skills course, a 2-day workshop which is designed to bring midwives up to speed on a variety of skills such as suturing, and examination of the newborn, as well as refreshing them around emergency situations such as shoulder dystocia and unexpected breech. I have to be honest and say that I initially received the idea of this compulsory requirement with a degree of scepticism. However, having now facilitated a number of the workshops, I feel much more optimistic. The most significant thing for me is that many of the midwives who arrive are clearly there under duress, but they seem to leave feeling positive and empowered, and hopefully ready to undertake further elective courses. It also helps them to formulate a concept of what is required for portfolio preparation, which is now also a requirement here. Other requirements include a breastfeeding update every 3 years and annual adult and neonatal resuscitation refresher courses (Midwifery Council 2006a).

In many ways, we migrant midwives can be seen to bring both positive and negative attributes to our new workplaces. On the one hand, we bring a variety of skills and experiences that could help to enhance the existing service. However, on the flip side of the coin, we can sometimes arrive with little understanding or cultural awareness of the society or the system here, which in my opinion is remarkably different from that of the UK and that of many other countries. I think that it is fair to say that not all midwives who choose to work in New Zealand are lured by the attractions of a ground-breaking maternity service. Some are undoubtedly primarily seduced by the amazing lifestyle opportunities on offer here and will simply try to emulate the midwifery that they knew and felt safe and comfortable with in their home countries. This could lead to a form of midwifery care that does not sit particularly comfortably within the New Zealand system, where the users are far more aware of their consumer rights. The Midwifery Council have attempted to address this potential for cultural discrepancy by making it a condition of registration for all overseas registrants to complete a course which explores the historical, legal, ethical and cultural dimensions of midwifery in New Zealand. It will be interesting to see if this has an impact on the service in terms of how many more emigrant midwives opt to become independent midwives and all that the true meaning of autonomy incurs. All overseas midwives additionally have to complete a Treaty of Waitangi course, which underpins much of the historical, political, and bicultural aspects of life in New Zealand. Additionally, because midwives in New Zealand have full prescribing rights, registrants from anywhere else in the world have to pass a fairly comprehensive pharmacology course. These courses can be accessed before arriving here by distance learning, or completed here within 18 months of registration with Midwifery Council.

So having reflected on the pros and cons of the system here, I guess that the obvious question is, do the benefits of working as a midwife in New Zealand outweigh the disadvantages? I think that I can give an affirmative response to that question with a resounding 'YES'. Many of the current anomalies within the system are currently being addressed and should be resolved within the foreseeable future. Both Midwifery Council and the New Zealand College of Midwives are fighting hard to ensure that every potential pitfall is accounted for in order to preserve the integrity of the hard-won battle to re-establish midwifery here. As a self-employed midwife, it is possible to have an amazing sense of autonomy, which, with privileges such as full prescribing and referral rights, surpasses that of even the independent midwives in the UK. No system is perfect but this system, in spite of its shortcomings, enables midwives to truly work within a framework of continuity and to be with woman in a holistic sense.

REFERENCES

Abbott L 2005 OMOM and IMA CMM: Two acronyms for radical change. AIMS Journal 17(3)

Department of Health (DoH) 1993 Changing childbirth: report of the Expert Maternity Group (Chairwoman J. Cumberlege), Vol. 1. HMSO, London

Department of Health (DoH) 2004 National Service Framework for children, young people and maternity services: supporting local delivery. HMSO, London, Online. Available: http://www.dh.gov.uk/PolicyAndGuidance/HealthAndSocialCareTopics/ChildrenServices/ChildrenServicesInformation/fs/en

Francis A, van der Kooy B 2004 21st-century midwifery: NHS community midwifery models. AIMS Journal 16(2)

Guilliland K, Pairman S 1995 The midwifery partnership – a model for practice. Department of Nursing and Midwifery, Monograph Series: 95/1

Health and Disability Commissioners (HDC) 2007 Online. Available: http://www.hdc.org.nz/ Accessed 12.1.07

Hunter B 2001 Emotion work in midwifery: a review of current knowledge. Journal of Advanced Nursing 34(4):436

Midwifery Council 2006a Online. Available: http://www.midwiferycouncil.org.nz/main/Workforce/

Midwifery Council 2006b Pre-registration midwifery review: Midpoint: July, p 3

Midwifery Council of New Zealand 2007 Reasons for working part time. Online. Available: http://www.midwiferycouncil.org.nz/content/library/Reasons_for_Working_Part_Time.pdf Accessed 21.1.07

Ministry of Health (MoH) 2007 Primary maternity services notice 2007. Online. Available: http://www.moh.govt.nz/moh.nsf/pagesmh/5845/$File/s88-primary-maternity-services-notice2007-v14.pdf Accessed 25.2.07

New Zealand College of Midwives (NZCOM) 1997 Questions to ask when you choose a midwife. NZCOM, Christchurch

New Zealand College of Midwives (NZCOM) 2006 First year in practice (MFYP) scheme. Online. Available: http://www.midwife.org.nz/index.cfm/MFYP Accessed 23.2.07

New Zealand Health Information Service (NZHIS) 2007 Online. Available: http://www.nzhis.govt.nz/ Accessed 12.1.07

New Zealand Immigration Services (NZIS) 2006 Long term skills shortage list. http://www.immigration.govt.nz/NR/rdonlyres/063ECB35-F5D5–44D8–8325–7041A727A9D5/0/1093.pdf Accessed 21.2.07

Primary Maternity Services http://www.midwife.org.nz/content/documents/187/guide-proposed-section88-maternity.pdf

Royal College of Midwives 2006 Cuts having dramatic effect on maternity services. RCM News. Online. Available: http://www.rcm.org.uk/news/pages/newsView.php?id=249

Womens Health Action 2007 Online. Available: http://www.womenshealth.org.nz/patientsrights/patients.htm

Topics for further reflection

- Several of the articles in this section describe the highs and lows of midwifery on a global scale and draw attention to the stark differences that exist between women giving birth in developing and developed countries. What strikes you most about the contrast between the area you work in and some of the areas described by the midwives whose articles are included here or in other sections of this book?

- Susan Burvill's article raises the issue of how, in some countries, traditional birthing customs – many of which, like the use of upright positions in labour, are conducive to normal birth – have been abandoned in favour of Western medical rituals. Although many of these medical rituals have now been abandoned in the West, their use continues in other areas of the world, which raises huge questions about the relativity of knowledge, as well as about the need to address the domination of Western medical ideals. How can we begin to separate the trends (whether traditional or modern) that are useful from those which are not? Are there any criteria which could be used to evaluate the usefulness of these in birth before they become ingrained to the point that it is hard to challenge them?

Stories and Reflection

A midwife reborn

Rosie Kacary

Following a long period of increasing dissatisfaction with my role as a community midwife, which was slowly but surely being destroyed, I finally decided last summer to throw caution to the wind, hand in my notice, return my lease car, wave goodbye to my regular pay cheque and become an independent midwife. My biggest worry was wondering whether or not anyone would ever call me, let alone choose to employ me and pay me for my services. However, 12 months on, I am happy to report that I have had the best year ever, feel totally rejuvenated as a midwife and really can't remember why on earth it was such a difficult decision to leave in the first place!

The first birth

On 31 July, just a few days after leaving, I attended my first birth: a planned home birth of 'an elderly primigravida', therefore classified by local guidelines as 'high risk'.

I had been what I can only describe as interviewed for the post of midwife by this woman, her partner and her parents, in whose home the birth was planned to take place. This involved some lengthy discussions around the kitchen table one Sunday morning, and I felt faintly amused when I thought of the likely reactions of some of my colleagues were they to be 'vetted' in this way. It struck me that all women should be able to choose their midwife, and that it would be a very good idea to have a system in place whereby all midwives were interviewed prior to being accepted by the woman.

A few days past the due date, my woman called me to tell me she was in labour. We laughed at how convenient this was since I had tickets the next day for a music festival I had been anxious not to miss! On my arrival, 'A' was clearly in early labour. I felt an almost heady excitement at the thought that I didn't need to carry out any routine procedures I deemed unnecessary, such as internal examinations. Now, for the first time since becoming a midwife,

I was answerable only to my woman, myself and to the NMC codes and rules rather than a whole entourage of labour ward guidelines, managers and medicalisation.

A was wonderful. She spent some time in the bath, the garden, tried a TENS machine and always remained positive and focused. During second stage, I was overawed by her strength and determination to birth her baby. She made my job easy, and when her eight-and-a-half-pound son slithered out that evening I remembered why I loved being a midwife.

During a longer third stage than any I had experienced – more than four hours – my independent midwife partner, Lynn, taught me more about third-stage management than I had learnt in the previous five years. Had I not been practising independently, local guidelines – together with my lack of appropriate support and knowledge – would have necessitated a transfer to (on this occasion) the hospital I'd just left! I must admit, I don't think I've ever been so pleased to see a placenta.

Night of the full moon

My next client was a traveller – and in case anyone out there is under the misapprehension that only rich women can afford independent midwives, let me tell you that this has certainly not been my experience. 'B' was fascinating, and I don't think I have ever encountered any woman like her before. When we met she told me she expected to have her baby, her first, on 12 August because that was the date she had worked out and it was a good one because there would be a full moon that night. She took me for a walk around a wildflower garden and showed me the old oak tree under which she planned to birth her baby. Sure enough, on 12 August, with a full moon and under the tree, she gave birth to her daughter – as she had told me she would.

My third birth came just three days later, another first baby to a couple who had originally planned to have a hospital water birth but became increasingly aware that the chances of this were very unlikely due to staff shortages and lack of appropriately trained midwives. Funny how all midwives are deemed competent to look after women with epidurals but panic at the thought of warm water.

At 37 weeks, 'C' phoned me while I was in the supermarket to tell me she had had a show. I think I may have been a little unimpressed, but she called back later that evening with the news that her waters had gone and she was contracting. When I arrived around midnight, C was anxious to get in the hurriedly assembled pool. Several hypnotherapy tapes and vials of lavender oil later, she, too, birthed her daughter beautifully. My earlier experience with a stubborn placenta stood me in good stead on this occasion, and it turned up eventually!

I suspect that if I hadn't been able to spend as much time postnatally with this family as I did, breastfeeding – which was a huge struggle initially – would never have been properly established. While the credit for persevering must obviously go to the parents, I felt enormously satisfied that I had no small part to play in it.

On 22 August, my fourth baby arrived, this time to a woman whose first birth had been complicated with an induction, an instrumental delivery and a PPH. She had had an elective caesarean the second time, although she resented the term 'elective' since she says she didn't elect for anything. Ten days past her due date, after several days of 'niggling', she had a quick, straightforward birth and is now planning another baby – having been adamant throughout the pregnancy that the third was definitely her last.

My last baby for the month arrived on the 30th – his mother's birthday, too! Technically another 'high risk' woman, she had birthed her first baby at home at 40 + 18 amidst incredible scaremongering tactics from her midwives, and had a PPH (although this was managed without oxytocics and it was only after booking in with the midwife during her second pregnancy that she was told she had had one at all). While achieving a homebirth with NHS midwives the first time, this woman knew she would have to fight to achieve what she wanted this time around. Therefore, despite living in rented accommodation and on a low income, she somehow managed to find the money to pay for independent care. Her 10-pound son arrived in the kitchen in between mouthfuls of birthday cake.

Expectations surpassed

Five beautiful homebirths in my first month as an independent midwife was more than I could ever have anticipated in my wildest dreams. I had expected perhaps six births in my first year, but have been privileged to have cared for more than 20 women and have advised many more. My knowledge has increased dramatically, since I now have time to research conditions thoroughly.

Twelve months ago I'd never heard of ankylosing spondylitis or Worster-Drought syndrome (neither of them mean you can't have a good homebirth!). I have witnessed a VBAC twin breech birth at home, something I doubt I would ever have seen in my former job since the supervisory structure necessary to support midwives in supporting women just wasn't there; and I recently attended a primip birth in a caravan in a field with no running water or toilet facilities, again dispelling the myth that only the wealthy can afford independent care.

I have learnt so much from the women I have cared for, who all shared a desire to give themselves the best possible chance of a normal birth. Sadly, perhaps shockingly, they believed their best chance was to stay well away from large, consultant-led units – and because many of the women seeking out independent care are classified 'high risk', unfortunately they cannot access the philosophy of normal birth more prevalent in small birth centre environments.

So have there been any frustrations?

Well, it's always frustrating when hospital managers deny women the choice of having a hospital birth and force them into homebirth against their wishes because hospital policies are so restrictive and inflexible. These hospitals seem only able to provide institutionalised, rather than individualised, care. I wish we could all remember that the service only exists because of women and is there for them, not for our own self-gratification. Maybe more of a 'let's see how we can accommodate this request' rather than an 'absolutely no way' attitude wouldn't go amiss.

However, there are one or two notable exceptions to this – the North Hampshire Hospital, Basingstoke, and The John Radcliffe, Oxford – two trusts that always bend over backwards to accommodate the most bizarre of requests, and where Lynn and I are always greeted with the utmost courtesy and respect rather than the suspicion we have sometimes encountered in other units. Such a shame that the majority of other units are unable even to consider our requests for honorary contracts – meaning that we frequently have to deny women access to independent care. Surely it is in everyone's interests for a woman to take her own midwife into hospital with her?

We have also experienced some excellent examples of supervision, but unfortunately the bad outweigh the good and there are still those who continue to confuse management with supervision. It's always irritating that the medical profession is allowed to get away with disseminating incorrect and outdated information. Will some GPs never learn that women need neither their permission nor their blessing to have babies at home, and will some obstetricians ever concentrate on those who really need them? The classic line that I think I'll take to my grave came from a consultant to a woman planning to home-birth with me: 'Well, of course, you know this midwife won't be able to listen to the baby's heartbeat properly, don't you? She'll only have a horn.' I assume she meant my pinnard stethoscope which, while I do have one (two, actually), isn't my only method of auscultation!

Happier and more confident

Twelve months on I cannot imagine ever returning to work within the current NHS. I'm happier and more confident. Friends tell me I smile more – I certainly cry less. I have regained a work–life balance, no longer having to work weekends and bank holidays unless I choose to, and I can take my holidays at times to suit my family and me rather than at times that suit an institution. I get to pick my children up from school, and the nightmare of asking for time off for the nativity play and sports day is a dim memory. I no longer suffer the constant nagging thought that to do my job with the commitment it deserves and with which I want to do it is a job for a single person.

While all this is wonderful, perhaps the most important fact is that for the first time I actually feel I am able to do my job properly and to the best of my abilities. I'm able to look after women and their families who truly value my skills, and my income now seems a fairer reflection of my worth. What price should we put on that?

I would urge all midwives and interested parties to contact their MP regarding the NHS Community Midwifery Model proposed by the Independent Midwives Association – accessible at www.independentmidwives. org.uk – as a real, viable addition to our current system. Who knows, it might just attract 8,000 midwives back to work and give all women a real choice.

The Practising Midwife 2005; 8(1): 53–54

Let's be realistic . . .

Caroline Flint

Thank goodness for realistic role models. I have had my fill of glamorous stars leaving hospital three days after their caesarean section looking as if they are going on a modelling assignment. I remember with great fondness the pictures of Princess Diana leaving hospital after Prince William's birth, obviously still wearing maternity clothes – presumably because, like most ordinary mortals, she could not get into non-maternity ones.

In January 2002, the harrowing pictures in the newspapers of Gordon Brown (Chancellor of the Exchequer) and his wife Sarah after the death of their baby Jennifer Jane were very sad, but very appropriate in reminding readers that childbirth does not always go without a hitch. Lovely to see the joy of the same couple following the birth of their son John in October 2003, following a very heavily supervised pregnancy and caesarean section.

Sophie, Countess of Wessex, was airlifted to hospital in 2001 with an ectopic pregnancy. Then, in November 2003, she was rushed to hospital with pregnancy complications, had an emergency caesarean and then stayed in hospital for 12 days, fuelling anxieties in the media that all was not well and that this birth had very much depleted this young mother. The baby girl, Louise, also stayed in hospital for two weeks, the Duchess being too ill to see her baby daughter for several days.

Media realism

In our culture of blame, where every baby has to be perfect and if it isn't then it must be someone's fault, it is good to see realism creeping into the media. Even today, one in every 100 babies dies (stillbirths and babies dying in the first month of life), and childbirth can be very gruelling for some women.

In our small independent midwifery practice (the Birth Centre), we are aware of how much pressure there is on modern women to 'perform' – that they should be able to tell their friends that they were going round Sainsbury's doing the weekly shop three days after the birth of their baby, or that they were entertaining 20 of their partner's relatives when the baby was only two days old, or that they took their baby into work when he was only 24 hours old to show their colleagues.

Sheila Kitzinger talks of a 'babymoon' – what a sensible idea for a woman who has been through one of life's greatest and most demanding experiences: she needs time to reflect and go over and over again the events surrounding her childbirth.

Rest and recuperation

In our practice, we recommend that all women stay in bed for 10 days following the birth of their baby. There are several reasons for this: so that they can get to know and fall in love with their baby in privacy and peace; so that they can establish breastfeeding in the comfort and quiet of their own bed; and so that they have time and space to recover and reflect on their labour and birth.

For people looking after the new mother, having her tucked up out of the way is also helpful. Grandmother or husband can get on in the kitchen without anyone bossing them around as to how 'we do things here'. Obviously, as midwives, we are aware of the danger of deep vein thrombosis, so the women we care for get up and walk around regularly to pass urine, to have a bath, to change the baby's nappy, etc.

For those who take advantage of our suggestion, their time of being mothered and cherished after the birth of their baby is remembered with great affection as a time of heightened sensitivity and fond memories. They are also relieved that the ordeal of labour is recognised as just that – something very demanding that they did brilliantly, but now they need to rest and recuperate after it.

No one likes lovely natural births more than I do, especially at home or in home-like surroundings. I love it when women can take up positions in which they are more comfortable, when they can tune into their very strong and active instincts, when they can make appropriate and helpful noises – roaring often helps significantly. Nothing is more gorgeous or more awesome.

However, the idea that labour is a difficult and sometimes dangerous process seems in danger of being forgotten. This week, I have had several rather difficult conversations with people who feel that their labour has gone wrong, that their midwives were at fault – that someone was to blame for labours that turned out differently from the labour that the parents had wished for.

Not an exact science

One couple have had a 'small for dates' baby; they are angry that the midwives missed this and that it was only picked up on an ultrasound scan when the couple were referred for an unstable lie. The fact that not only their midwives had failed to pick up the smallness of their baby but also three experienced obstetricians seems to cut no ice with the couple – their midwives let them down and they had a caesarean section when they had wanted a Birth Centre birth. Sorry, midwifery is not an exact science, and this happens.

The other couple had an undiagnosed breech and ended up, to their great disappointment, with an emergency caesarean. They pointed out (rightly) that had they known earlier they could have tried techniques to turn the baby. I pointed out that even after nearly 30 years as a midwife, I have had two undiagnosed breeches in the past 18 months: one came out at home unscathed; and one was picked up on scan prior to the labour, solely because the mother had had an undiagnosed breech in

her last pregnancy and I didn't want that shock again so I had recommended a scan – just in case. The obstetrician who was scanning and I were both convinced that the baby was cephalic – we were shocked when the scan showed us a breech again.

Striving for natural birth

In our midwifery practice, we have an 85 per cent completely natural birth rate. I'm sure it would be even higher if we didn't practise in central London where most hospitals have a 30 per cent-plus caesarean section rate for primigravidae. In some of the hospitals we transfer into, a caesarean section is almost seen as a therapeutic exercise for any situation – I sometimes think even bunions might qualify!

However, at this moment I am feeling weighed down by expectations of perfect births – people who tell me that the birth would have been perfect if only I had had more patience, been more skilful, tried this or that way of moving/standing, etc. Parents quote Michel Odent at me – me, who could almost quote verbatim every word he has written! Sorry, folks, but some births are horrible – however lovely, patient or knowledgeable the midwife. They are too long, too painful, too demanding, and the baby doesn't come out without assistance.

Most births are magical, miraculous and the most joyful, emotional, sweaty, passionate experiences we can ever go through – but some births are an ordeal to be got through as quickly as possible with every modern aid used and every path tried. Thank goodness for epidurals, Syntocinon, intravenous infusions and caesareans. Sometimes – not often, but just sometimes – they are a godsend and necessary.

The Practising Midwife 2004; 7(3): 4–5

The birth of Nuno

Becky Reed

Nuno was born in January, a first child for Motoko and Seth. From the start of pregnancy they were both determined to have their baby at home provided all went well. This is the story of Nuno's birth, a beautiful normal home birth which in a hospital setting would undoubtedly have been deemed to require interventions of one sort or another.

A long pre-labour

Labour – or pre-labour – started at 4.30am on Sunday, and Nuno was born at 11pm on Tuesday. It was a long and at times difficult labour; his parents certainly thought so, and even advertised those hours of hard work on his birth announcement. Motoko was at term, her pregnancy had been straightforward and she was planning a waterbirth. Mary (her primary midwife) and I were anticipating an easy and enjoyable birth – at least for the midwives! However, Nuno had other ideas, and he had done what so many babies seem to do – wiggled himself into a position of slight asynclitism. 'Slight' is a misleading word here; as all midwives know, a tiny tilt in a baby's head position can lead to a huge difficulty during birth.

Pre-labour continued for two days, with Motoko contracting every three to five minutes for much of that time. Mary visited three times and twice she left again, having established that all was normal and that this was indeed not active labour. A vaginal examination (VE) on Monday morning confirmed a 2cm dilated cervix, and a diagnosis was made of possible asynclitism. Mary wrote in the notes at this point: 'We discuss findings – in view of pattern of contractions and ?asynclitic head, discuss doing lots of different positions esp. stairs/slow dancing/rocking to try to move head. Also to do what Motoko's body wants to do: bath/rest/eat/drink/wee, etc."

By the third visit on Monday evening Motoko was needing more support; contractions were still every three to five minutes, lasting a minute and quite intense. By 10pm the cervix felt less well applied to the head, the os was 3cm dilated and definite asynclitism was diagnosed, with sutures just palpable under the cervical rim. The membranes were felt intact and bulging. Contractions spaced out after this, and Mary would have liked to go home to sleep; however, a baseline tachycardia developed, and Mary recommended monitoring at the hospital. Motoko and Seth, imagining their longed-for home birth going out of the window, were understandably reluctant, but agreed when the registrar on call suggested they could return home if and when the tachycardia settled.

In hospital

Monday night was spent on the labour ward, with CTG monitoring and obstetric input. By 3.15am the CTG was satisfactory, and by 6am Motoko was ready to return home to get on with her labour. With the registrar's blessing she left hospital and by 7am she was back at home, still contracting every three to four minutes. Membranes remained intact and the fetal heart was normal. Mary went home to bed and I took over being on call.

Labour at last

At some time on Tuesday morning Motoko's body swung into action at last. I arrived (with Denise, a visiting student midwife from Scotland) at 12.30pm, and was immediately impressed with what was happening. Motoko was in the pool, quite obviously in good strong labour. In view of the long pre-labour I suggested doing a VE to check my diagnosis was correct, and so that Motoko could pace herself if necessary; she was happy with this. The cervix was effaced and thin, the os was central and

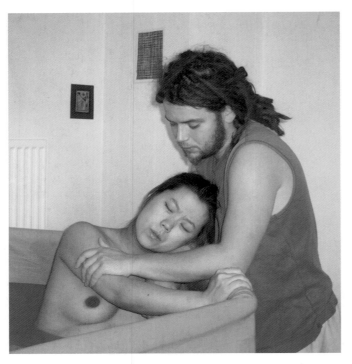
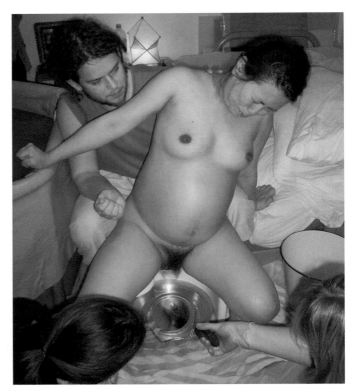
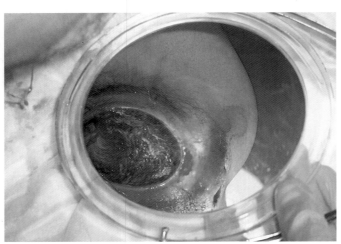
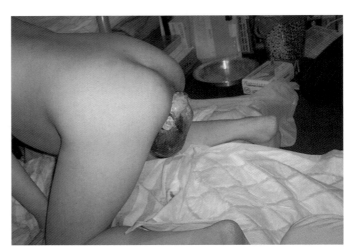
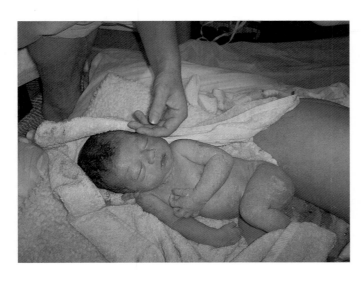
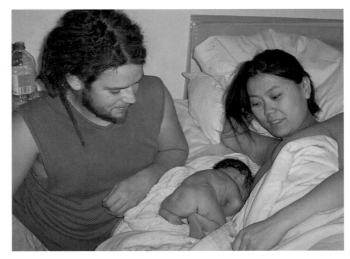

7cm dilated, stretching during a contraction. The membranes were intact and bulging, and I found it difficult to define the position of the head. It didn't matter – we were in business! I wrote in the notes: 'Good established labour at last.'

After this we stayed with Motoko and Seth until their baby was born. They spent a long time on their own together in their birthing room, while we drank tea in the kitchen with their flatmates Mizue and Tomoko. We checked the heartbeat every 15 to 30 minutes. A quick VE in the pool at 3.30pm showed normal progress: 8 to 9cm dilated, with no cervix felt posteriorly, an anterior lip and a rim of cervix at the sides. Mary came back at 4pm and I left for a while. By 8pm the anterior lip was still present but impossible to push back. At 9pm I returned, and suggested that Motoko get out of the pool and sit on the birthing stool; this upright position with good gravity might help to correct the baby's position and finally achieve full dilatation. On the birthing stool the membranes ruptured spontaneously with clear/blood-stained liquor, and half an hour later, with Motoko pushing hard, I was able to ease the lip of cervix gently over the last bit of Nuno's wonky head. Fifteen minutes later Seth could just see the top of his baby's head in the mirror at the height of a contraction. Over the next hour the asynclitism gradually corrected itself, although Nuno's head was born in the oblique, never having managed to rotate to a direct AP position.

The Practising Midwife 2005; 8(4): 18–20

Second stage

Because of an expectation of a slow and maybe difficult second stage, we suggested that Motoko stay out of the pool, using the birthing stool, the toilet and deep squatting to encourage good descent. When Nuno's head really began to stretch the perineum we encouraged Motoko to move onto her knees and gently blow her baby's head out to minimise perineal trauma. Nuno gasped immediately he was born, and we laid him on a warm heating pad in front of Motoko, where he gently began to breathe. I wrote in the notes: 'He's obviously been lying in a difficult position – lots of caput, clearly asynclitic head. We feel he's a bit shocked by his difficult birth.'

Five minutes later we gave Nuno an Apgar score of eight, as he was still not very active or responsive, although he was breathing normally, with a good heart rate and colour. He opened his eyes and looked around, reassuring his parents that all was well. The cord stopped pulsating but before we had a chance to cut it the placenta slipped out into the bedpan.

Blood loss was minimal, and Motoko felt fine; she went to lie down on her bed with Nuno snuggled next to her, grunting slightly but otherwise in good condition.

An hour later he had stopped grunting and was warm, alert, responsive and ready to breastfeed. Both his parents were exhausted but elated, and delighted to have had the home birth that meant so much to them.

Sitting in judgement – a personal reflection

Anonymous

During the past 12 months, the first year of my training, I have taken part in a wide variety of aspects of maternity care. I have shared the excitement of a long-awaited pregnancy, the emotions and tears of childbirth, the trepidation and rewards of parenthood. I have been there for the couple who have undergone in-vitro fertilisation; for the woman desperate to have a normal birth, only to end up having an emergency caesarean; for the woman determined not to breastfeed who changed her mind the minute she held her newborn. I have worked with women from a variety of socio-economic backgrounds and of varying educational standards, age groups, faiths and cultures.

So whose experience shall I reflect on? Whose psychological needs in pregnancy were met so well that she cannot wait for her next ovum to be fertilised? Whose sociological requirements were so well catered for that she now has a nice new home, designer clothes for her baby and enough formula to sell to the entire estate? Forgive me for being cynical, but this is a reflection of my experiences, my feelings and how I see my future.

I have chosen to adapt the Gibbs (1988) model for this reflection, and will be writing in the first person throughout. It is based on a series of events that culminated in the last six weeks of my first year. I will describe the events that prompted this writing, how these made me feel and if any sense can be made from them. I will also consider what actions I shall take should these events happen again.

I should like to reassure the reader that I have retained an ethical stance – therefore, all names and identifying features have been changed in order to maintain client confidentiality.

Sitting in judgement

I first noticed it during the second week of my first clinical placement. Having arrived for my shift on the postnatal ward, I sat in the office with the midwives and other ward staff as 'handover' was carried out. Then it started: 'Room A, para 2, second day, normal delivery, bottle-feeding . . .' and so on, as a summary of the woman's physical condition, personality, capability and overall judgement of her relationship and life was delivered to an expectant audience, red pens poised. I remember wondering to myself if I had been scrutinised and judged in the same way by the midwives at the hospital where I had given birth to my son. After all, at the time I was unmarried, a 'mature' mother and my now husband was 10 years my junior.

Then it came. The 'juicy bit' we had all been waiting for. The woman in room A was a drug addict! Not any old drugs, but heroin and methadone. The room was a blur of red pens; there were audible gasps of 'how could she?'. And so it went on. I have never pre-judged anyone intentionally or formed an opinion based on appearance, and I have worked with 'Joe Public' since leaving school. Nevertheless, here I was, gasping with the rest of them, condemning a woman on whom I had never laid eyes. I was shocked by my reaction.

I was even more shocked a short while later when I was awarded the dubious honour of being the one to 'give her a once over' before the doctor arrived on the ward. Why was I shocked? Because on meeting the woman, scared out of my wits, expecting to find a crazy, dirty, syringe-wielding person, I was greeted by a lovely young woman. With her in the room were her three other children, each well-dressed and non-swearing; her husband was equally well groomed and pleasant in manner. I spent an enjoyable 15 minutes or so with the family as I carried out my duties.

I vividly remember sitting down for a coffee later that morning with the other staff members. I brought up the subject of the 'druggie woman' and voiced my opinion of what a lovely family they were. I mentioned that under normal circumstances I would not have considered them any different from any of my neighbours. I will never forget being told, 'Don't talk ridiculous! They're druggies . . . tell you what you want to hear, show you what you want to see! Stay still long enough and they'll have your jewellery off!'

So that was it. My first conscious experience of stereotyping, labelling, judging – call it what you like, but it was there. It was not restricted to that particular ward, either. It could be found in various guises on the delivery suite, sometimes positive but usually negative, always resulting in an inequality of care. It was evident in the community setting: one midwife, a self-confessed 'snob', could be seen to turn up her nose on entering some women's accommodation.

Each time it happened, I found myself taking part in the sarcastic comments, the judgemental chats, the distasteful looks, as I became more accepted within the culture of the maternity care providers. I'm still not sure whether I made a conscious decision to act in this manner (remembering the first 'don't talk ridiculous' incident) or if I just did the same as many people do – imitated my peers in order to gain acceptance. I do know, however, that recently I forced myself to look at how my behaviour and attitudes had changed and I found that I did not like the person I had become.

Different ward, same attitudes

On my last placement of the year, I was working on another postnatal ward – different staff, different layout; same attitudes, same inequalities. A young woman was admitted to the ward following the birth of her daughter. I did not see her arrive on the ward, and had no idea who she was. A short time later, my mentor asked me to undertake a postnatal examination of the woman and to prepare her discharge notes as she was staying for only six hours. Off I went, performed the necessaries and completed her records, before returning to the office to begin her discharge notes.

The woman had a large and very obvious love-bite on her neck and, while I like to think I'm quite liberal in my views, even I considered this distasteful. I made the mistake of mentioning the love-bite to the other staff present. 'The dirty bitch!', 'That's disgusting!', 'Sick, more like!' and 'Perverted!' were among the nicer comments. I was asked how old the woman was; she was not yet 21. 'I might have guessed. No morals, the youngsters today,' was one reply.

The next question concerned the number of children she had – now totalling four. A unanimous guess was made that she lived in the less desirable area of the district; they were correct. Her notes were then taken from me as someone said, 'Let's have a look, I bet they've all got different dads!'. The children's names proved to be a

source of great amusement. 'Oooh, look! The first one's called Denzel. I bet his dad's black! The next one's called Carlos! Bet she went to Ibiza for her holidays that year!' The more it went on, the more I joined in. Comments were made about her personal hygiene, guesses made about her source of income ('fiddling' welfare benefits and prostitution being the most popular), the health and welfare of her other children questioned, suggestions made that she should be sterilised.

Then I ceased to join in this 'friendly' banter. I sat there and looked around the room. I looked at these women, with whom I had built up a working relationship which I respected and relied on to develop my clinical skills. I looked at myself. I looked and, to be blunt, I wondered who the hell we all thought we were. Which one of us was so perfect that we could sit in judgement in this way? Of the six people in the room, only the midwife who had admitted the woman to the ward and I had actually seen this client. Yet here she was, being accused of all sorts, labelled a 'slag' and allegedly typical of a woman from the area in which she lived.

I just sat there and said nothing, did nothing. I should have left the room but I stayed. I should have said something in her defence but I remained silent. Maybe I was scared of being ridiculed again. Maybe I was scared of being ostracised from the unit community. Maybe, as a student, I felt too weak and insecure to challenge the ways of my superiors. In order for me to make sense of my (non) actions, I needed to revise and expand my knowledge of psychosocial issues in pregnancy.

Care according to social class

Research by Sheila Hunt in the late 1980s and early 1990s suggests that the social class of the client is an important aspect of the care that midwives give. Her studies suggest that women of a higher socio-economic background are given more information, and that an elaborated code of speech is used by the midwife. In contrast, women from lower socio-economic backgrounds are treated as deviant, and a restricted code of speech is employed (Hunt and Symonds 1995). This certainly seems to have been the case in the many situations I have personally witnessed. Heptinstall (2000) points out that this fitting into categories according to social class has indeed led to class stereotyping of women using the maternity services. She says that: 'The stereotype portrays women in a negative light and assumptions are made by the midwives and doctors about women's understanding and their wants'.

Again, this sounds all too familiar, but in the case of the woman in my last example, stereotypical assumptions were initially based purely on the area in which she resided. The woman's notes stated that she was employed as a cleaner. Not the most 'professional' of jobs, I agree, but at least she was working. She might be working to provide the best she can for her children; maybe she works as a way to socialise with people other than her children. The fact that she works possibly gives her self-esteem a boost; maybe working gives meaning and routine to her life. Whatever her reasons, it was not our place to judge her but to provide the same care and support that we might to a teacher or solicitor.

I personally feel a great deal of respect for this young mother. She had her first child at the age of 16, and has gone on to have three more. Not yet 21, with four children and a job . . . I really do not know how she copes; I certainly could not. However, it would seem that I am in the minority, as the general opinion appears to be that young women living in disadvantaged circumstances deliberately get pregnant in order to make financial and material gain – for example, council housing and welfare benefits (Clement 1998). Likewise, it was assumed that because this young woman in our care was unmarried, then she must be a lone parent – another reason to be stigmatised.

It is a widespread belief that lone mothers are part of the 'dependency culture' in that they cost society a great deal of money in welfare benefits (Kent 2000). Is the same then true of the teacher who is a lone parent by choice, but in receipt of state maternity benefits and child benefits? It is true that the woman who caused me to take a closer look at myself was unmarried. She did, however, have a partner who was the father of the new baby. They might be living together; I did not get the chance to find out. He may be her long-term partner and the father of the other three children – it is not that difficult to imagine.

One client whom I met while working with the community midwives is 23 and has six children, the first born when she was 14. She is still with the father of the first child – indeed, he is the father of all the children. He has a good job within the public sector. They live together in a house they have bought from the local council, but are not yet married – they are waiting for the latest child to take her first steps before they 'name the day', so that all the children can be involved in the wedding as either bridesmaids or pageboys. She loves her life, loves being a mother, loves looking after her children, and says that is the reason she was put on this earth. When her youngest is old enough to attend nursery, she is going to college to become a registered childminder. Is she part of this dependency culture also?

The midwife's duty

I know that my opinions are personal and insignificant, and I realise that my voice will not be heard. I do know,

however, that the Code of Professional Conduct (NMC 2002: 3) states that a midwife should at all times '. . . act in such a manner as to: safeguard and promote the interests of individual patients and clients; serve the interests of society; justify public trust and confidence; and uphold and enhance the good standing and reputation of the profession'.

I also know that it is the duty of the midwife to act as advocate for the client, protecting and promoting the woman's interests and supporting any decisions she may make, and to respect the client's autonomy when making choices concerning her own life. Furthermore, I know that all registered practitioners must be non-judgemental when providing care to a client. A midwife must: '. . . recognise and respect the uniqueness and dignity of each patient and client; and respect their need for care, irrespective of their ethnic origin, religious beliefs, and personal attributes, the nature of their health problems or any other factor' (UKCC 1996: 25).

The unit in which I do my clinical training is situated within a small district general hospital. The hospital is located in a predominantly white area in which only small pockets of social deprivation can be found, and is staffed by predominantly white women. It would be interesting to compare experiences with my fellow students who are training within the larger, inner-city hospitals where social deprivation and ethnic minorities are the norm. I wonder if they encounter the same stereotyping – or maybe in their experience it is the white, middle-class woman who is stigmatised and receives unequal care.

I know that I cannot change the system – the 'banter' that goes on behind closed doors. I can, however, change my own attitudes and practice. I could risk ridicule by voicing disagreement when clients are being criticised, judged or labelled; I could remain silent. At this time, I do not know the answer. The only solution I can see for now is tactfully to remove myself from all situations in which I feel a woman is being pre-judged, stigmatised or labelled. In the event that I feel the care the woman receives is negatively affected by socio-economic or psychological stereotyping, then I shall seek advice and direction from one of the supervisors of midwives located within the hospital and from a relevant tutor within the university.

However, I think I can gain some comfort from the fact that I have recognised my flaws and intend to act positively on them. By making myself aware of the individuals (as well as of the groups) who make up our society, by providing individualised, woman-centred care and by following the guidelines laid down in the midwives' code of conduct, who knows – perhaps one day I will be able to make a difference.

REFERENCES

Clement S (1998). Psychological Perspectives on Pregnancy and Childbirth, Edinburgh: Churchill Livingstone.

Gibbs G (1988). Learning by Doing: A Guide to Teaching and Learning Methods, London: FEU.

Heptinstall T (2000). 'The sociological context of childbirth'. In: Mayes' Midwifery: A Textbook for Midwives, 12th edition. B Sweet with D Tiran D (eds). London: Ballière Tindall.

Hunt S and Symonds A (1995). The Social Meaning of Midwifery, London: Macmillan.

Kent J (2000). Social Perspectives on Pregnancy and Childbirth for Midwives, Nurses and the Caring Professions, Buckingham: Open University Press.

NMC (2002). Code of Professional Conduct, London: Nursing & Midwifery Council.

UKCC (1996). Guidelines for Professional Practice, London: United Kingdom Central Council for Nursing, Midwifery and Health Visiting.

The Practising Midwife 2004; 7(4): 21–23

Managing cord prolapse at a home birth

Claire Patterson

I have been working as a community midwife for over four years, actively supporting women in their choice to give birth at home. I participated in an ALSO (Advanced Life Support in Obstetrics) course in 2002 and recently had the opportunity to put some of the theory into practice when one woman, booked for a home birth, had a cord prolapse at home.

Onset of labour

It was about 4.30am when Joanne phoned to say that she thought she was in labour. I'd got to know Joanne well over the course of this, her third pregnancy, and I knew that her baby was by now a week overdue. She had had two previous 'normal' births, although both were very medicalised experiences in hospital. This time Joanne was hoping for a calm, quiet physiological labour and water birth and I had been supporting her in this. Joanne had decided to give birth at a close friend's house and had prepared a room (affectionately known as 'The Shed') in the garden, with cushions, a heater and a pool. The room was warm and spacious and a perfect environment in which to labour.

Straightforward pregnancy

With the exception of one episode of reduced fetal movements, the pregnancy had so far been straightforward. One week previously, Joanne had attended an antenatal appointment and was found to have a high mobile cephalic presentation that was able to swing into the oblique. As a para two it was not entirely unexpected that the presenting part would be high, but if the head did not descend before the membranes ruptured, the possibility of a cord prolapse was a concern. I discussed a plan with our consultant midwife and we decided that the most appropriate approach would be to perform an abdominal palpation at the onset of contractions and monitor descent

abdominally during labour. Joanne and I talked this through and also discussed what she should do in the event of spontaneous rupture of membranes (SRM) and a cord prolapse in the absence of any trained support.

A week later Joanne contacted me to inform me that she had started to have some contractions. In view of the plan that we had made previously I immediately went to assess descent of the presenting part. I arrived at about 5am to find Joanne having frequent, irregular, short contractions that were strong to palpate. An abdominal palpation confirmed Joanne's feeling that there had been descent of the presenting part into the pelvis. The head was in fact 3–4 fifths palpable and in the left occipito anterior position. The fetal heart was auscultated and all was well. We decided that a vaginal examination was not indicated in view of the descending head on palpation so we sat back to await events.

At 5.58am Joanne felt a gush of fluid and a copious amount of clear liquor was draining. Immediate auscultation of the fetal heart found the baseline to be 120 beats per minute but descending rapidly to about 70 beats per minute.

Cord prolapse?

The possibility of a cord prolapse came to mind and so a vaginal examination was quickly performed. Initially I could feel a small bumpy protrusion that I considered could be a compound presentation of fingers against the head but, as the next contraction started, a loop of cord fell through the 2cm cervical os into my fingers. As soon as I told Joanne that I could feel the cord she turned into the knee-chest position, just as I had described to her a week earlier.

Relief

Much to my relief I felt the fetal head fall out of the pelvis and away from the cord. Listening in proved that the position was effective as the fetal heart was back up to 120 beats per minute. I did not remove my fingers; even though the maternal position was excellent there was significant descent whenever there was a contraction or when Joanne vomited. I contacted the maternity unit using my mobile phone to ask for an ambulance and advise them of our impending arrival. All we could do was wait. Joanne's partner and friend prepared for our transfer to hospital by packing up my equipment, creating space for the ambulance crew and jotting down a few notes for me as my hands were full!

Ambulance support

The ambulance seemed to take an age but was actually only about 15 minutes. The crew were shocked by my request that we transfer to hospital without losing our position. Working out how to get to the ambulance was a problem: the Victorian narrow hallway and corners couldn't accommodate a stretcher. Being in the garden meant that we could use the side gate but the stretcher couldn't negotiate the tight bend from the passage through the gate. The ambulance crew brought the board more commonly used for transfer of spinal injury patients onto stretchers, and we were able to slide this, in two halves, under Joanne's knees and lock it into place.

I was lucky that we had two strong crew who were able to lift the board through the garden and manoeuvre it out onto the stretcher.

We got into the ambulance and headed for the unit. When we arrived, the midwives and obstetricians were in theatre waiting for us; a quick ultrasound confirmed a normal fetal heart-rate and a healthy baby boy was delivered by caesarean section (under general anaesthetic) at 6.45am.

The whole episode had only lasted 47 minutes but it felt like a lifetime for all of us.

Mother and baby doing well

I have seen mother and baby back at home and, apart from feeling bruised under the ribs (presumably from the effect of the maternal position), Joanne is recovering well. The baby is a very calm, relaxed little boy, none the wiser about his adventure. Incidentally, not only did the cord

prolapse but it was wrapped around the baby's neck three times and, on examination, I found that the umbilical cord contained a true knot – a perfectly tied knot about half-way down the length of the cord!

Hospital vs home birth

Afterwards the registrar who performed the caesarean section asked me if this meant that I would now want to return to practise in the hospital and I have been reflecting on this. 'What if?' and 'just in case' are phrases used regularly when discussing home birth; rather than leaving me feeling anxious and nervous about the next home birth I attend, I feel inspired. I am lucky that I work for a unit that believes in regular ALSO-type skill drills and this is an outcome that I have managed dozens of times in theory. When the unexpected did happen, I was able to put theory into practice without a second thought.

Discussion

This case has subsequently been discussed at the unit perinatal mortality meeting. An interesting suggestion made by a consultant obstetrician was to fill the bladder with 500ml of saline using a foley catheter. This is put forward as a suggestion by ALSO, although it is described as having only 'some success' in working as a tocolytic and pushing the presenting part up and away from the prolapsed cord (Eisinger 2001).

We are now debating whether all community midwives should carry catheters specifically for this purpose. It is difficult to envisage how a community midwife can single-handedly insert a catheter, draw up and insert 500ml of normal saline, call for help and prepare for transfer. Perhaps given a very long transfer, an extra pair of hands and appropriate equipment that befitted the purpose well, it could be attempted. In a hospital with CTG machines, scan machines and lots of spare pairs of hands it would be feasible. But, as uncomfortable as the alternative of the knee-chest position and an assistant taking the pressure off the cord is, I think in a similar situation, in a town centre back garden, I wouldn't reach for the catheter: I would do exactly the same again. I think the outcome speaks for itself . . .

REFERENCE

Eisinger S (2001). Advanced Life Support in Obstetrics Provider Manual (4th edition), Kansas: American Academy of Family Physicians.

Celebrating the 'art' of midwifery

Tricia Anderson, Lorna Davies

Children are naturally creative beings. We are born with an ability to use many different forms of self-expression. If you offer a three-year-old a selection of poster paints and a piece of paper, they will proudly present you with their masterpiece without a modicum of self-consciousness. If you offer an adult in higher education the same tools, the majority will feel at best challenged and at worst patronised.

Our mainstream educational system continues to elevate the status of the scientific and undermines the value of the aesthetic during our developmental years. Literacy and numeracy are the core features within the national curriculum. Although primary school children may be 'allowed' to spend time using art, this time becomes increasingly rationed throughout the school years. By the time they are 14, the vast majority of children have chosen to 'drop' art, unless of course they have 'talent' and have opted for a 'specialist' arts-based programme in order to pursue a career in an arts-based area.

Where does art fit in?

Midwifery is a profession that combines both art and science, yet it is currently more 'science' than 'art'. Midwives know this phenomenon first hand as the 'super-valuation' of the scientific and technocratic: the supremacy of the rational, medical model (Davis-Floyd and Mather 1993).

There is a lot of talk among midwives about challenging this medical model and humanising birth. But if we are to challenge the supremacy of the scientific – and don't forget that most of us have been educated within this scientific, medical model – we need to give value, space and time to exploring alternative ways of expression, thinking and being.

In our lives prior to our entry into midwifery, we both studied for degrees in arts-related subjects. We believe that midwifery education has failed to capitalise on the power, energy and sheer fun of the arts to enable midwives to explore their emotions, passion and experiences of being involved in the extraordinary world of birth. The power and beauty of a woman giving birth under her own steam can be breath-taking; the sight of a woman strapped up in lithotomy stirrups can be devastating. Yet, how often do we encourage midwives and students to explore their emotions in bearing witness to these things?

Developing humanity

The scientific, medicalised component is well-established within midwifery education; however, little emphasis is put on providing appropriate education for student midwives on the more sensitive, caring side of midwifery. Students need to develop appropriate attitudes, empathy and understanding, and the depth of articulate emotional responses required of a skilled, sensitive midwife. This area is more subtle and complex than technical skills, and is harder to teach and assess.

It is for their humanising gifts that women value midwives: skilled communication, support and empathy are values that women seek in their carers. Yet, little attention is paid in contemporary midwifery education to how to develop and strengthen these skills. The first step must be to help students open their hearts to the experiences of women, babies and new families, and artistic expression is one way to facilitate this.

The arts can also contribute to education as a learning activity, helping students to acquire communication and interpersonal skills, emotional literacy, team skills, problem-solving, lateral thinking, flexibility and adaptability. These are the very skills we now recognise as essential for today's midwives – skills that will help to develop the critically thinking, autonomous midwife required for current and future practice.

Grant (1998), a pioneer in this approach to education who is leading its development at South Bank University in London, suggests that the main purpose of studying the arts is to enable healthcare professionals to take better care of their patients and better care of themselves.

Art has the power to confront and challenge dogma and ideology. The arts can also be used for empowering oneself and others as catalysts for change. Through art, the neglected imagination is watered and flourishes. In our opinion, it is a wasted opportunity for midwives who are privileged enough to be involved in birth – the ultimate act of creation – not to be given the opportunity to explore and unleash their own creative potential.

Unleashing the creative force

When invited to participate in artistic activity – be it painting, singing, dancing or theatre work – most midwives and students alike will generally proclaim, 'But I'm not creative!'. However, create a permissive and safe space for them to do so and, to use a Stateside expression, Wow, do they rock!.

We co-facilitate a weekend residential workshop called 'Sex, Birth and Rock & Roll', where we use the power of the arts to convey a more holistic view of midwifery practice. At a point during the weekend, the participants are invited to take some paints and paper and to sit for an hour or so and create an image that represents childbearing for them. It is not art therapy, but simply a space for women to engage in a form of self-expression that may have been denied to them for some considerable time. The results are amazing.

What the painting seems to do is to give the participants the confidence to move beyond the cognitive, into less tangible areas of their being. England and Horowitz (1998) describe how painting is used to encourage parents to move into their right brains, the less rational, more primal brain space. Rogers (1983) talks about the concept of 'whole-person' learning, in which both hemispheres of the brain engage. The left hemisphere is logical, linear and deals in ideas that are clear-cut and defined. The right hemisphere functions in a different way, grasping the essence before it understands the details and can make creative leaps. It operates in metaphors, and can take in what Rogers calls the whole gestalt, the total configuration. To help students become skilled reflective practitioners, able to use professional artistry in their decision-making, the right hemisphere needs to be stimulated as much as the left. Using art is a direct route into this 'whole-brain' thinking.

Accessing the 'affective' domain

Learning needs to take place in both the affective (emotional) and the cognitive (rational) domains. Bloom (1965), a cognitive theorist, draws a clear distinction between the two, both of which need to develop in a parallel pattern of growth to facilitate the highest possible level of genuine learning. Too often in institutionalised education, the emphasis remains firmly on the cognitive. Bloom's taxonomy incorporates in the affective domain at its base level the notion of 'receiving' – paying attention to stimuli, observing and developing awareness. This is followed by 'responding', in which students are encouraged to formulate a response to the stimuli. Working with art helps students develop this skill of first observing and then articulating a personalised response. Unlike cognitive approaches, there is little opportunity for surface learning; students engage with the material on a deeply personal level.

We talk a great deal about holism in midwifery practice, but what does it really mean? The Concise Oxford English Dictionary (2002) defines holism as 'the tendency in nature to form wholes that are greater than the sum of the parts through creative evolution'. However, in midwifery the word appears to have taken on a vague, nebulous character and smacks of empty rhetoric, because the 'physical' takes precedence at every step. How can we care for a woman's emotional and spiritual well-being if we are not emotionally literate ourselves? Something is missing – perhaps the rejection of the arts in midwifery education could be this missing link.

We need to debate seriously the greater inclusion of arts subjects in our curricula. In New South Wales, Australia, they have recently introduced a core theme in the midwifery curriculum entitled Creative Arts and Midwifery (Jackson and Sullivan 1999). The aims are for students to demonstrate an understanding of midwifery as art; develop an understanding of the artistic and scientific components of clinical practice; examine images of concepts such as pain, suffering, parenting and caring through a variety of artistic media; and show sensitivity to the intricacies of human relationships through exploration of what it is to be human.

The work submitted by the students includes poetry, prose, collage, sketches, photographic essays, needlework and quilting, and is of a high quality. Students appreciate being able to look at the wider issues of midwifery and explore their own ideas and feelings in a creative way. Through creating artwork and then telling its story, they are able to make sense of previously irreconcilable events and develop a deeper understanding of the context of midwifery, including such concepts as 'love', 'pain' and 'loss'.

Jackson and Sullivan state that on completion of the course, students are able to conceptualise pregnancy and birth in a more holistic way. They recommend this approach as a way to help students develop insights and understanding into a range of human conditions and experiences to which they may previously have had little exposure (Jackson and Sullivan 1999).

At Bournemouth University there is now a similar option unit for pre-registration students entitled 'Using the humanities to learn about birth', which explores existing birth art and poetry and encourages students to produce their own. At Anglia Polytechnic University, there are several modules that promote the arts in midwifery, such as 'Images of Women and Childbirth'. An 'arts thread' is also woven into the fabric of the curriculum, and is used primarily to support personal growth and development.

Conclusion

The value of storytelling is now gaining credence in academia (Fairburn 2002), but why not poetry, dance, music and, of course, painting? We need to set aside our prejudices, feel the fear and do it anyway.

In the process, we may be offering access to a window to the soul that midwives have long been denied; it has the potential to alter the meaning of midwifery care beyond recognition.

REFERENCES

Bloom B S (1965). Taxonomy of educational objectives, London: Longman.

Davis-Floyd R and Mather F S (2002). 'The technocratic, humanistic, and holistic paradigms of childbirth'. MIDIRS Midwifery Digest, 12 (4), 500–506.

England P and Horowitz R (1998). Birthing From Within, Albuquerque: Partera Press.

Fairburn G J (2002). 'Ethics, empathy and storytelling in professional development'. Learning in Health and Social Care, 1 (1), March 2002.

Grant J (1998). 'Different ways of knowing'. The Practising Midwife, 1 (11): 41.

Jackson D and Sullivan J R (1999). 'Integrating the creative arts into a midwifery curriculum: a teaching innovation report'. Nurse Education Today, 19: 527–532.

Rogers C (1983). Freedom to Learn for the 80s, Colombus, Ohio: Charles E. Merrill Publishing Co, Bell & Howel.

The Concise Oxford English Dictionary (2002), Oxford: Oxford University Press.

Quotations from: www.quotationreference.com

The Practising Midwife 2004; 7(6): 23–25

Four labours and a Mars Bar

Phil Logan

She wakes me up at 2.22am. Her waters have broken. Oh, God. I stare at her stupidly for a second before reacquainting myself with the well known 13th Herculean task of putting trousers on in an emergency. 'Are you, are you . . .'

Yes, she nods, concentrating hard. The contractions are coming every five minutes and she's having one right now, so shut up. Oh, God, every five minutes . . . That's good, that's good. No it's not . . . we live 30 miles from the hospital. I'm trying to remember if the car is pointing the right way. I'm trying to remember the drill, even though we don't have a drill because we've done this three times before and everybody knows it's like not forgetting how to fall off a bike. Oh, God . . . 'Shall I ring the hospital, shall I ring the neighbours, shall I, shall I . . .?'

'Just let me get ready,' she says calmly, trying to talk me down from the ceiling. 'Why don't you set up the camp bed?' But before I have a chance even to forget what she has just told me, she's into the airing cupboard and pressing a bottle of Mr Muscle into my useless hands. 'You'd better clean the toilet.' The toilet is spotless, but I pretend it looks like a French one because she's kneeling over a chair and breathing in that funny way and probably not in the mood to discuss things too deeply.

Oh, God. What happened to the usual 12 hours' notice? What happened to leisurely contractions once an hour with time to hire a video, defrost a box of Birds Eye chocolate eclairs and listen to womb music from a Radox bath?

I leap into the air as our six-year-old suddenly materialises behind me. 'Look, Dad!' he yells, holding out the shiny new pound coin the tooth fairy has left him. 'It's the middle of the night,' I say as gently as ripping your ear off on a newly installed Ikea towel hook allows. I frogmarch him back to his cell, but he follows me out again. 'Dad, why are you and Mum getting dressed?'

I stick him in our bed and quickly explain the situation without using any verbs or recognised syntax. Now he's

really awake. 'Read your book,' I hiss, ducking out to check on the other two, whose teeth luckily haven't fallen out today, and who are snoring upside down in their beds.

In the kitchen, my wife has made coffee and is busy breathing again. I phone next door. No answer. I rush out into the street to see if their lights are on. Nothing. What's wrong? I gave them at least four seconds to get to the phone . . . I rush back in, just as my wife is replacing the receiver. 'She's on her way,' she says.

As our good neighbour arrives, I load the car with a king-size Mars Bar and other essentials and we're off. The motorway is eerily black, without a single other vehicle to crash into. The inside of the car is silent, too. 'You OK?' I whisper, not wishing to intrude, merely to establish that I remembered to pack her. She's probably contracting like mad. Why doesn't she moan like other people? Silence. I glance in the mirror. She's hunched over the seat. Good, fine, good, fine, good . . . Twenty-five minutes later, we come to a skewed halt outside the maternity doors. I grab everything from the boot and we stagger to the lifts. My wife refuses to take two of the bags off me, pointing out that old bottles and newspapers for recycling are not the obvious sine qua non of a smooth birth.

At 4.10 she is lying on a bed strapped to one of those machines, damp-haired and steaming. I make myself useful with a cooling flannel. The midwife announces a five-centimetre dilation situation and lets her off the leash. My wife immediately goes off to a corner where she squats quietly. 'Are you sure this woman is having a baby?' quips the midwife cheerfully, and trips off for an unearned cup of tea.

I'm just thinking about starting my Mars Bar when my wife enters her famous roaring phase. Aaaaaaaargh, she bellows. Oh, God, we've only been here an hour. Shall I get the, the . . .Rrrrrrnnnnnnnnnnnnnn. I think that was a yes.

The midwife arrives and is amazed that we have started without her. We load my wife on to the bed on all fours. There's a bit of grunting, then suddenly the net splits open and the catch comes slithering out all over the deck, a beautiful red snapper, its mouth wide open in surprised protest. Fantastic. I murmur something fatuous and shallow while my wife, whom nature has suddenly re-endowed with her senses, scoops up the slippery one and treats it to a nice fat nipple. It's a boy.

'Thank you, God,' I say, grinning like an idiot.

'That's OK,' comes the reply. 'May the fourth be with you.'

The Practising Midwife 2004; 7(1): 29

'There is a foot!'

Sonia Richardson

'Quick, she is fully dilated, it's her second baby.' I am called to be second midwife at a home birth.

When I arrive at the flat there is a typical home birth atmosphere: lovely! Dim lights, it's warm and it's peaceful. Everybody talks, if at all, in a quiet tone of voice.

Melissa, their first daughter, has fallen asleep by the television, defeated by tiredness, waiting for the birth.

There is also a subtle smell of cannabis in the air as I introduce myself to Maiko, who is Japanese and Michael, a tall Caribbean with a Rastafarian ponytail. 'What an interesting match,' I find myself thinking.

Not long to go before the baby's arrival now.

Maiko is on all fours on the couch and hiding her face between Michael's knees. She's gently pushing. The membranes bulge at the perineum and the baby's head is visible.

Sue, the first midwife, kneels at Maiko's side, occasionally listening to baby's heartbeat, and nods approvingly.

I sit in a corner, away from where Maiko is pushing strongly and read her notes.

Her first baby had been born at home; her Hb is 8.6. She declined iron supplementation, declined prenatal diagnosis including ultrasound, and wishes for a physiological third stage.

The head crowns, Maiko starts to pant . . . pant . . . head is out! The newborn spits and cries even before the rest of the body is born. Another contraction, a final push and . . . here he is! Welcome, little Japanese-Caribbean baby! Sue passes him between Maiko's legs, who immediately hugs him in her arms, wet and slippery as he still is. Michael is smiling.

It's a magical moment: Sue dries him, the calico cat comes close, smells him, mews approval and turns away. I've a stupid ecstatic smile on my face like a student midwife witnessing her first birth.

Not over yet

But Maiko hasn't the facial expression typical of a woman who has just become a mother and complains that 'underneath' it is still burning a lot. 'It's normal,' I say, and at that precise moment Sue says the words that I will never forget:

'There is a foot!' She carries on: 'It's twins!'

'WHAT?' I look down at that little foot kicking out of Maiko's body and I soon see another little foot appear. We stare at each other, 10 seconds of complete bewilderment and then we act automatically. We clamp and cut the cord of the first baby, and call an ambulance:

'Ambulance please . . . yes, yes . . . booked home birth . . . flat n . . . Yes, the baby is out . . . Actually, I mean, it is not out . . . No, not bleeding. Yes, there is a presenting part. No, she is not crossing her legs preventing birth: what kind of questions is . . .? Yes . . . yes . . . I do understand: I said the baby was out . . . No, I'm not contradicting myself! One is out and the other is not! No, not the same baby – it's twins! No, I'm not panicking!! Just come quickly, please!'

We help Maiko onto all fours again and get everything ready in case we need to resuscitate baby: Maiko is amazing: although shocked as we are she is still calm and concentrated. Michael is enthusiastic: 'Two babies? Cool! I always dreamt of having twins one day. Let's hope it's another boy!'

Sue tells me she has never seen a breech birth before. I've seen one, when I was a student. Heeeeeeeeeeelp!

In the meantime, the little one has managed to make his way as far as the umbilical cord: it's another boy. I take a deep breath, concentrate and simply let the body hang. I'm trying to remember every detail of my last drills and skills update and, as if by magic, they all come back to my mind. 'Sit on your hands, do not interfere, give the baby time to rotate and come down properly . . .'

Waiting

Time is ticking away, the contractions stop, five minutes go by, then a whole minute more and no contraction. The baby is not advancing.

In the meantime the ambulance arrives, but we can only wait.

The baby stops moving, he becomes blue, then white. Maiko breastfeeds the first twin with the hope of stimulating contractions. My face burns as if it were on fire, my hands are shaking and I need to throw up.

I feel the baby's cord, then the chest; I can't feel a heartbeat. Sue massages Maiko's uterus. A contraction comes – a mild one, but it'll have to do. I gently insert two fingers and manage to pull down an arm; the other arm comes by itself. I leave the body hanging again, but no: the head is not coming and by now I feel I'm holding a rag doll, rather than a baby. 'It's not coming,' I hear myself saying, and hope the others have not heard the desire in my voice to cry and run away. I insert my fingers again, aiming at the cheekbones, but only managing to locate the mouth and so stick my middle finger in. With my other hand, I reach the occiput and try to flex the head downwards. I feel the cord loosely around the neck. I pull, gently, and hear the jaw 'click'. ' I've broken it!' I say. The urge to vomit increases. I pull again, but nothing happens. I'm desperate.

The textbook drawings of obstetric complications come to my mind. I remember when I studied them, then think of the horror stories, told by senior mentors during quiet night shifts, probably just to scare us.

I take one more deep breath. I look at Sue who, miraculously, smiles at me, although I can see the same fear in her eyes that must be in mine. I try again. I pull gently downwards. It's much more difficult than on the dummies. And then, slowly, the head is finally moving . . . it's coming . . . it's born! A totally flat baby, white, no heartbeat. It looks dead.

We immediately start resuscitation. Two puffs, five compressions, two puffs, five compressions, dried, stimulated . . . 'Come on, baby, come on, please.' Maiko is sitting on the couch, feeding the first twin; Sue is dealing with the placenta. Michael is now paralysed with shock.

Five minutes go by. I place the stethoscope on the baby's chest and I hear the most wonderful sound. 'TUM-TUMTUMTUM': 110 beats per minute. 'Yes – there is a heartbeat!' I say, and then shut my mouth because I feel ready to vomit again! Soon after, Twin Two starts to pink up, to move his extremities and suddenly opens his eyes wide and looks me directly in the eyes – not with a 'near-to-death' look on his face, more like a curious one!

The ambulance leaves with Michael and Twin Two and we remain with Maiko and Twin One who, bless him, is still sucking at the breast. We're exhausted, but so excited. We help the new mum get comfortable in bed and enjoy her baby, and then we leave her alone for a while. I go to the toilet and look at myself in the mirror: I'm all sweaty and my face is red like after a whole day at the beach, my jeans are splattered with blood all the way to my sandals. Sue is in no better condition; her hair in a mess and her mascara smudged under her eyes. We look at each other and we hug. Gosh, what an experience!

My mobile phone starts ringing. I answer it: a newborn baby is crying in the background and then I hear Michael's voice: 'He's doing great – started screaming even before we reached hospital!'

The boys are identical twins. They weighed 2750g and 2150g. The surprise arrival stayed in hospital only that first night and was discharged as a 'live and healthy' newborn. Maiko, calm and peaceful as always, breast-feeds them both. Michael is the proud father of twin boys, like he always wanted.

Afterwards

When I got home later I was finally able to vomit in the privacy of my bathroom. Sue and I now have something else apart from the weather to talk about.

I completed an incident form and statement describing every detail of that special night (avoiding writing about my constant nausea) and my excited community manager rewarded me with a cup of tea.

And now? I still love home births, all women who give birth, all babies who are born and my wonderful profession.

The Practising Midwife 2004; 7(6): 49–50

An education in training

Sandy Kirkman

Midwives well advanced in years, like me, will remember that their training (and it was a training rather than an education) was in two six-month parts. Part one was hospital based, and part two community based. Some lucky pupils (as we were called) did the whole of part two in the community attached, loosely or tightly, to a teaching midwife. Uniform was worn at all times, and first names were not used either for mothers or for staff.

The Central Midwives Board (CMB), the forerunner of the National Boards, set rules and standards for training that involved many numbers. So many 'witness cases', so many babies to be delivered, and a number of mothers and babies to be looked after postnatally. So many episiotomies to be made (yes!), so many instrumental deliveries to be witnessed and so many lectures to be attended. These were given by medical staff, (obstetricians, anaesthetists, paediatricians), and took place from 9–10am.

The morning after the night before

As a pupil could not 'pass' part one without the requisite number of lecture attendances, one was obliged to go to them after night duty. If one missed a lecture, it had to be 'made up' by attending another, on any subject, as long as the numbers added up. I have sat in such lectures inflicting mighty bruises on myself by pinching my arms to stop me dropping into a deep slumber after a busy 10-hour night shift!

Apart from the lectures, pupils had the odd study day taught by magnificent, uniformed and bosomy midwife teachers. One made me laugh out loud by remarking lugubriously that, if the ovum was not fertilised, it passed harmlessly out of the body 'to be heard of no more'! We had one textbook (Myles) and one midwives' dictionary (Da Cruz). We had a test every week and could recite large chunks of material such as the landmarks of the pelvis and the denominators. The teachers had just 'gone

metric' and struggled to teach us the dimensions of the pelvis in centimetres. This led to a very confused friend trying out her own method of conversion in a test and triumphantly multiplying the centimetres by 2.5 then calling the result inches. Thus, the 30+ inch brim.

Neither the textbooks nor the lectures were referenced. We had no access to a professional library, and no databases. As a young midwife teacher in the mid-1970s, I began to frequent the medical library, and remember giving one reference during a lecture on diabetes in 1974–75.

Evidence, what evidence?

During my own midwife teacher's course, our main anatomy textbook was by CWF Burnett. It was certainly authoritative, but I doubt that it was evidence-based. I used to recommend Llewellyn-Jones to my student midwives, written for medics but readable and referenced. The first midwife-written, fully referenced textbook was 1992's The Art and Science of Midwifery, a marvellous book by Louise Silverton that arose from her teaching on the Advanced Diploma in Midwifery (ADM) course at Swansea University. I keenly await an updated version. (I told her so, and she very politely suggested that I should do it myself if I was so keen!)

I never recommend textbooks to students today: they seem, however, to go out and buy either Mayes or Myles. My main complaint about the single textbook, with the exception of Henderson and Jones, is that they claim multiple authorship but most of the multiple authors are indeed midwife teachers. I like Henderson and Jones because they have a chapter on sociology written by a sociologist, a chapter on pharmacology by a pharmacologist, etc. My other beef with the 'M and Ms' is that they claim to be heavily referenced, but many of the references are old – and to other textbooks. I would recommend the wonderful new book edited by Soo Downe, Normal

Childbirth, Evidence and Debate, because my copy has been stolen and replaced three times and I would prefer the culprits to supply their own.

Looking back over three decades has made me realise how far we have come from those dusty old lectures delivered by bored registrars to top up their salaries. We are fortunate indeed to have such easy desktop access to excellent databases and libraries. Students need not take notes in lectures but can retrieve the whole presentation on the intranet (we use 'Blackboard'). Prospective students can look for recommended book lists on Amazon rather than buying what they are told to buy, as we were.

I do wonder what the future holds: possibly journals and news media in online format only; perhaps books, too, will become virtual, with students paying a fee to download a chapter or a section as they need it. I am old-fashioned enough to enjoy the feel of a book, but the 400-year phase ushered in by Caxton may be drawing to a close. Or is that unthinkable?

The Practising Midwife 2005; 8(9): 50

Midwifing my daughter, receiving my grandson

Becky Reed

'Mum, would I be able to book you?' My daughter Laura, nine weeks pregnant with her first baby and my first grandchild, was sitting opposite me at the table. She tells me now that there was never any question that she would want me to be her midwife, but at the time I remember so many questions in my own mind . . . Would she want her mum to be her midwife, too? Would I want to? Might I prefer to be 'just' the grandma? Yet, when she did ask me it seemed as though I didn't even need to answer – it was the normal and right thing to do.

Laura was 11 when I started my midwifery training, and she remembers clearly how I hated so much of it – the sausage-machine mentality of the labour ward, the fragmentation of care. I became an independent midwife as soon as I qualified, providing continuity of care to local women and doing mostly home births – and, of course, talking about all this endlessly at home. Laura was interested but not fascinated, and she certainly wasn't sure about finding the occasional placenta in the freezer or bloods in the fridge! I remember thinking when she was a teenager that maybe she would choose an epidural or a caesarean when she came to have babies of her own. But now she was 27 and pregnant, and definitely choosing a home birth – preferably in water – and for her mum to be her midwife.

When I officially 'booked' her at 16 weeks, I wrote in the notes, 'Nothing can describe how wonderful it is to be Laura's midwife!.' And it's true, nothing can. Any midwife who has been there will understand; others can only imagine.

What was so fascinating, as I began to tell everyone, was the complete spectrum of reactions, from 'You can't do that' (consultant obstetrician, friendly but misguided) to 'But, of course, there's no other choice' (a friend from Senegal). My absolutely favourite comment was from my own GP, a woman who has known me and my family for very many years. When I told her Laura was pregnant and wanted me to be her midwife, her response was, 'Oh, Becky, what an honour!.'

It did feel like an honour, but at the same time this feeling was mixed with many other emotions. I felt so close to Laura and her partner, Tim; I felt so privileged to be sharing this experience so very closely with them; and I felt unbelievably responsible. I know that responsibility is part of what I do, I know that in my normal practice I deal with it every day, but this definitely felt like a different dimension. However, when I talked about this feeling with Laura she brought me down to earth completely with her comments, 'Mum, you'll be fine; you do this every day. It's what you know.'

A little extra support

She was right, of course. I do know how to be a midwife: it's my life and I do it all the time. However, for this very special experience I knew I wanted support from someone who lived locally to Laura (she and I are about an hour apart) and who, if necessary, could 'mother' me as I mothered my daughter. After all, I had no idea how I was going to feel: whether I would be able to be midwife and mother together; how I would cope if Laura had a difficult labour or birth. I rang Jane Evans, a local independent midwife, who responded perfectly, offering to be there for me in whatever capacity I wanted or needed her. We agreed that she would meet Laura and Tim later in the pregnancy and, if they were happy, be there at the birth.

I also needed to go through the formalities of being a midwife away from my normal area of practice. I am an NHS midwife in south London, and rather naively assumed that I would be able to practise in another NHS Trust. However, this was not the case. I submitted my Intention to Practice form, and requested an honorary contract at Laura's local hospital, in the event of her needing to transfer in labour, or indeed needing any other hospital-based care. In spite of a positive reply from the RCM ('The RCM would hope that Trusts would assist midwives seeking to care for friends or family outside their normal area of work by providing an honorary contract'), the contract was flatly refused. The letter from the Trust states: 'Although you are very welcome to be with your daughter as a birthing partner, we are bound by law to have a midwife present for her delivery and postnatal care.' Needless to say, I found this insulting and very frustrating. However, the door was closed, so we all hoped that Laura would have her planned home birth, and I told myself that if things didn't work out and we needed to transfer to hospital then maybe I would prefer to be with her as her mum rather than as her midwife.

Part of the magic

In the end my beautiful daughter did it all perfectly! After a threatened miscarriage at seven weeks, Laura had a wonderfully enjoyable pregnancy, with no problems at all apart from heartburn. We saw each other lots, and the rest of the family also became very involved in the magic and the excitement of this little person growing inside her. Laura's best friend from school (also called Laura) was pregnant at the same time and asked me to be her midwife, too. At about 36 weeks we had a video evening, with the two Lauras and their partners watching films of births and focusing on how it might feel for everyone involved. Jane and I also had a 'birth talk' evening with Laura and Tim, discussing how labour might start, the normal progress of labour, when Laura and Tim might want me there, and all our different roles. I felt very clear that if all seemed to be going well, Laura and Tim should be on their own for as long as they wanted. I would come only when called, however difficult this might feel at the time.

In the event it all worked out beautifully. We hadn't fussed about due dates (there was a confusion between Laura's period date and the date from the scan she had at seven weeks), but were thinking about early August. After a couple of false starts, labour started gently on 10 August: Laura texted me in the morning to tell me she had 'backache and boredom'! By 2pm she was contracting regularly every 10 minutes and feeling fine, with no show or SROM. By 4pm the contractions were closer together, and she and Tim went off for a walk.

By 6.15 things were hotting up, contractions were longer and stronger, and about every five minutes. I took a deep breath and asked them to call me when they wanted me, knowing they were about an hour away, but also completely trusting my daughter to know the right time for me to come.

And, of course, she did, about two hours later, with regular strong contractions every three minutes.

Feeling elated

I was more than ready to leave, unbelievably excited and not remotely anxious – in fact, I felt an emotion close to elation as I drove there, stopping on the way to take a photo of the beautiful sunset, and singing aloud to a CD all the way. Tim was grinning round the curtains when I arrived, and Laura, obviously in good strong labour, greeted me with, 'We're having fun, as you can see!.' From then on it was fun: Laura and her baby were clearly fine, and she and Tim were both enjoying themselves. I felt relaxed, happy and confident in my daughter. I remember actively revelling in the moment and thinking, 'This is how birth should be.'

A few days later I wrote an email to Nicky, a midwife friend in Australia: 'Yes, I'm a grandma!! Laura had a beautiful little boy last Wednesday and it's all so exciting . . . She has been amazing – no more than I expected but, still, when you're the midwife you have to face all sorts of 'what ifs' . . . But she laboured wonderfully – powerfully and positively – and after about an eight-hour labour she gave birth to little William in the pool at home. No problems, no difficulties, just a lovely young woman enjoying the experience! And her mum managed to enjoy it, too . . . Actually, I didn't worry at all, it just felt very right to be there supporting her. Jane Evans came as my support person, and she says she found it all very 'refreshing' (!!). I think [she] was interested to see how matter-of-fact Laura was about it all . . . no hanging around before cutting the cord (which had stopped pulsating almost instantly) as she wanted Tim to hold William, and then asking me to just pull the placenta out (we did that together!). Lovely photo of the three of them sitting on the sofa afterwards – Laura sitting with her legs crossed looking as though she's at a coffee morning! . . .'

Normal, straightforward and fun

And that's how it was – normal, straightforward and fun. An everyday miracle, as we so often say. I can't remember when I first felt like a grandma, though I know it wasn't straight away. During the birth I definitely felt like a midwife, although I was also acutely aware of my love for Laura, Tim and their baby. During second stage Laura also became acutely aware of me, asking if I was all right ('just checking you're not too overwhelmed'), and, a bit later, as her baby's head was advancing, saying, 'Are you jumping up and down, mum? Thought you were . . . I am – in spirit, obviously!' When William was born, and Tim and I 'received' him together, it all just felt right, a completion of our plans and dreams. And when the rest of the family arrived to celebrate with us an hour later, it felt, for me, like the icing on a very special cake.

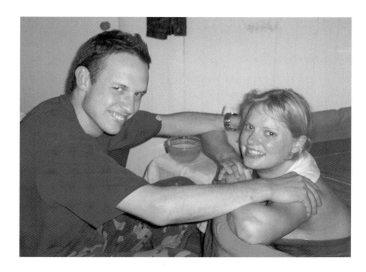

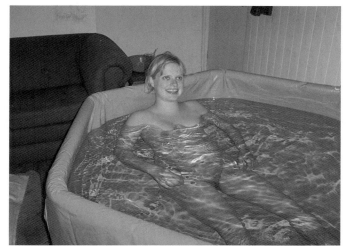

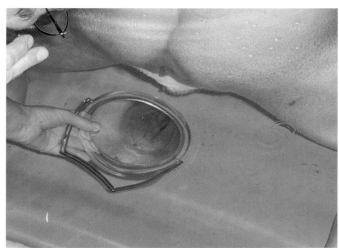

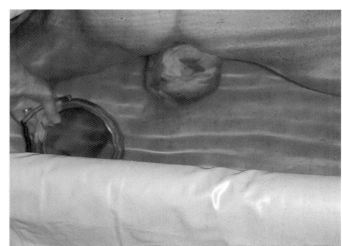

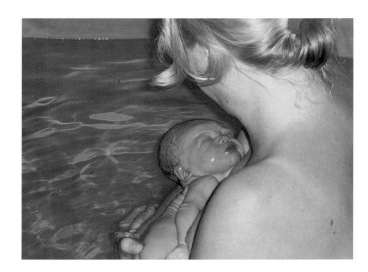

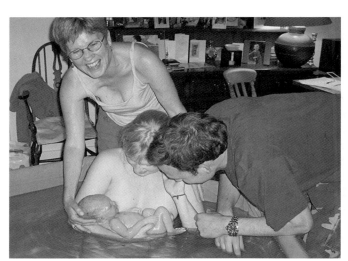

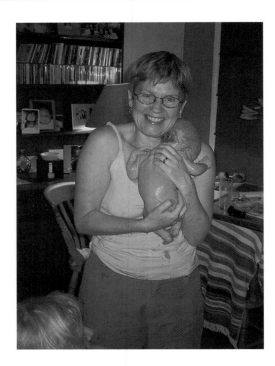

At the end of Laura's birth notes I added; 'What an incredible night! – impossible to describe the emotions involved. I feel so proud of my beautiful daughter and her wonderful man, so honoured and privileged to have been with them as their midwife as well as their mum. And so in love with my beautiful grandson – it has been unbelievably special to be part of his coming into the world.'

Laura's story

For almost as long as I can remember my mum has been a midwife, and pregnancy and birth have been imprinted overwhelmingly in my subconscious as positive experiences.

When I finally did a positive pregnancy test myself, the first person I rang was my mum. I was desperate to share my excitement, and I knew from the beginning that she would look after me in both a mothering and midwife capacity. My trust in her abilities as a midwife extended to my partner Tim. He believed that, as she obviously had my best interests at heart, no one else could provide such loving care! It wasn't until later in my pregnancy when I had spent more time with other expectant mums that I realised just how fortunate I was. My upbringing surrounded by midwives and the women for whom they cared had ingrained in me a confidence in my body and a firm belief that birth was a natural and wonderful thing and not something to be feared.

During my pregnancy my mum was a fantastic source of information, and I think she particularly enjoyed being involved from the start. In the beginning she remarked that she didn't normally see women this early in their pregnancies, and so when we heard my baby's heartbeat at 11 weeks it was especially exciting. We talked endlessly about the baby and its development, and I got the real feeling that through me (rather than anyone else she had looked after) she was reliving her own pregnancies – and especially the first, which had been me. It was through books and the internet that I gained my factual information, but it was my mum who brought the experience alive with tales (endless at times!) of other pregnancies and other birth stories.

By the time I was 40 weeks I was incredibly excited and terribly impatient. Unlike the other pregnant women with whom I had made friends, I was looking forward to the birth and eagerly anticipating the first contractions. Although we had talked a lot about coping with a difficult birth, I was filled with confidence that things would go smoothly, and that if they didn't we would all cope and my mum could be my support if it was no longer possible for her to be my midwife. She had arranged for a second midwife to be present at the birth as a supporting role for her in the event that she was overwhelmed by difficult circumstances or emotion. I had never worried about how my mum would behave during my labour: I felt she would slip into her role as midwife and guide me as she would any other mother.

The 'real thing'

On 10 August 2004 my labour pains began, and I knew this was the 'real thing'. Tim and I spent a wonderful afternoon alone together as the excitement and contractions built. My mum was in phone contact but we had agreed she would not come until I needed her. By eight o'clock that evening I felt she should be leaving London as I live about an hour's drive away and my contractions were coming hard and strong. She said she would be leaving shortly, but almost immediately I asked Tim to check and my dad said she had already left. I felt this was an immensely positive sign – even though she was not here, she seemed in tune with my needs. It was wonderful to see her arrive so calm and confident and just let us get on with the first stage. I found my labour very much as I had expected, with the contractions getting harder to deal with but plenty of time in between to enjoy the atmosphere.

My baby was born into the birthing pool at home at 1.50 the next morning. I have strong memories of my mum guiding me through second stage, talking to me firmly about breathing and blowing and trying to ease my baby's head out gently. In my head her voice was comforting and supporting, and it is hard for me to imagine how it would feel to have a stranger helping you through this process.

After my baby was born there are photos of my mum holding him close, and to me she looks just like his grandma. When I am asked how it felt to have my mum as my midwife, I can only ever answer that it felt right. It was a privilege to join the many other women she has looked after, and to understand what a remarkable occupation she has chosen.

The Practising Midwife 2005; 8(5): 29–32

Spreading some magic

Tricia Anderson

If we are educating midwives, then the philosophy of normal birth is in everything we do: it is our raison d'être. What defines a midwife is her belief in the normalcy of birth. If she does not hold that belief, she is not practising midwifery but obstetrics (Kennedy et al 2003). So the question is not so much how do we go about educating midwives to facilitate normal birth but, more simply, how do we go about educating midwives?

I wish we could get rid of the word 'student'. It tends to have such a derogatory, impersonal overtone in the NHS: 'She's only a student,' 'There are three midwives on today . . . oh, and a student' (to be said with a sneer as if you'd just sucked a lemon). Such a put-down, so interchangeable . . . Already the socialisation process has begun where the aspiring midwife learns she is not a person with unique skills but a replaceable, faceless grade.

All midwives need to be able to defend their professional position with confidence. This should be a core requirement for professional registration and included in the curriculum, with appropriate research, statistics, role play and so forth – even assessed with a viva. If faced with a GP who says, 'I won't allow my patients to have a home birth,' or a paediatrician saying, 'Birth centres are death-traps for babies,' each midwife needs to be practised in immediately responding in a professional and well-informed way. A good way to learn these skills is by learning basic assertiveness and improvisational comedy techniques – great fun, too!

Arts and learning

I've written before about the importance of the arts in the midwifery curriculum: one way to develop our human side is to use poetry, literature, art and music to delve deeper into women's reproductive life experiences. How else can we support women through the many experiences we may never know ourselves? How else do we

start seeing a woman as a human being like us – not a 'girl', 'lady', bump, number, cervix, condition, perineum, discharge, 'mum'.

Providing inspiration

Aspiring midwives need to be inspired: by teachers who remain excited by the magic of birth, by midwives who are pushing the boundaries of practice, by supervisors and managers who are championing midwifery and who are prepared to stand up for what they believe. How else will they find their own strength? They need to be taught by midwives who are doing it, living it, breathing it. They quickly 'suss' if they are being taught home birth or water birth by people who are teaching out of textbooks, not experience. Bring expert midwives, community midwives, independent midwives into the classroom; help lecturers get back into practice at home births or in birth centres.

The well-known US midwife educator Elizabeth Davis talks about the power of women's truth circles: women sharing thoughts, feelings, experiences honestly; learning to talk, to listen and to respect; to feel at home in a welcoming, supportive and skilfully facilitated group. As women relax and learn to trust each other, they release oxytocin. Midwives need to experience this themselves so they can in turn incorporate it into their practice.

They need to be touched: so much of midwifery education engages the brain, but not the heart. They need to see images of beautiful births from around the world – again and again. They need to read poetry and look at paintings and understand how birth crosses cultures and centuries. The best teachers of all are women: pregnant women, new mothers, grandmothers. Bring women into the classroom so that others hear the triumphant voices of those who have given birth normally and learn just how much it means to them . . . and the silent tears of women who have not, to understand their sense of loss.

Hour upon hour of PowerPoint lecture must be interminably boring. Activities with the body, the hands, stick in the brain far longer. Painting, drama, role play, crafts . . . Teach midwives to trust birth: the human race is resilient, and women have been giving birth for centuries without CTGs, drips, catheters. Teach them that on the rare occasion when a birth is not going well they will see signs. Provide a deep understanding of physiology: how the female body works, how the emotions and the environment affect it. They need to travel, be it to the other side of the county or the other side of the world, to open their minds to different ways, different styles, to see that birth can happen safely in a bus, in a cottage, in a high-rise, in a birth centre, in a hospital . . .

Don't fear the bogeyman

Tackle the fear head on – it's very real. Just what are the statistics around the big bogeyman, Mr Litigation, against midwives? Actually, they're very small. Teach midwives over and over what they need to do in an emergency until they feel confident and can put those fears to one side.

Finally, support them to make trusting relationships with women, accompanying them through their pregnancy journey via caseloading schemes. One third-year student said to me after this experience, 'Now I finally understand what midwifery's all about.'

REFERENCE

Kennedy H P, Rousseau A L and Low L K (2003). 'An exploratory meta-synthesis of midwifery practice in the United States'. Midwifery, 19, 209–214.

The Practising Midwife 2005; 8(4): 17

Index